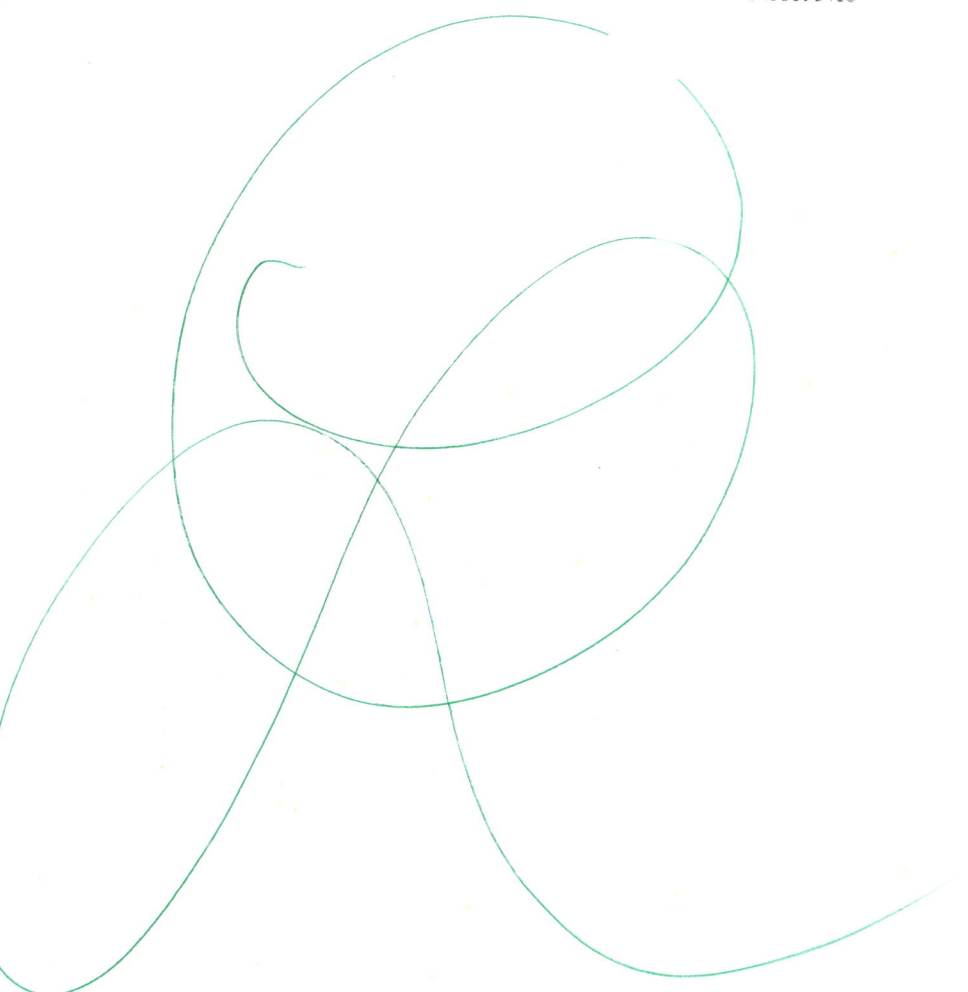

Personality Psychology

David M. Buss Nancy Cantor
Editors

Personality Psychology
Recent Trends and Emerging Directions

With 15 Illustrations

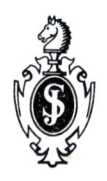

Springer-Verlag
New York   Berlin   Heidelberg
London   Paris   Tokyo

David M. Buss
Nancy Cantor
Department of Psychology
University of Michigan
Ann Arbor, Michigan 48109, USA

Library of Congress Cataloging-in-Publication Data
Personality psychology: recent trends and emerging directions/
editors, David M. Buss, Nancy Cantor.
　　p.　cm.
Papers from a conference held at the University of Michigan, Ann
Arbor, April 15-17, 1988.
Includes bibliographies.
ISBN 0-387-96993-4
1. Personality—Congresses.　I. Buss, David M.　II. Cantor,
Nancy.
　　[DNLM: 1. Personality—congresses.　2. Personality Assessment—
trends—congresses.　3. Psychological Theory—congresses.　BF 698
P4679 1988]
BF698.P3713　1989
155.2—dc20
DNLM/DLC
　　　　　　　　　　　　　　　　　　　　　　　　　　　　89-6442

Printed on acid-free paper.

© 1989 by Springer-Verlag New York Inc.
All rights reserved. This work may not be translated or copied in whole or in part without the written permission of the publisher (Springer-Verlag, 175 Fifth Avenue, New York, NY 10010, USA), except for brief excerpts in connection with reviews or scholarly analysis. Use in connection with any form of information storage and retrieval, electronic adaptation, computer software, or by similar or dissimilar methodology now known or hereafter developed is forbidden.
The use of general descriptive names, trade names, trademarks, etc. in this publication, even if the former are not especially identified, is not to be taken as a sign that such names, as understood by the Trade Marks and Merchandise Marks Act, may accordingly be used freely by anyone.

Typeset by TCSystems, Inc., Shippensburg, Pennsylvania.
Printed and bound by R.R. Donnelley & Sons, Harrisonburg, Virginia.
Printed in the United States of America.

9 8 7 6 5 4 3 2 1

ISBN 0-387-96993-4 Springer-Verlag New York Berlin Heidelberg
ISBN 3-540-96993-4 Springer-Verlag Berlin Heidelberg New York

Preface

Scientific disciplines sometimes reach critical junctures in their development–points of departure that can radically alter their subsequent course. We believe that the field of personality psychology has reached such a juncture.

In the 1930s, the seminal books by Allport (1937) and Murray (1938) set an agenda for decades to come. The 1940s and 1950s were marked by talented researchers carrying out that broad agenda. The study of personality flourished, and a basic textbook by Hall and Lindzey (1957) established personality psychology as an essential part of psychology's curriculum. During the 1960s, however, fundamental assumptions of the field were questioned, and limitations in predictability from trait measures were noted. The decade of the 1970s and the early years of the 1980s were marked by internal debate consisting of defenses of the basic paradigm, further attacks, and yet more defenses.

During the 1980s, however, the intense internal debate waned, and new approaches to substantive issues in the field began to emerge: new middle-level units of analysis were advanced; new forms of personality coherence were proposed; advances in assessment yielded more powerful methods. A dimensional structure began to receive consensual endorsement, and the explanatory tools used by researchers expanded beyond their earlier confines to include neighboring disciplines such as cognitive psychology, evolutionary biology, and sociology.

In 1988, we decided to organize a conference to articulate these emerging issues in personality psychology. Four goals were central to the conference: (1) to identify interesting and promising emerging issues; (2) to stimulate debate and intellectual exchange among active researchers in the field; (3) to begin to consolidate the otherwise scattered gains in the field; (4) to reinforce our burgeoning group identity and shared sense of purpose.

To accomplish these goals, we decided to invite only young personality psychologists. Informally, the conference was referred to as "the small fry conference." Unfortunately, financial constraints imposed a limit of twenty-five participants. Clearly, there are many more outstanding young personality psychologists, here and abroad, and we regret that our limited resources forced this restriction.

The conference, which took place over three days (April 15–17, 1988), provided several formats: (1) symposia with brief presentations; (2) workshops and round table discussions; (3) free-wheeling coffee breaks, lunches, dinners, and parties. We believe that the sense of excitement shared by the participants augurs well for accomplishing our goals. Of course, the true test of success can only be evaluated in the next decade by accomplishments in the field.

To realize a conference of this scope requires dedicated teamwork. The Chair of the Department of Psychology at the University of Michigan, Professor Al Cain, gave intellectual support to the conference from its inception, and provided the financial support needed to make it a reality. Judy Mackey, our Personality Area Secretary, provided the structural core of the conference. Without her tireless efforts, organizational expertise, social skills, and imperturbable good humor, the conference could not have occurred.

Our personality area faculty functioned as a team in preparing this conference, and deserve special recognition: Abigail Stewart worked closely with us from the outset; David Winter and Warren Norman transported people, as well as ideas throughout; Don Brown, Janet Landman, Mel Manis, Hazel Markus, Dick Nisbett, Carolyn Phinney, George Rosenwald, Mac Runyan, Claude Steele, and Joe Veroff added valued support.

The nuts and bolts of the conference were assembled by the tireless devotion of our graduate students. Their contributions, which spanned many months, began in our graduate seminar, continued throughout the actual conference, and beyond. We would like to extend special thanks to: Scott Bunce, Armen Asherian, Mike Botwin, Rose Pacini, Bill Peterson, Richard Doty, Kaz Kato, Ethel Moore, Jeanne Oggins, Chris Langston, Sabrina Zirkel, Will Fleeson, Avonne Mason, Liisa Kyl-Heku, Doug Leber, Dave Ametrano, Cheryl Peck, Rob Sellers, Steve Byers, Eric Stone, and Mike Morris.

Finally, we thank the twenty-five participants who provided the intellectual core of the conference. This book is the product of their efforts.

David M. Buss
Nancy Cantor

Contents

Preface v
Contributors xi
Introduction... 1
DAVID M. BUSS and NANCY CANTOR

Part I   **New Middle-Level Units in Personality Psychology**

Chapter 1   Personal Projects Analysis: Trivial Pursuits, Magnificent Obsessions, and the Search for Coherence 15
BRIAN R. LITTLE

Chapter 2   Exploring the Relations Between Motives and Traits: The Case of Narcissism............................. 32
ROBERT A. EMMONS

Chapter 3   Cognitive Strategies as Personality: Effectiveness, Specificity, Flexibility, and Change... 45
JULIE K. NOREM

Chapter 4   An Alternative Paradigm for Studying the Accuracy of Person Perception: Simulated Personalities.. 61
JACK C. WRIGHT

Part II New Forms of Personality Coherence

Chapter 5 On the Continuities and Consequences of Personality: A Life-Course Perspective 85
AVSHALOM CASPI

Chapter 6 Life Paths of Aggressive and Withdrawn Children 99
DEBBIE S. MOSKOWITZ and ALEX E. SCHWARTZMAN

Chapter 7 Emotional Adaptation to Life Transitions: Early Impact on Integrative Cognitive Processes 115
JOSEPH M. HEALY, JR.

Chapter 8 Performance Evaluation and Intrinsic Motivation Processes: The Effects of Achievement Orientation and Rewards 128
JUDITH M. HARACKIEWICZ

Chapter 9 The Problem of Life's Meaning 138
ROY F. BAUMEISTER

Chapter 10 Conditional Patterns, Transference, and the Coherence of Personality Across Time 149
AVRIL THORNE

Chapter 11 The Development of a Narrative Identity 160
DAN P. MCADAMS

Part III Advances in Assessment

Chapter 12 A Process Approach to Personality Psychology: Utilizing Time as a Facet of Data 177
RANDY J. LARSEN

Chapter 13 Metatraits: Interitem Variance as Personality Assessment 194
DIANNE M. TICE

Chapter 14 Socially Desirable Responding: Some New Solutions to Old Problems 201
DELROY L. PAULHUS

Chapter 15	Accuracy in Personality Judgment and the Dancing Bear	210
	DAVID C. FUNDER	
Chapter 16	Construct Validity in Personality Assessment	224
	DANIEL J. OZER	

Part IV   **Advances in Identifying the Structure of Personality**

Chapter 17	Why I Advocate the Five-Factor Model: Joint Factor Analyses of the NEO-PI with Other Instruments	237
	ROBERT R. MCCRAE	
Chapter 18	The Optimal Level of Measurement for Personality Constructs...	246
	STEPHEN R. BRIGGS	
Chapter 19	Towards a Taxonomy of Personality Descriptors......	261
	OLIVER P. JOHN	

Part V   **Expansion of Levels of Explanation in Personality**

Chapter 20	Identity Orientations and Self-Interpretation............	275
	JONATHAN M. CHEEK	
Chapter 21	Using Traits to Construct Personality.....................	286
	SARAH E. HAMPSON	
Chapter 22	Personality Theory and Behavioral Genetics: Contributions and Issues.....................................	294
	DAVID C. ROWE	
Chapter 23	A Biosocial Perspective on Mates and Traits: Reuniting Personality and Social Psychology	308
	DOUGLAS T. KENRICK	
Chapter 24	The Evolutionary History of Genetic Variation: An Emerging Issue in the Behavioral Genetic Study of Personality...	320
	STEVEN W. GANGESTAD	

Chapter 25 Levels of Explanation in Personality Theory 333
            JEROME C. WAKEFIELD

            Subject Index.. 347

Contributors

ROY F. BAUMEISTER
Department of Psychology, Case Western Reserve University,
Cleveland, Ohio 44106, USA

STEPHEN R. BRIGGS
Department of Psychology, University of Tulsa,
Tulsa, Oklahoma 74104, USA

DAVID M. BUSS
Department of Psychology, University of Michigan,
Ann Arbor, Michigan 48109, USA

NANCY CANTOR
Department of Psychology, University of Michigan,
Ann Arbor, Michigan 48109, USA

AVSHALOM CASPI
Department of Psychology, Harvard University,
Cambridge, Massachusetts 02138, USA

JONATHAN M. CHEEK
Department of Psychology, Wellesley College,
Wellesley, Massachusetts 02181, USA

ROBERT A. EMMONS
Psychology Department, University of California, Davis,
Davis, California 95616, USA

DAVID C. FUNDER
Department of Psychology, University of Illinois at
Urbana-Champaign,
Champaign, Illinois 61820, USA

STEVEN W. GANGESTAD
Department of Psychology, University of New Mexico,
Albuquerque, New Mexico 87131, USA

SARAH E. HAMPSON
Oregon Research Institute, Eugene, Oregon 97401, USA

JUDITH M. HARACKIEWICZ
Department of Psychology, Columbia University,
New York, New York 10027, USA

JOSEPH M. HEALY, JR.
Psychology Department, Wesleyan University,
Middletown, Connecticut 06457, USA

OLIVER P. JOHN
Institute of Personality Assessment and Research,
University of California, Berkeley,
Berkeley, California 94720, USA

DOUGLAS T. KENRICK
Department of Psychology, Arizona State University,
Tempe, Arizona 85287, USA

RANDY J. LARSEN
Department of Psychological Sciences, Purdue University,
West Lafayette, Indiana 47907, USA

BRIAN R. LITTLE
Department of Psychology, Carlton University,
Ottawa, Ontario, Canada K1S 5B6

DAN P. MCADAMS
Department of Psychology, Loyola University of Chicago,
Chicago, Illinois 60626, USA

ROBERT R. MCCRAE
Personality, Stress and Coping Section, Gerontology Research Center,
The National Institute on Aging,
Baltimore, Maryland 21224, USA

DEBBIE S. MOSKOWITZ
Department of Psychology, McGill University,
Montreal, Quebec, Canada H3A 1B1

JULIE K. NOREM
Department of Psychology, Northeastern University,
Boston, Massachusetts 02115, USA

DANIEL J. OZER
Department of Psychology, Boston University,
Boston, Massachusetts 02215, USA

DELROY L. PAULHUS
Department of Psychology, University of British Columbia,
Vancouver, British Columbia, Canada V6T 1Y7

DAVID C. ROWE
School of Family and Consumer Resources, University of Arizona,
Tucson, Arizona 85721, USA

ALEX E. SCHWARTZMAN
Department of Psychology, Concordia University,
Montreal, Quebec, Canada H3G 1M8

AVRIL THORNE
Department of Psychology, Wellesley College,
Wellesley, Massachusetts 02181, USA

DIANNE M. TICE
Department of Psychology, Case Western Reserve University,
Cleveland, Ohio 44106, USA

JEROME C. WAKEFIELD
The Columbia University School of Social Work,
New York, New York 10025, USA

JACK C. WRIGHT
Hunter Laboratory of Psychology, Brown University,
Providence, Rhode Island 02912, USA

Introduction

The field of personality psychology, while consolidating earlier gains, is expanding in important directions, many of which are highlighted in the following chapters. In this introduction our purpose is to extract the major issues that emerged at the conference.

New Middle-Level Units in Personality Psychology

Allport (1937, 1958) posed a fundamental question that all personality psychologists must address in their theoretical and empirical work: What units shall we employ? Although a wide variety of units have been proposed over the past five decades, the field of personality psychology has concentrated primarily on two: *traits* (or dispositions) and *motives*, which correspond to the units championed by Allport (1937) and Murray (1938) respectively.

The choice of units has fundamental consequences for theory and research since it implies a conceptual decision about how to parse the phenomena of personality. Script units (Abelson, 1981), for example, chunk actions that are temporally contiguous (e.g., the restaurant script). Trait and motive units, in contrast, subsume actions dispersed over time and context, intercalated with actions not conceptually relevant to the unit. The power motive, for example, may subsume such diverse and temporally distant acts as monopolizing the conversation, purchasing prestige possessions, and running for office.

Units of analysis also carry consequences for causal explanations. Motives, by their very nature, imply causal forces within persons that energize, direct, and select behavior (McClelland, 1980). Trait units, however, can be causally neutral, and serve a descriptive function that calls for, but does not provide, an explanation of observed behavioral consistencies.

Measurement operations are also affected by whatever units are adopted: some require observations extended over weeks or months;

some require daily sampling; some require reliance on self-report; others virtually dictate the use of external observers.

Two new units of analysis emerging in the 1980s are personal projects (Little, 1983) and personal strivings (Emmons, 1986). These units bear a conceptual affinity to Floyd Allport's concept of teleonomic trend, but differ in scope and measurement operations. Whereas teleonomic trends refer to themes that dominate a person's entire life (Captain Ahab in Melville's Moby Dick, for example, was obsessed throughout his life with the white whale), personal projects and personal strivings, in contrast, focus on a person's conscious articulations of what they are trying to do or what they are engaged in or currently concerned about (see also Klinger, 1977). Little focuses on a range of personal projects, from the immediate (e.g., putting the cat out) to the grand (e.g., changing Western thought). Emmons's concept of personal striving tends to focus on the intermediate level, i.e., on what people are trying to achieve. A benefit of both approaches is forceful attention focused on the everyday texture of people's lives.

Another set of new units are life tasks and strategies (Norem; see also Cantor & Kihlstrom, 1987) and evolutionary tasks and tactics (Kenrick; Gangestad; see also Buss, 1986). The former approach identifies important tasks in the lives of individuals (e.g., achieving at school, forming good relationships), and focuses on alternative construals of those normative tasks, and on the cognitive strategies people construct to try to deal with *their* tasks. Defensive pessimism, for example, is posited to be one cognitive strategy that entails generating "worst case scenarios" of possible outcomes. It carries a functional component in that it calms the self with the knowledge of forethought, and has a motivating effect on behavior so that worst cases are actively avoided.

Evolutionary life tasks are problems that individuals typically must have solved in the past in order to survive (e.g., obtaining food, defense against predators) and reproduce (e.g., competing for mates, selecting mates, retaining mates). Broadly-based strategies (e.g., forming reciprocal alliances) and subsumed tactics (e.g., making friends with important people; providing help when needed) are used by individuals to solve these evolutionary life tasks. Personality, in all of these goal-based frameworks, is viewed roughly as a set of problems, projects, or tasks toward which human action is directed, as well as the strategies, tactics, and acts employed to pursue them.

Complementing these approaches to the intentional side of personality, other researchers have been exploring the conditional, contextualized nature of individuals' characteristic responses. The notion of "conditional dispositions" has been forcefully developed by Wright and Mischel (1987). Rather than viewing dispositions as summaries of act trends (e.g., Buss & Craik, 1983), Wright focuses on the environmental conditions (e.g., frustrating events) that predictably elicit classes of acts (e.g., aggression). This approach to dispositions carries the promise of conceptual insights into eliciting conditions, as well as increases in the predictability of behavior.

Thorne argues persuasively for *interpersonal* contexts as critical elicitors of dispositional displays, particularly when individuals' goals are repeatedly frustrated in certain types of relationships. In her perspective, individuals have characteristic forms of relationships, and their patterns of bonding provide a core definitional context for the self. Cheek presents compelling evidence of both intrapersonal and interpersonal contexts for self-development, and argues that people also differ in the relative weight they give to the personal and social definitions of identity. Others, Caspi and Healy in particular, highlight the social-structural and social role constraints on personality development, and the impact that turning points in social involvements can have on emotional well-being and personality functioning. Caspi, in fact, argues that it is precisely those changes in the social structure or social milieu of an individual's life that serve as the conditions for display of dispositionally driven behavior. In all of these models of identity and dispositions, the critical self-characteristics that comprise personality are themselves deeply and intimately embedded in, and are, in large part, defined by context; consequently these are also middle-level units of personality description.

An intriguing agenda for the next decade centers on the relations among these new middle-level units. How are cognitive strategies linked with conditional dispositions? What are the critical interpersonal or role constraints on personal projects? How do life periods shape the pursuit of personal strivings? What are the links between the conscious articulation of projects and strivings and evolutionary life tasks? And how do all of these units relate conceptually and empirically to traits and motives as traditionally conceived and measured? Briggs and John both present compelling cases for the integration of Big-Five factor models with these more contextualized and goal-based middle-level units; each proposes this task of integration as a worthwhile project for personologists to embrace.

New Forms of Personality Coherence

Consistency and coherence have been central issues in personality psychology since its inception. Early studies (e.g., Hartshorne & May, 1928) focused on cross-situational consistency by examining inter-act correlations. The decade of the 1970s and the early years of the 1980s focused heavily on the temporal stability of personality characteristics, as well as on cross-situational consistency. A central emerging issue is a focus on the *coherence,* rather than simple consistency, of personality.

Caspi coined the term "interactional continuity" to describe one form of coherence over time. In a compelling longitudinal study, Caspi found coherent links between assessment of "ill temper" in children and later life outcomes, such as lower educational level, lower military rank, divorce, and job problems. This is not consistency in any simple sense, but rather demonstrates a temporal coherence to manifestations of personality through a series of life transitions.

In a longitudinal study of the development of children, Moskowitz and Schwartzman used the construct of a *life path* to highlight a similar form of personality coherence. They found coherent links between aggressiveness or social withdrawal at age 7, 10, and 13 years, and a host of topographically distinct outcomes five to seven years later, such as pregnancies, abortions, and poor school performance.

Healy focused even more explicitly on life transitions using Stewart's (1982) four-stage model: receptivity, autonomy, assertion, and integration——stages that subsume both emotional and cognitive components. Healy found links between emotional adaptation and cognitive skills involving information integration and simultaneous processing, and thus documented a form of personality coherence in the context of major life change.

Harackiewicz studied the links between the trait of achievement motivation (measured through Jackson's Personality Research Form) and values adopted in the context of performance evaluation. She found that subjects scoring high on achievement orientation tended to value competence, cared more about doing well in competitive tasks, and generally valued those factors that enhance intrinsic motivation.

Emmons posed the problem: What is the relationship between traits and motives? Using a study of narcissism, he demonstrated that personal strivings provide one integrative bridge between traits and motives.

Little used the methods of "right and left laddering" to identify links between personal projects, the acts that carry out the projects, and the terminal values that the projects represent. These methods yield a form of personality coherence from the low-level units (acts) to high-level units (values), with conscious project articulation providing the bridge between them.

Baumeister, Thorne, and McAdams provide alternative conceptual frameworks for identifying personality coherence by focusing on how people make sense of their own lives. McAdams develops the concept of a "life story." Identity, according to McAdams, is created through the life story, which serves to configure the self, to provide a sense of sameness and continuity, and to yield a sense of purpose to an individual's life.

Baumeister adopts a similar stance, but proposes four essential needs underlying an individual's search for meaning: a sense of purpose (where present is related to future); a sense of efficacy (the belief that one's actions will bring about that future); a sense of legitimation (moral and positive values); a need for self-worth (the feeling that you are better than other people).

Thorne anchors personality coherence in the self-views of individuals' most characteristic social relationships, thus elaborating an "interpersonology." Rather than looking for personality coherence in private meanings (as do McAdams and Baumeister), Thorne views personality coherence as a feature of those recurrent interactions with others. At the same time, she suggests that individuals have special insight into these key relationship forms, and provides fascinating data from studies of the "play-by-play" analyses of dyadic conversations between introverted and extroverted participants. The private knowledge of the most operative social contingencies for one's behavior can indeed be made public——when, for example, an introvert reveals that her jealous behavior in the company of extroverts is not solely contingent on the extroverts' behaviors, but rather on a recurrent image of her mother pushing her to be outgoing with those extroverts. Personality coherence emerges somewhere in the merging of self-views and social contingencies.

Another form of coherence is revealed in analyses of personality *processes*——the ebb and flow of thoughts, feelings, and actions, as individuals work on tasks, confront crises, interact with others (e.g., Carver & Scheier, 1981; Kuhl, 1985). Several conference participants adopted this process emphasis. Larsen, for example, traces the patterning of human moods by abstracting characteristic cycles of variation through intensive repeated measures observations. Harackiewicz takes an indepth view of the unfolding motivational processes that mediate the effects of reward on persistence and performance for highly motivated individuals on intrinsically interesting tasks. She traces the strands of behavior that represent an individual's *involvement* in a task; some people intensely involved in their ongoing performance and the pursuit of competence; others side step some of those self evaluations in favor of an appreciation of the task activity itself. Importantly, her results show that both kinds of involvement promote, rather than diminish, intrinsic motivation.

In these examples, coherence exists both in the characteristic patterning and recursive cycling of an individual's thoughts and feelings in situations, and in the consistency between the individual's goals and intentions, and his or her way of responding. Coherence also emerges in the matching of characteristic modes of thinking and of feeling, as when Healy finds a compelling complementarity between underlying emotional stances to life transitions and the more manifest aspects of information-processing. When individuals feel emotionally-overwhelmed by a life change, their cognitive skill in integrating information and structuring simultaneous input also becomes swamped and burdened. When the dynamics of time are added, this cognitive-affective blending is reconstituted repeatedly as the individual adapts in progressively more refined ways to change. As Larsen, Norem, and Hampson suggest, coherence is not a static, but rather a dynamic feature of personality.

These various approaches to the study of personality coherence present a range of important research directions. They highlight the notion that personality is complex and multifaceted, and that personality theories must come to terms with individuals both as they *construe* their worlds and as they *function* in those worlds. A simple focus on personality consistency, whether cross-situational or temporal, does not capture the personality coherence suggested by these approaches.

Advances in Assessment

Related to the study of new forms of personality coherence are advances in personality assessment, which come in two forms: (1) as a consequence of a conceptual advance that drives the search for new assessment techniques; (2) as an increase in the understanding of existing assessment tools. The advances in assessment shown in the following chapters represent blends of impetus from both forms.

Larsen focuses on time in personality and proposes that fluctuations over time can be considered features of personality. Using a single case assessed across occasions, he documents the features that can be compared with other cases, including (in the context of mood) mean level, standard deviation, skew, and kurtosis. Larsen shows that inclusion of time permits spectral analysis, auto-regression, and factor analyses of temporal patterning of emotions, and he raises the intriguing possibility that the number of factors found might reflect emotional complexity, thus showing how an assessment advance can yield a conceptual advance.

Tice tackles the problem of increasing the prediction of behavior and proposes "metatraits" as a concept that can do this. The concept of metatrait refers to the Allportian notion of whether or not a trait applies to an individual. Those who are "traited" (the trait of having the trait) will display behavior predictable from that trait; the behavior of those who are "untraited" (the trait of not having the trait) will be less predictable from the trait.

Paulhus and Funder make contributions towards understanding the two most frequently used methods in personality research: self-report (Paulhus) and observer-report (Funder). Paulhus proposes that social desirability, sometimes a bias in self-report personality measures, is actually composed of two distinct facets: (1) impression management, which does not correlate with substantive personality characteristics and is linked with the deception of others; (2) self-deception, which is linked with substantive personality characteristics. One implication for assessment is that the first facet should be controlled or eliminated, whereas the second facet should be retained.

Funder focuses on observer accuracy in personality assessment. He proposes two criteria for accuracy: interjudge agreement and behavioral prediction. Empirically, he finds that some personality characteristics show consistently good agreement among observers, whereas other characteristics show consistently poor agreement. One important implication is that assessment methods (in this case, observers) should focus on substantive domains in which they perform well, and that alternative methods should be sought for assessing those domains in which they perform poorly.

Wright has developed the "simulated personalities" paradigm in order to further specify the sensitivities of and the limitations on social perception. He asks whether observers can distinguish sets of behavior-context pairs that follow the actual contingencies of real individuals' responses in different contexts from those that violate those contingencies. As in Funder's work, Wright's paradigm presents the hope not only of answering general questions of observer accuracy, but, more importantly, of delineating the precise parameters of social sensitivity. Whereas observers may be good at identifying "mutation" conditions based upon violations in the behavioral elicitors of actions (e.g., Jimmy will not turn violent when praised but will be aggressive when threatened), judgment may be less sensitive to violations in the interpersonal conditions for actions (e.g., Jimmy is violent when threatened by peers and passive when threatened by adults).

Ozer, in an intriguing examination of construct validity, poses the problem of what to do with method variance when substantive traits and the methods best for assessing them co-occur. Self-esteem, for example, is best assessed by self-report methods, whereas agreeableness is, perhaps, best assessed by observer-based or peer-based methods. When examining correlations between different traits, does shared method variance inflate relationships, or does this linkage artificially deflate observed links between traits assessed through different methods? Although he offers no definitive solution, Ozer points to an important assessment agenda in understanding the method variance associated with our most common assessment techniques. He concludes by suggesting that reflexively invoked criteria for construct validity may substantially impede progress in the field.

Taken together, these contributions point to an increasing sophistication among researchers in basic assessment methodologies. Rather than merely invoking cries of social desirability response (SDR) set, Paulhus has tried to identify what SDR means substantively and methodologically. Instead of simply calling attention to problems in observer-assessment, Funder has contributed to an understanding of precisely how this data source can and cannot be used. Tice and Larsen suggest conceptually driven assessment advances, whereas Ozer highlights a substantive issue in the construct validation of personality measures. Combined, these contributions point to an increase in the precision and incisiveness of the tools of our trade in the coming decades.

Advances in Identifying the Structure of Personality

A central issue in personality psychology has been identifying the most important ways in which individuals differ. A plethora of alternative and seemingly irreconcilable structures have been proposed over the past several decades. Eysenck proposes three, Cattell 16, Gough 20, and so on. In the 1980s, researchers employing different theoretical perspectives have converged on a five-factor model of personality, initially articulated by Norman (1963): Surgency, Agreeableness, Conscientiousness, Emotional Stability, and Intellectance-Openness.

McCrae and Costa have been among the most vigorous proponents of the five-factor model in the 1980s. In a compelling series of studies, McCrae demonstrates that this five-factor structure is robust across methods (e.g., bipolar adjective scales, inventory item statements), data sources (e.g., self-report, spouse-report), time, instruments, and different theoretical approaches. He demonstrates that many alternative systems can be reduced empirically to these five dimensions.

Briggs endorses this five-factor model, but advocates a focus on what he calls the "primaries"——those narrower and more homogeneous elements of personality subsumed by each large Big-Five factor. He argues that because a scale works does not mean that we understand *how* it works, and proposes that a focus on primaries provides the best route to cumulative advances in understanding.

John views the five-factor model as an integrative, heuristic model for personality researchers. Like Briggs, John sees the five factors as large, superordinate categories that subsume most or all of the important smaller sub-traits, and his work on category breadth provides an empirical demonstration of this. The superordinate category of Extraversion (Surgency), for example, subsumes the progressively more narrow categories of sociable and talkative. John also addresses several objections that have been raised to the five-factor model, and illustrates a research agenda whereby the Big Five can be discerned in existing assessment techniques (e.g., ACL, Q-Sort).

Not all personality psychologists agree that the five-factor model provides an adequate description of the major ways in which individuals differ. Nonetheless, it has received enough independent replications by investigators using different methods to warrant serious attention. The five-factor model remains atheoretical, but the next decade of research should move towards anchoring the five factors in theory, and developing a deeper understanding of precisely what they represent. Buss for example, sees the five factors as categories of social judgment that correspond to the most important adaptive questions humans need to answer about someone with whom they will interact (see also Goldberg, 1981). In this view, the five factors are shorthand extractions or summaries of the most important features of a person's "adaptive landscape," to be linked, perhaps, with dimensions of evolutionary significance, as in Kenrick's analysis of the adaptive constraints on social cognition. Such approaches also provide important avenues for theoretical integration between trait-based and goal-based accounts of personality, as illustrated in both Emmon's and Little's chapters (see also Pervin, in press).

Expansion of Levels of Explanation in Personality

The problem of explanation is central to personality——what accounts for observable regularities in human action? Wakefield argues that at least three forms of explanation are needed: intentional, dispositional, and functional. Intentional explanation deals with beliefs, desires, and wishes that people hold——the cognitive-affective psychological mechanisms. In answer to the question "Why did Sue attend the concert?" an intentional explanation would invoke a desire to hear rock music along with a belief that attending the concert would satisfy that desire.

Wakefield views dispositions as stabilities in the intentional system and distinguishes primary from secondary traits. Primary traits are basic intentional stabilities that do not rely on other intentional states for their maintenance; secondary traits are stabilities that depend on other intentional states. A stability in talkativeness, for example, might depend on the belief that talking a lot is a way to increase one's being liked. The discovery that the belief is wrong could, however, dramatically decrease talkativeness. Hence, primary traits are essential stabilities in the intentional system, whereas secondary traits attain their stability through reliance on other intentional states.

Functional explanation provides a third element in Wakefield's tripartite system, and refers to the adaptive problem solved. Sexual jealousy provides an example in Kenrick's chapter. Consider the question: "Why does Sally habitually become enraged when another woman flirts with her boyfriend." A functional explanation would have recourse to evolutionary biology, and would, perhaps, posit that jealousy solved the adaptive problem of retaining one's mate (e.g., Daly, Wilson, & Weghorst, 1982). Wakefield stresses that such functional explanations should not be confused with intentional explanations, as is sometimes the case in the sociobiological literature, and he argues that all these forms of explanation are necessary in personality psychology.

Several chapters invoke specific forms of these explanatory levels. Cheek invokes the concept of self with two components—personal identity and social identity. (In Wakefield's scheme, these components of identity would be stabilities in the intentional system.) As Cheek demonstrates, people's reactions to social life pressures and group situations vary in predictable ways according to their differing orientations to self-identity. Individual differences in the intentional system can be quite useful as road-maps to social behavior.

Hampson views personality as a social construction. She uses the dramaturgical metaphor, and posits two essential components to social construction—the actor and the observer. Beliefs about the self and others would be stabilities in the intentional system. Hampson's proposal raises the intriguing possibility that two intentional systems (self and observer) may be needed for an adequate depiction of the construction of personality.

Norem focuses on cognitive strategies for solving life tasks, and emphasizes the flexibility of adaptive solutions. The defensive pessimism strategy, for example, may represent a stability in the desire-belief intentional system. But, if the belief that "framing worst case scenarios increases positive outcomes" turned out to be false in certain contexts, then the strategy might shift flexibly as a function of this new information. Thus, defensive pessimism could be viewed as a secondary disposition in the intentional system.

Rowe focuses on another level of explanation—that genetic variation within our species accounts for personality differences. He highlights the advantages of behavioral genetic methods for understanding both genetic and environmental causes of personality. On the environmental side, he emphasizes that behavioral genetic studies have pointed to the importance of non-shared environmental influences. The next decade of research should reveal concrete information on precisely which aspects of nonshared environments carry causal force for personality development.

Kenrick and Gangestad focus on functional explanation, and use explanatory accounts from evolutionary biology to account for regularities in behavior. Kenrick proposes that traits are integral to understanding mate selection. His studies suggest that dominance, and traits linked with dominance, are sought by females in mating contexts. His research also highlights an important contextual cause—that of short-term versus long-term mating contexts.

Gangestad has developed a research program that attempts to understand individual differences in how close a relationship must be before it becomes a sexual one—a difference he refers to as "sociosexuality." He draws upon work in evolutionary biology on the conditions under which females should have more daughters (when monogamous) and/or more sons (when polygynous), and generates specific predictions from his model. Gangestad's work provides an intriguing bridge between behavioral genetics and evolutionary biology by providing a functional explanation for existing genetic variability.

These different approaches to explanation highlight the fact that personality psychologists are expanding their explanatory search. Cognitive psychology, behavioral genetics and evolutionary theory, lifespan development, and social-structural analysis, in particular, seem to have provided personality research with new directions. That personality psychology should encompass all these levels of explanation is appropriate, for this field is unique among the branches of psychology in its integrative and wholistic focus.

Future of Personality

We believe that the chapters that follow portend an exciting future for the field of personality psychology. The new middle-level units, new forms of personality coherence, advances in assessment, advances in identifying the structure of personality, and expansion of the explanatory tools pose an intriguing agenda for the 1990s.

The future of any field rests with the spirited young. We believe that this collection indicates that the present generation of personality psychologists is not mired in the problems of the past, but rather extracts the best from the past while pushing optimistically towards the future.

The chapters that follow differ radically from one another: they reflect disagreement and divergence in the participants' visions of the field; in what phenomena each view as important; and in the future direction of personality psychology. But the conference from which these papers derive was permeated with a spirit of cooperation and enthusiasm, and the disagreements clarified the issues rather than clouding them. As we emerge from the strident debates of the 1970s and early 1980s, we believe it is best to let a thousand flowers bloom. The chapters in this collection represent the buds of those flowers.

References

Abelson, R.P. (1981). Psychological status of the script concept. *American Psychologist, 36,* 715–729.

Allport, G.W. (1937). *Personality: A psychological interpretation.* New York: Holt.

Allport, G.W. (1958). What is a trait of personality? *Journal of Abnormal and Social Psychology, 25,* 368–372.

Buss, D.M. (1986). Can social science be anchored in evolutionary biology? Four problems and a strategic solution. *Revue Européenne des Sciences Sociales, 24*(73), 41–50.

Buss, D.M. & Craik, K.H. (1983). The act frequency approach to personality. *Psychological Review, 90,* 105–126.

Cantor, N. & Kihlstrom, J.F. (1987). *Personality and social intelligence.* Englewood Cliffs, NJ: Prentice-Hall.

Carver, C.S., & Scheier, M.F. (1981). *Attention and self-regulation: A control-theory approach to human behavior.* New York: Springer-Verlag.

Daly, M., Wilson, M., and Weghorst, S.J. (1982). Male sexual jealousy. *Ethology and Sociobiology, 3,* 11–27.

Emmons, R.A. (1986). Personal strivings: An approach to personality and subjective well-being. *Journal of Personality and Social Psychology, 51,* 1058–1068.

Goldberg, L.R. (1981). Language and individual differences: The search for universals in personality lexicons. In L. Wheeler (Ed.), *Review of Personality and Social Psychology, 2,* 141–165. Beverly Hills, CA: Sage Publications.

Hartshorne, H., & May, M.A. (1928). *Studies in the nature of character. Volume 1. Studies in Deceit.* New York: Macmillan.

Hall, C.S., & Lindzey, G. (1957). *Theories of personality.* New York: Wiley.

Klinger, E. (1977). *Meaning and void: Inner experience and the incentives in people's lives.* Minneapolis: University of Minnesota Press.

Kuhl, J. (1985). From cognition to behavior: Perspectives for future research on action control. In J. Kuhl & J. Beckmann (Eds.), *Action control from cognition to behavior.* New York: Springer-Verlag.

Little, B.R. (1983). Personal projects: A rationale and method for investigation. *Environment and Behavior, 15,* 273–309.

McClelland, D.C. (1980). Motive dispositions: The merits of operant and respondent measures. In L. Wheeler (Ed.), *Review of Personality and Social Psychology, 1,* 10–41. Beverly Hills, CA: Sage.

Murray, H.A. (1938). *Explorations in personality.* New York: Oxford Press.

Norman, W. (1963). Toward an adequate taxonomy of personality attributes: Replicated factor structures in peer nomination personality ratings. *Journal of Abnormal and Social Psychology, 66,* 574–583.

Pervin, L. (Ed.) (1989). *Goal concepts in personality and social psychology.* Hillsdale, NJ.: Erlbaum.

Stewart, A.J. (1982). The course of individual adaptation. *Journal of Personality and Social Psychology, 42,* 1100–1113.

Wright, J.C., & Mischel, W. (1987). A conditional approach to dispositional constructs: The local predictability of social behavior. *Journal of Personality and Social Psychology, 53,* 1159–1177.

Part I
New Middle-Level Units in Personality Psychology

CHAPTER 1

Personal Projects Analysis: Trivial Pursuits, Magnificent Obsessions, and the Search for Coherence

Brian R. Little

I. Introduction: Personal Projects and Social Ecology

Personal projects are extended sets of personally relevant action, which can range from the trivial pursuits of a typical Tuesday (e.g., "cleaning up my room") to the magnificent obsessions of a lifetime (e.g., "liberate my people"). They may be self-initiated or thrust upon us. They may be solitary concerns or shared commitments. They may be isolated and peripheral aspects of our lives or may cut to our very core. Personal projects may sustain us through perplexity or serve as vehicles for our own obliteration. In short, personal projects are natural units of analysis for a personality psychology that chooses to deal with the serious business of how people muddle through complex lives (Little, 1987a).

In 1983, a theoretical and methodological framework for the study of such personal projects was proposed (Little, 1983) and empirical evidence was presented that scores from Personal Projects Analysis Methodology (PPA) successfully predict indicators of emotional well-being (Palys & Little, 1983). These publications had developed out of several years of preliminary research on both theoretical and empirical explorations of person-environment interaction (e.g., Argyle & Little, 1972; Little, 1972, 1976; Little & Ryan, 1979). More recently, I presented data on the content and structure of personal projects in adolescent development (Little, 1987b) and on the distinctive psychometric assumptions of the method in the context of counselling psychology (Little, 1987c). In the present chapter, I wish to review the progress of recent research and to chart some of the more promising directions that Carleton University's Social Ecology Laboratory, and others, have taken.

One of the major thrusts of our research has been the development of a social ecological model of personality in which the analysis and enhancement of human well-being is a central concern (Little & Ryan, 1979). Under this model, individuals stand at the intersection of several converging sets of influence emanating from biological, environmental, social, and cultural systems. A central and continuing task of the human condition is that of integrating or forming some coherent balance between these disparate, and often conflicting, sources of influence. One of the ways in which we do this is through the planning and enactment of personal projects. The substance and style of these endeavors, and how they are individually constructed and collectively managed, will reflect each person's specialized orientations and competencies (Little, 1972, 1976). They will equally reflect the specialized resources and constraints of the ecosettings within which the individual is embedded. The analysis of personal projects, in short, comprises an inherently interactional perspective on personality (Little, 1987a).

One of the practical implications of accepting this assumptive framework is that personal projects may serve as the focus for interventions intended to enhance well-being. While the biological and cultural determinants of our projects are acknowledged, the personal project system can be seen as a kind of final common pathway for these influences, thus offering greater tractability for change and development. Before reviewing initial attempts in this area, several basic research questions need to be posed and answered, and to do this it is necessary to outline the methodological tools we have developed to examine personal projects. Personal Project Analysis (PPA) breaks with a number of assumptions in assessment methodology and is designed to meet fairly stringent measurement criteria that go beyond the usual psychometric verities.

II. Personal Projects Analysis: Method and Strategy

A. Propaedeutic Criteria: Toward Coherent Units of Analysis

Human assessment is ultimately concerned with the ascription of valid psychological predicates to people. Depending upon one's assessment goals, different types of assessment unit (e.g., act trends, life tasks) can serve as the vehicle for such ascriptions. Assessment goals, in turn, reflect one's philosophical assumptions about what constitutes a satisfactory explanation of human conduct. Unless the measurement process is explicitly related to the explanatory assumptions undergirding it, the possibility of a coherent account of human conduct will be compromised (Little, 1972, 1976). In essence, the assumptions underlying a project analytic orientation emphasize that human conduct is subject to systemic influences of both an intentional and contextual nature. It is therefore necessary to examine both the reasons underlying personal conduct and the contexts within which it is embedded before an adequate account of its meaning can be proferred (Little, 1987a, 1987b). Detailed examination of the implications of these assumptions led us to propose a set of measurement criteria that can be regarded as propaedeutic to psychometric evaluation. While it is beyond the scope of this paper to show in detail how personal projects meet each of these criteria (see

TABLE 1.1. Propaedeutic measurement criteria underlying personal projects analysis.

Criterion	Brief explanation
Personal Saliency	Are the units expressed in the idiosyncratic language of the respondent or are they "provided" by the experimenter?
Reflexivity	Does the unit apply reflexively both to the conduct of investigators and those traditionally investigated?
Ecological Representativeness	Does the unit elicit information that reflects the local ecosystem in which the respondent's projects are embedded?
Temporal Extension	Is the unit restricted to a "snapshot" picture of human conduct or does it allow for temporal extension?
Joint Individual and Normative Level Measurement	Does the unit allow access to both idiographic and normative assessment?
Systemic measurement	Can the measurement of different variables radiate from the use of the same unit or are different "tests" required for each variable?
Modularity	Can different measurement operations be added in modular fashion via the unit or is it "fixed" and unmodifiable?
Integrative	Are the units such that cognitive, affective and behavioural aspects of human conduct are constitutive elements or are the units restricted to a particular domain (e.g. the cognitive?)
Indicator Status	Are the assessment units useful as social indicators above and beyond their utility as devices for the ascription of predicates to people?
Direct Applicability	Do the units have an ontological status of their own such that they can serve as the direct focus of intervention efforts or are they only oblique referents for psychological variables?

Little, 1987c), several examples will emerge in what follows as we discuss the empirical research carried out with PPA.[1]

B. Project Elicitation Lists: The Content of Commitments and Concerns

The opening module of PPA is the Personal Projects Elicitation List (or Project Dump as we call it less formally). Generically, it calls for the listing of a respondent's personal projects. Given the modular, open-ended nature of project analytic measurement, it is possible for this listing to be done orally or in writing, and it may be done with or without examples. In the most frequently used variant in our laboratory, we give

---

[1] While we feel it is important to explicate the assumptive base upon which our measurement units are constructed, we do recognize, of course, that these criteria are tailor-made to display the virtues of our own assessment technique. Personal projects are not, however, the only units which fare well on them. As will be seen in a later section, a whole new family of units in personality research (including life tasks, act trends, current concerns, and personal strivings) also meet many of these criteria. Comparative analyses of these units is an ongoing priority for research (e.g. Emmons, in press; Little, 1988).

an elicitation list accompanied by a brief description of the nature of personal projects and several examples selected to show a diversity of levels and contents of project (see Little, 1983). One might also prime individuals in order to elicit particular categories of project (e.g., generate projects that are in the service of some academic or social life task (Cantor & Kihlstrom, 1987)) or to generate personal goals falling into prespecified time frames (Zaleski, 1987). In addition, for clinical or counselling purposes, other priming procedures are found to be useful (Little, 1987c). For research purposes, however, we have tended to allow the respondents free reign to generate the full diversity of projects currently active in their system. This diversity is shown in Table 1.2, which displays a sampling of some of the personal projects generated by university student respondents.

While we do not specify how many projects are to be listed in the instructions, the mean number typically found is close to fifteen. These projects constitute the assessment units that are then used by each of the PPA modules to form an increasingly detailed picture of individuals in context and to generate indices that can be used for both predictive and explanatory purposes. It should be noted that PPA is primarily, but not exclusively, a self-report method and subject to the limitations inherent in such techniques. It is possible, however, for third parties to provide information about the key respondent's projects. A variant on this procedure will be taken up in Section II E.

Beyond their central status as the prime assessment units of PPA, the project descriptions generated during Phase I of PPA offer rich data for analysis in themselves. In particular, category analysis of personal project labels generated in Phase I of PPA has been examined in a number of investigations (e.g., academic, interpersonal, health, recreation projects). We have found very satisfactory interjudge agreement with a twelve-

TABLE 1.2. Examples of personal projects generated by university students in phase 1 of PPA.

finish my history essay
set time aside for spiritual life
watch Toronto beat up on Detroit
meet new friends
develop a philosophy of life
gain more cerebral friends
get laid
be more attentive to my brother
lose 15 pounds
care for my dying aunt
let fingernails grow
get wasted over Christmas
write the GRE
figure out mom and dad

category system using subcategories with the higher frequency categories (Little, 1988). In addition to category analysis, it is possible to examine other features of the written description of projects such as syntactic complexity or social desirability, and some of these will be illustrated below.

C. Project Rating Matrices: Basic and Special Dimensions

The core module in PPA is the Project Rating Matrix, which comprises a matrix of the individual's personal projects down the left hand side and a set of rating dimensions (for example, how "stressful" each project is) across the top. Respondents are asked to rate each of their listed projects on a 0 to 10 scale for each of the dimensions. The projects, then, are treated very much like test items in orthodox personality assessment, except that they meet the propaedeutic criteria discussed above, such as personal saliency and ecological representativeness.

It is possible to score each dimension of the matrix by summing the ratings in that column across each of the projects. Again, while PPA is meant to be a flexible methodology rather than a fixed test (more like ANOVA than an MMPI), we have tended to select *ten* projects from those listed on the Project Elicitation List, which individuals then rate on a number of dimensions chosen for their theoretical and applied relevance. While the initial versions of PPA (e.g., Little, 1972) involved only five dimensions, new columns were added to the matrix as different research questions were addressed. Column 2 of Table 1.3 lists the dimensions that comprise the basic PPA instrument, which are routinely scored in our laboratory. As shown in Column 1 of Table 1.3, we see the project dimensions as being subsumed by five core conceptual domains of project meaning, structure, community, efficacy, and stress. Project meaning dimensions tap whether one's pursuits are seen as worthwhile or worthless. Project structure dimensions assess the extent to which projects are organized or in disarray. Project community dimensions evaluate the extent to which projects are both known and supported by others. Project stress dimensions question whether the demands of our projects exceed our capacity to cope with them. Project efficacy dimen-

TABLE 1.3. Standard rating dimensions used in PPA and five theoretical factors.

Theoretical factors	Ratings dimensions on PPA
MEANING	Enjoyment, Value Congruency, Self-Prototypicality, Absorption, Importance
STRUCTURE	Initiation, Control, Time Adequacy, Positive Impact, Negative Impact
COMMUNITY	Visibility, Others View
STRESS	Stress, Challenge, Difficulty
EFFICACY	Progress, Outcome

sions probe whether one's undertakings have been, and will continue to be, progressing well.[2] To anticipate our later discussion, we believe that well-being will be enhanced to the extent that individuals are engaged in personal projects that are meaningful, well-structured, supported by others, not unduly stressful, and which engender a sense of efficacy. Conversely, depressive affect is expected to be experienced by those whose projects are meaningless, chaotic, isolated, stressful, and futile——a state of misery which, I keep assuring students, is not restricted to attempts at completing doctoral dissertations.

While ratings on these dimensions form the core of Phase II of PPA, they are often augmented by ad hoc dimensions that are regarded as relevant for a particular adoption of PPA Methods. Several examples can be given from our laboratory (see Little, 1987d for an annotated bibliography of these and related studies). Laura Goodine and I, in examining the project systems of anorexic and bulimic patients, used a dimension of depressive affect associated with each project. Pam Burgess created dimensions of "financial load" and "experienced guilt" to examine the conflict between academic and domestic projects in "student mothers." Brian Mavis asked men to rate "how old you feel when you are engaged in this project" to examine feelings of youthfulness associated with projects during middle age. Pit-Fong Loh used a dimension of "difficulties involving language" associated with each project in examining the ability of South East Asian "boat people" to adapt to their new, Canadian homes. In adopting PPA for use with women's interest groups, Susan Phillips created several new dimensions, including the extent to which each project received sufficient "human resources support" and sufficient "financial support."

As well as the standardized and ad hoc rating columns, the Project Rating Matrix has what we call Open Columns that require the respondent to describe aspects of the social context within which the project is embedded. Two questions that appear in our standard format, for example, are Where? (is the project carried out) and With Whom? (is it undertaken). Several measures has been derived from these columns, including measures of social network diffusiveness (e.g., Palys & Little, 1983; Bowie-Reed, 1984; see also Ruehlman & Wolchik, 1988) and category analysis of eco-settings within which projects are undertaken (e.g. Little, Pychyl & Gordon, 1986).

D. Phrasing Level Analysis: The Inner Context of Projects

One of the most interesting aspects of personal projects is their capacity to capture aspects of the hierarchical nature of human action. Projects can

---

[2] We have also used the project column matrices as input for Modal Profile Analyses (Skinner & Lei, 1980) which extract high frequency patterns of project dimension scores. We have presented evidence that these project profiles offer alternative routes to life satisfaction (Horley, Carroll & Little, 1988).

range from relatively molecular level, subordinate acts (such as "return the ladder to my neighbour") to highly molar level superordinate activities (such as "Challenge the rise of Australian realist philosophy"), though not surprisingly, most projects occupy a kind of middle class molarity between these extremes. Even within particular content categories, however, highly similar projects can be phrased at different levels—for example one person may list her project as "finish Chapter 8 of my Physics text," while her lab mate may list his as "grapple with the concept of superconductivity." We have been particularly interested in trying various methodological routes to measuring the hierarchical placement of projects and in looking at the correlates of phrasing level.

Some of our early studies (Little, Lavery, Carlsen, & Glavin, 1984) explored the use of what we called left and right laddering procedures for the analysis of the hierarchical level at which projects were phrased. Starting with the project as listed in the Project Dump (e.g., "finish my thesis"), respondents were asked to write down "Why" they were engaged in this project (e.g., "in order to get a job") to the left of the project description. This first-rung ladder was itself laddered by a further "why?" question and so on, until a terminal point was reached (e.g., the respondent maintained that a core value had been reached). In parallel fashion, a set of laddered, iterative, "How?" questions was also asked for each of the projects, which called for writing down to the right of each project the means through which it would be accomplished. Each response was laddered here until it reached a criterion of what we call "schedulability" (i.e., could it be scheduled into a fifteen minute time slot?). Our assumption was that projects were middle-level units of analysis hierarchically lodged between overarching values, core concerns, strivings, justifications, reasons or goals, on the one hand, and molecular level acts or operations on the other. For successful project management, it would be necessary to jointly optimize the manageability and the meaningfulness of projects. We assumed that the greater the distance between projects and their superordinate justifications the less meaningful were they likely to be. The greater the distance between projects and schedulable acts, the less manageable they were assumed to be.[3]

---

[3] While laddering may still be an appropriate methodological probe for examining the hierarchical nature of projects, some problems emerged in our recent explorations with this method. First, it is apparent that most projects are hierarchically organized, not in a ladder fashion, but more in terms of a lattice; that is, for each project there are multiple reasons and multiple means for carrying them out at the same level in the action hierarchy. This led to explorations with a project latticing technique (Little, 1988) which proved superior to the laddering procedure. Our most recent research, however, has tried to cut the Gordian knot by direct ratings of the molarity level of a personal project. We shall give examples drawn from this research in a later section.

E. Cross-Impact Matrices: The Outer Context of Projects

Personal projects have an outer face as well as an inner one. They have impacts upon each other within a single individual's project system, and they have impacts upon the outer ecology, including other people's project systems (Little, 1988). My trivial pursuits may play havoc with your magnificent obsessions, and both may end up as missions impossible.[4] Here is where the social ecological nature of personal projects comes into sharp focus. Methodologically, we can assess these contextual features with the Open Columns discussed earlier, and with the Personal Project Cross-Impact Matrices. Cross-impact matrices were introduced to reflect the fact that projects do not exist in vacuo, but form systems with attendant properties such as conflict and facilitation (Little, 1983). By rating the impact of each project on every other one in the system, we can calculate measures of overall project system conflict and cohesion as well as unpack which specific projects create the greatest systemic conflict for the individual.

The Joint Cross-Impact Matrix is a simple generalization from the single subject case. Here one gets two or more individuals to rate the impact of the other persons' projects on their own. Again, measures of joint project cohesion or conflict can be easily calculated.

To summarize, Personal Projects Analysis offers a window on the everyday plans, pursuits, and passions of people in context. Its modules offer an inward look at the hierarchical structure of projects and an outward look at their ecological impact. The indices that can be derived from the various modules are unconstrained: both new columns and modules can be added as theoretical or applied concerns dictate. Some of these indices have turned out to be important in studying aspects of human well-being, and will be briefly reviewed.

III. Personality, Personal Projects and Human Well-being: Alternative Routes to Coherence

We have recently completed a series of studies on the content, structure, and dynamics of personal project systems and the mediating role they play between personality and emotional well-being. The extensive set of

---

[4] It is important to note that triviality and magnificence are subjective construals rather than objectively discernible characteristics of personal projects. One of my students, for example, took umbrage with my use of the example "let my nails grow" as a fairly trivial project (a rather off-handed comment that landed me in hot water). She presented me with a four page history of nail cultivation in Western civilization. Clearly, for her, nail growing was a magnificent obsession. I was appropriately disarmed.

findings is available elsewhere and will not be summarized here (Little, 1988). I would, however, like to focus on one recurring pattern that emerged from our studies—the pervasive role that perceived *efficacy* vis-a-vis one's projects (hereafter termed "project efficacy") plays in linking project dimensions with orthodox personality variables and in providing a major path through which well-being and ecological competency are enhanced (Bandura, 1977).

It will be recalled that project efficacy was assessed by two project columns: the progress that respondents felt they had made on each of their projects, and their expectation that there would be a successful outcome to their projects. We refer to these components of project efficacy as project *progress* and *outcome* respectively. First, the links between personal project dimensions and personality will be examined, and then the relationships with measures of well-being. Finally, some emerging evidence relating to social competency and project management will be reviewed.

A. Big Five and other Correlates of Personal Project Indices

Results of a study of the correlations between normative scores on each of the standard personal project dimensions and four personality measures revealed some interesting patterns, particularly with respect to project efficacy. The NEO-PI (Costa & McCrae, 1986) is a multiscale inventory for the appraisal of what is now referred to (following Norman, 1963) as the Big Five domains of Neuroticism, Extraversion, Openness to Experience, Agreeableness, and Conscientiousness. Specific facets are also measured for each of the first three domains (for details on the meaning and measurement of the domains and facets see Costa & McRae (1986) and also McCrae (this volume)). With a composite sample of undergraduate respondents, a strong pattern of relationships was found with two of the major NEO domains: neuroticism and conscientiousness. Neuroticism scores were significantly correlated with project stress, difficulty, and negative impact, and (negatively) with project control, progress and, particularly, project outcome. Conscientiousness was significantly correlated with enjoyment, control, time-adequacy, outcome, self-identity, and progress in one's projects (Little, 1988).

Given the interdependencies within both facet and project variable sets, a clearer picture results from a canonical correlational analysis between the project dimensions and NEO facets (plus the single domain scores of Agreeableness and Conscientiousness). While it had been expected that several distinct dimensions of covariation would link the personality and project domains, one highly significant canonical variate emerged: inspection of structure coefficients reinforces the conclusions from the correlational analysis. Variation on the personality side centered on conscientiousness ($-.73$), self-consciousness ($.51$) and assertiveness ($-.51$), with the highest structure coefficients on the Projects side being outcome (−.73) and progress (−.59). It appears that the key axis of covariation between personality traits and project dimensions is epitomized by the contrasting images of Assertive Reliables pushing their projects through to completion and the Self-Consciously Timorous muddling along with, but not quite through, their projects.

Similar results were found with Paulhus' (1983) Spheres of Control measures, where, with another sample of university respondents, significant correlations were found between the Personal Control scale and project control, outcome, self-identity and, in particular, progress. Of considerable theoretical interest, however, is that these relationships were even higher with the *Interpersonal* Control scale, suggesting that social competency may play an important role in the negotiative aspects of project management (see Cantor & Kihlstrom, 1987).

The same general pattern also appeared when project dimensions were correlated with Scheier and Carver's (1985) recently developed measure of dispositional Optimism. Once again, project outcome was a key correlate, as was project control. Interestingly, progress in one's projects was not significantly correlated with Optimism, thus supporting the notion that the Optimism scale measures a future-oriented expectancy rather than a generalized gloss on one's achievements, past and present.

Finally, Antonovsky's (1983) Sense of Coherence (SOC) Scale afforded us a chance to examine directly our assumption that personal projects could provide routes towards the discovery of coherence, defined by Antonovsky as a belief "that things will work out as well as can reasonably be expected" (Antonovsky, 1979, p. 123). Here, too, substantial and theoretically interesting correlations were obtained, with overall coherence showing the strongest associations with the two project efficacy dimensions of progress and outcome.

Taken together, these studies provide converging evidence that personality factors and ratings of personal projects are linked largely through the pervasive connections between project efficacy and the personality dimensions of conscientiousness, control, optimism, and perceived coherence. This shown, we can now examine the links between personal projects and life satisfaction, with the expectation that efficacy might again prove to be a key link—this time between what we are doing and how we are feeling.

B. Project Dimensions and Well-being: Quantitative Synthesis

In Carleton's Social Ecology Laboratory, we have collected data on the relationship between life satisfaction and personal project dimension ratings with twenty-four separate samples of respondents (Little, 1988).

Deborah Wilson and I have been carrying out a quantitative synthesis of these studies through metaanalysis, and the first stage of the study can be briefly summarized. The three dimensions that show the greatest mean effect sizes in predicting life satisfaction are stress (negative), outcome, and control. Of these, stress and outcome show sufficient variation in effect sizes across studies that a search for moderator variables seems warranted. Our initial examination suggests that mean age of sample may play a key role, at least with respect to stress. For younger samples, the relationship between stress and well-being is greater than with older samples. It is not yet clear what sample characteristics mediate the relationship between project outcome and well-being, although we suspect an age × gender interaction may prove illuminating.

One of our recent studies confirms the importance of these variables and allows us to examine the relationship between project variables and depressive affect as measured by the CES-D depression scale (Radloff, 1977). With 290 students, project outcome, stress (negatively), and difficulty (negatively) had the highest correlations with life satisfaction. With depression scores, outcome (negatively) and stress, again, were the highest correlates, together with control (negatively) (Little, 1988).

While dimensions within each of the major theoretical domains of meaning, structure, and community show significant correlations with well-being, it is in the domains of stress and efficacy that satisfactions and disaffections with life are centered. The single best predictor of both life satisfaction and depressive affect is, once again, project outcome—the extent to which people feel their projects are likely to be successfully completed. Not only does our sense of efficacy in bringing our personal projects to successful completion provide the major link with personality factors, it also seems to be a pivotal factor in whether we thrive emotionally or lead lives of perhaps not so quiet desperation.

C. Project Scale, Spin and Social Competency: New Directions

We alluded earlier to the fact that we are now directly assessing the molarity level of personal projects generated in the Project Dump. Some early results from this research have yielded promising new directions for understanding project systems and the subtleties with which they need to be managed. There are two distinguishable components of phrasing level——linguistic complexity and ecological load. Personal projects rated high on linguistic complexity are phrased abstractly, with a high degree of verbal hedging and contingency (e.g., "try to be a better person"), while those rated lower are more concrete and direct (e.g., "stop smoking"). While complexity can be assessed in an absolute sense, ecological load is assessed by using benchmarks within certain project domains. It refers to the level of onerousness or demand associated with a project. Thus, "get a Ph.D." would score higher on load in the academic domain than would "get a cover for my history essay," even though they are identical in terms of linguistic complexity.

Stephen Szawlowski and I have run a preliminary study on phrasing level (restricted to linguistic complexity) which yielded an interesting pattern of results (Little, 1988). Higher phrasing level was associated with projects that were seen as more difficult, more time constrained, and less likely to be successfully completed (outcome). These high level molarity projects were also more likely to be seen as challenging, and as having others view them as important. In short, a trade-off seems to be involved with respect to the scale at which projects are mounted—the higher the phrasing level the less manageable projects are, but the more challenging and meaningful they appear to be (at least in others' eyes). These results dovetail with the perspective of Vallacher and Wegner (1987) on action identification, where a similar trade-off between meaning and manageability is postulated.

The scale at which projects are mounted is only one of a number of features of projects which, to invoke a recent media term, we might generically refer to as *project spin*. Project spin is the communicative form or style within which individuals wrap their projects. The same project "go away with Dan for a weekend" may be communicated differently depending upon whether one was talking to Dan or Dan's spouse. Beth MacDiarmid and I are starting to examine gender differences in project spin, in the light of evidence that women rate their projects as more important than do men.

We assume that socially skilled individuals will be able to spin their projects such that they have greater likelihood of generating social support, and that this may involve flexible shifting of phrasing level according to the situational demands or type of person receiving the communication. We also recognize that the same skills are particularly well-honed in Machiavellians and card-carrying psychopaths.

Len Lecci and I explored, in some detail, the social competency aspects of personal project management by developing a social competency scale based on act-frequency methodology (Buss & Craik, 1984), and by examining project system correlates of scores on this scale (Little, 1988). Again, a pattern we have now come to expect emerges clearly. Social competency is particularly associated with being engaged in personal projects that are high in outcome expectancy. Nevertheless, social competency scores were *also* highly correlated with *other people's* view of the project's importance. The socially competent person seems to be engaged in projects (or is able to spin projects) such that personal meaning and manageability are not reciprocally traded off but jointly maximized. We plan to continue this line of research this year in examining the skills with which individuals successfully negotiate life transitions between the educational and work domains.

IV. Enhancing Coherence: Individual and Contextual Applications of PPA

Several lines of applied work have developed out of our basic research on personal project systems, including an individual level intervention program for enhancing project systems (CAPPA), the development of short project system screening measures, and of a data bank of project profiles for use in community development and policy research. While the first two have been treated in more detail elsewhere, the third can be very briefly described.[5]

SEAbank (for *S*ocial *E*cological *A*ssessment data *bank*) takes the projects perspective up from the individual level of analysis to that of the social ecological or community context. Essentially, SEAbank is the cumulative set of data gathered in our laboratory formatted and designed for use by social agencies, community workers, government planning departments etc.. To adopt Cronbach's (1975) terms, SEAbank provides a resource through which we can pin down the contemporary facts about what people are doing. For example, at the project level, personal projects have been stored in SEAbank as strings containing both the project description (e.g., "lose ten pounds") and ratings on each of the core and special dimensions. Extensive demographic information, emotional and physical well-being indices, and individual difference scores on standard inventories are also stored for the individual case. By storing the

---

[5] CAPPA (Counsellor (or Computer) Assisted Personal Projects Analysis (Little, 1987) comprises a set of counselling modules which assist the counselor and client to detect possible problem areas relating to the content, scope, dynamics, and impact of personal project systems. Modules have been designed to help clients enhance the degree of meaningfulness, structure, community, and efficacy of their project systems and to decrease stress associated with their projects.

It should be noted that CAPPA provides a systemic framework within which a diverse set of social or life skill components can be integrated in a coherent fashion, thus decreasing the likelihood that benefits in one area (e.g., achieving greater control over one's projects) will be undermined by another (e.g., decreasing the likelihood of social support).

Brief screening measures have been developed in both Project System Q-Deck and Project System Rating Scale formats. Lisa Carver and I have been able to show that brief global ratings on project system meaning, structure, community, efficacy, and stress can serve as adequate proxy measures for the larger PPA assessment, and can be used as a preliminary screening device (for example in a counselling context) prior to more intensive assessment (Little, 1988).

data archivally at the individual project level, we are able to address an intriguing array of practical questions: What specific projects are seen by the rural elderly in Ontario as particularly stressful?; What categories of project have shown the greatest changes in perceived control for women from 1977 to the present?; Are the health projects of extraverts related more to recreational projects than they are for introverts?; What projects seem to offer the greatest sense of enjoyment and challenge to depressed students? SEAbank, in short, can provide fertile ground for conceptual trawlers of different orientation as well as those who wish to plan and deliver community services.

Both individual and social ecological levels of intervention with personal projects analysis emphasize the search for more coherent ways of living lives. CAPPA aids in providing a synoptic view of the full set of concerns and pursuits of individuals and promotes a more global consideration of life concerns than is typically found in counselling methodologies. SEAbank is designed to promote coherence by providing planners and caregivers with information about what people are up to and how things are going. This allows them to tailor the delivery of recreational, social, educational, and other programs to the specific project system profiles of target groups. In short, to borrow a phrase from green politics, projects analysis promotes coherence by enabling us simultaneously to think globally and act locally.

V. Big Five versus PAC10 Units in Personality Research: Reflections on Two Conferences

As part of this conference, we had the opportunity to exchange views on the likely trajectory of personality psychology as we approach the end of the century. One issue I raised, with which I would like to conclude, is the rise of a new generation of units of analysis in personality psychology, which, I feel, offers a genuine alternative to the Big Five traits that continue to figure so importantly in our field. These new units are middle-level rather than molar or molecular constructs, and they include current concerns (Klinger, 1977), life tasks (Cantor and Kihlstrom, 1987), personal strivings (Emmons, this volume), and our own personal projects, among others. While these units take somewhat different slants on personality, they share a concern with depicting human action in terms of its hierarchical structure, its intentional nature, and its contextual embeddedness.

The Big Five rubric always conjures up for me images of glory days on the personological gridiron. I propose, therefore, that these new emerging units in personality psychology form their own competing conference, which we might label the PAC10—where PAC stands for Personal Action Constructs and ten refers to a not entirely arbitrary guess as to how many basic dimensions (such as meaning, structure, efficacy etc.) will eventually emerge from the burgeoning work in this area.[6]

One of the key agenda items for personality psychology in the next few years will be the comparative analysis of these emerging units, their range and focus of convenience, and their relationship to the more conventional units in the field (Buss & Craik, 1983; Emmons, in press; Little, 1987a, 1988).

As our field prepares a new personology for the next decade, project analysts and other PAC10 research teams will want to be in the thick of things. We will be working to extract meaning, impose structure, attract support, modulate stress, and enhance efficacy both in our own projects *about* projects and in the lives of those individuals whose search for coherence falls short of successful completion. Whether the venture turns out to be mundane or magnificant, trivial or triumphant, it will be but one more manifestation of the enduring human project of searching for coherence.

Acknowledgements. The research reported here was supported by grants from the Social Sciences and Humanities Research Council of Canada, which is gratefully acknowledged. I also wish to thank the current members of our Social Ecology Laboratory, particularly Barb Watkinson, for their continuing support and collegial involvement.

References

Antonovsky, A. (1979). *Health, stress, and coping.* San Francisco: Jossey-Bass.

Antonovsky, A. (1983) The sense of coherence: Development of a research instrument. *Tel Aviv University Newsletter and Research Reports, 1,* 1–11.

Argyle, M., & Little, B.R. (1972). Do personality traits apply to social behaviour? *Journal for the Theory of Social Behaviour, 2,* 1–35.

Bandura, A. (1977). Self-efficacy: Toward a unifying theory of behavioral change. *Psychological Review, 84,* 191–125.

Buss, D.M., & Craik, K.H. (1983). The act frequency approach to personality. *Psychological Review, 90,* 105–126.

Buss, D.M., & Craik, K.H. (1984). Acts, dispositions, and personality. In B.A. Maher & W.B. Maher (Eds.), *Progress in experimental personality research: Normal personality processes:* Vol. 13. New York: Academic.

Cantor, N. & Kihlstrom, J.F. (1987). *Personality and social intelligence.* Englewood Cliffs, NJ: Prentice-Hall.

---

[6] Aficionadoes of NCAA football will recognize other reasons for coining the term (as will political activists). One senior psychologist at this conference let it be known sotto voce that if the Big Five played in a conceptual bowl game it would most likely be called the Dust Bowl. I propose that the PAC10 plays in a Coherence Bowl. Here the major goal is not descriptive empiricism about hypothetical traits, but explanatory accounts of intentional action (Little, 1988).

Costa, P.T. & McCrae, R.R. (1986). *Manual for the NEO-PI*. Odessa, Fla: PAR.
Cronbach, L.J. (1975). Beyond the two disciplines of scientific psychology. *American Psychologist, 30*, 116–127.
Emmons, R.A. (1989). The personal striving approach to personality. In L.A. Pervin (Ed.), *Goal concepts in personality and social cognition*. Hillsdale, NJ: Erlbaum.
Klinger, E. (1977). *Meaning and void: Inner experience and the incentives in people's lives*. Minneapolis: University of Minnesota.
Little, B.R. (1972). Psychological man as scientist, humanist and specialist. *Journal of Experimental Research in Personality, 6*, 95–118.
Little, B.R. (1976). Specialization and the varieties of environmental experience: Empirical studies within the personality paradigm. In S. Wapner, S.B. Cohen, & B. Kaplan (Eds.), *Experiencing the environment*. New York: Plenum.
Little, B.R. (1983). Personal projects: A rationale and method for investigation. *Environment and Behavior, 15*, 273–309.
Little, B.R. (1987a). Personality and the environment. In D. Stokols & I. Altman (Eds.), *Handbook of environmental psychology*. New York: Wiley.
Little, B.R. (1987b). Personal projects and fuzzy selves: Aspects of self-identity in adolescence. In T. Honess & K. Yardley (Eds.), *Self and identity: Perspectives across the life span*. London: Routledge & Kegan Paul.
Little, B.R. (1987c). Personal Projects Analysis: A new methodology for counselling psychology, *Natcon, 13*, 591–614.
Little, B.R. (1987d). Annotated bibliography of studies on personal projects and social ecology. Social Ecology Laboratory, Department of Psychology, Carleton University, Ottawa, Canada.
Little, B.R. (1988). Personal Projects Analysis: Method, Theory and Research, Final Report to Social Sciences and Humanities Research Council of Canada (SSHRC), Ottawa, Canada
Little, B.R., Lavery, J., Carlsen, N. & Glavin, G. (1981). *Personal projects across the life span*. Final Report to SSHRC. Ottawa, Canada
Little, B.R., Pychyl, T.A., & Gordon, C.C. (1986). What's a place like this doing in a project like me? In J.A. Teske (Chair), *People acting in places*. Symposium, Eastern Psychological Association Conference, New York.
Little, B.R., & Ryan, T.M. (1979). A social ecological model of development. In K. Ishwaran (Ed.), *Childhood and adolescence In Canada*. Toronto: McGraw-Hill.
Norman, W.T. (1963). Toward an adequate taxonomy of personality attributes: Replicated factor structures in peer nomination personality ratings. *Journal of Abnormal and Social Psychology, 66*, 574–583.
Palys, T.S. & Little, B.R. (1983). Perceived life satisfaction and the organization of personal project systems. *Journal of Personality and Social Psychology, 44*, 1121–1230.
Paulhus, D. (1983). Sphere-specific measures of perceived control. *Journal of Personality and Social Psychology, 44*, 1253–1265.
Radloff, L.S. (1977) The CES-D Scale: A self-report depression scale for research in the general population. *Applied Psychological Measurement, 1*, 385–401.
Ruehlman, L.S. & Wolchik, S.A. (1988). Personal goals and interpersonal support and hindrance as factors in psychological distress and wellbeing. *Journal of Personality and Social Psychology*, (in press).

Scheier, M.F. & Carver, C.S. (1985). Optimism, coping and health: Assessment and implications of generalized outcome expectancies. *Health Psychology, 4,* 219–247.

Skinner, H.A. & Lei, H. (1980). *Manual for modal profile analysis.* Toronto: Addiction Research Foundation.

Vallacher, R. & Wegner, D. (1987). What do people think they're doing? Action identification and human behavior. *Psychological Review, 94,* 3–15.

Zaleski, Z. (1987) Behavioral effects of self-set goals for different time ranges. *International Journal of Psychology, 22,* 17–38.

CHAPTER 2

Exploring the Relations Between Motives and Traits: The Case of Narcissism

Robert A. Emmons

Personality psychology has never suffered from a shortage of theoretical constructs. Terms such as motive, trait, value, wish, attitude, goal, belief, schema, and need represent a mere sampling of the conceptual units that have been employed in the pursuit of understanding the human personality. Of these, motives and traits have clearly received the lion's share of the attention, and most personologists would agree that these two are the primary tools existing in our conceptual armamentarium with which to attack emerging issues in personality. One of the emerging issues confronting the field today is mapping the conceptual and empirical relationships between trait-based and motive-based structures. The purposes of this chapter are to address the issues involved in this mapping, and to provide an example of how it may be possible to address the interrelations between these units of analysis empirically.

The trait concept has recently been the target of a conceptual overhaul (Buss & Craik, 1983; Read & Miller, 1989) and the motive concept has similarly benefited from creative reanalyses (Cantor & Kihlstrom, 1987; Emmons, 1987; McAdams, 1985). For the purpose of this chapter, traits will be broadly defined as stylistic and habitual patterns of cognition, affect, and behavior. Motives can be defined as a disposition to be concerned with and to strive for a certain class of incentives or goals. Traits are descriptive units and account for repetitive, habitual behavior, while motives are invoked to explain directional behavior (Maddi, 1989).

Many theorists, especially those identified with the motive tradition, have argued for a separation of these concepts. Murray (1938) drew a distinction between needs and need-integrates, the latter representing stable, habitual behavior in the service of needs. McClelland (1951, 1981, 1985) has maintained that personologists need to pay attention to three types of variables: motives or needs, schemas or beliefs, and traits or skills. In his "logical geography" of personality, Alston (1970, 1975) excavated two units of analysis, traits in a summary-frequency sense and motives as purposive-cognitive concepts, and argued that it is possible to understand the former in terms of the latter. Since one objective of the science of personality is to distinguish the parts and subsystems and to understand them in relation to the whole system, we must consider the relationship between two of the major parts, motives and traits. These are weighty issues, and do not lend themselves to a cursory treatment. Therefore, the remainder of this chapter is devoted to an empirical example of how it might be possible to attack the problem of the relationship between trait-based and motive-based units of analysis.

There are many ways to explore this relationship, and some are likely to be more profitable than others. It will probably not be useful to correlate lists of motives with lists of traits, because lists of motives often turn out to be nothing more than disguised trait inventories. This approach would also shed little light on the processes linking motivational and trait structures. On the other hand, one could study motivation at different levels of depth, ranging from greater to lesser accessibility to awareness, and focus on the motivational underpinnings of a single trait as it is manifested in the lives of individuals. That is the tack that will be followed here, using narcissism as an example.

Few personality traits have captured the attention of as diverse a group of scholars as has narcissism. Psychologists, psychiatrists, psychobiographers, social critics, historians, poets, and writers, to name but a few, have sought to understand the dynamics underlying what may be the most talked about personality characteristic of our time. Ironically, until recently, little was known about the role of narcissism in personological functioning. Fortunately, Raskin & Hall (1981) developed a multidimensional individual difference measure of narcissism, the Narcissistic Personality Inventory (NPI), and much of the talk has now been translated into action: a number of studies have documented the construct validity of the NPI, in both clinical and non-clinical samples (see Raskin & Terry, 1988 for a review). Narcissism can be defined as "Self-admiration that is characterized by tendencies toward grandiose ideas, exhibitionism, and defensiveness in response to criticism; interpersonal relationships are characterized by feelings of entitlement, exploitativeness, and a lack of empathy" (Raskin & Terry, 1988, p. 896).

Why focus on narcissism? Not all traits are equally worthy candidates for exploring the links with motivation. For example, temperament characteristics such as neuroticism or emotional intensity are less likely to be directly involved in goal-directed activity. Narcissism, however, is a rich, multifaceted construct consisting of attitudes toward the self and others, characteristic interpersonal orientations, and chronic emotional reactions. Therefore, narcissism should have considerable relevance for understanding the motivational facets of a person's life. What sorts of motivational concerns should a narcissistic individual display? In order to formulate these hypotheses, it is first necessary to consider the major motivational systems that have been outlined in the motive literature: achievement, affiliation, intimacy, and power.

Achievement motivation can be defined as a recurrent preference or readiness in thought and behavior for experiences of attaining excellence——of competing with a standard of excellence (McClelland, 1985). Achievement-oriented individuals are highly self-motivated persons who persist when faced with obstacles, and who are concerned with achieving excellence as an end in itself. Narcissistic individuals have been described as possessing intense ambition and experiencing fantasies of success (Akhtar & Thomson, 1982). At the same time, their aspirations are often unrealistic, and they lack the internal motivation required to bring long-term projects to completion. It has also been suggested that the achievement-related behaviors are employed more in the service of recognition and admiration rather than an end in themselves. Given this mixed evidence, a positive relationship, though not a large one, was expected between narcissism and achievement.

Affiliation motivation can be defined as a recurrent preference in thought and behavior for experiences of establishing, maintaining, and restoring a positive affective relationship (Atkinson, Heyns, & Veroff, 1954). Affiliation-oriented individuals have a strong concern with being liked and a fear of being rejected; they tend to report high levels of negative affect when not interacting with others, yet do not show a corresponding increase in positive affect when interacting with others (McAdams & Constantian, 1983). Narcissistic individuals are exhibitionistic, are highly concerned with being liked, crave attention and admiration, and are highly sensitive to criticism (Akhtar & Thomson, 1982; APA, 1980). Based upon these findings, narcissism was expected to show a positive relationship with affiliation-motivation.

Intimacy motivation can be defined as a recurrent preference in thought and behavior for experiences of warm, close, and communicative interactions with others. The preference is for interpersonal exchange as an end in itself, rather than as a means to another end (McAdams, 1980). Intimacy-oriented individuals are concerned with establishing and maintaining close interpersonal relationships and report positive emotions in the presence of others (McAdams & Constantian, 1983). McAdams (1980) found intimacy motivation to be negatively correlated with peer reports of dominance and self-centeredness. Narcissism should be negatively correlated with intimacy: one of the prototypical features of narcissism is a lack of empathy and concern for others (Watson et. al., 1984). Other characteristics of narcissistic individuals that make a negative relationship likely include the inability to remain in love, a tendency to devalue others, interpersonal exploitation, and a superficiality in interpersonal relations (Akhtar & Thomson, 1982; Kernberg, 1976).

Power motivation can be defined as a recurrent preference in thought and behavior for experiences of feeling strong and having impact on others. Among other correlates, power-oriented individuals are concerned with attaining status and prestige; they choose as friends persons low in power motivation and are highly promiscuous in heterosexual relationships (Winter & Stewart, 1978). Narcissism is characterized by fantasies of wealth, power, beauty, and brilliance——the "narcissistic pursuit of power" (Kernberg, 1976). Narcissistic individuals report engaging in disinhibition-related activities, such as drinking, gambling, and casual sexual encounters (Emmons, 1981). Based on these findings, narcissism is predicted to be positively associated with the need for power.

Of course, these four motives do not exhaust the possible ways in which narcissistic individuals strive for goals in their everyday lives. Other needs, such as striving for perfection, self-presentation, and self-sufficiency (Raskin & Terry, 1988) could also be added. Nevertheless, these constitute four well-developed major motivational systems about which considerable evidence exists (McClelland, 1985).

Motivational themes are most commonly assessed through content analysis of imaginative stories written to TAT pictures. McClelland (1981) refers to these stories as "operant" measures—spontaneous thoughts and actions that are not necessarily in response to clearly identifiable stimuli; they are distinguished from "respondent" measures, such as items in a questionnaire.

There are several assumptions behind the use of the TAT; one is that individuals are not able consciously to report on their motives; another is that all individuals can be characterized by a common set of motives. While there may be some truth in both of these assumptions, there is also reason to believe that such an approach fails to capture the complexity and discriminativeness with which motivational concerns impact on the lives of individuals. Therefore, Emmons (1986, 1989) developed the concept of a "personal striving," which he defines as the types of goals a person typically or characteristically seeks in his or her everyday behavior. Personal strivings can be thought of as idiographic representations of the major motives, and are one example of the "new look" in middle-level units of analysis (Buss, this volume; Little, this volume). Examples of strivings are shown in Table 2.1. In addition to asking what motives narcissistic individuals possess, the personal strivings approach

TABLE 2.1. Striving examples and content categories.

Category	Example
Achievement	"Work toward higher athletic capabilities"
Affiliation	"Be friendly with others so they will like me"
Intimacy	"Help my friends and let them know I care"
Power	"Force men to be intimate in relationships"
Personal Growth/Health	"Develop a positive self-worth"
Self-Presentation	"Be concerned about my physical appearance"
Autonomy/Independence	"Be myself and not do things to please others"

asks: What is a narcissistic individual trying to do? The approach also assumes that the person can, when probed, consciously report on what they are trying to do. Both motive dispositions and personal strivings were assessed in this study.

Fifty subjects were administered the NPI and the TAT, and generated lists of their personal strivings. From the NPI, the total scale score and scores on seven subscales (Authority, Self-Sufficiency, Superiority, Exhibitionism, Exploitativeness, Entitlement, and Vanity) were derived. After the striving lists were obtained, strivings were coded into the content categories shown in Table 2.1 by two trained coders, whose level of agreement was 88%. Discrepancies were discussed until resolved. The TAT was administered in the standard group format in which subjects have five minutes to write a story in response to each of six pictures (described in McAdams & Constantian, 1983). Protocols were scored according to the standard training manuals for achievement, intimacy, and power (affiliation was not scored), and scorer agreement with the manuals ranged from 88 to 94%.

Subjects provided names and addresses of up to ten peers, whom each of were sent letters asking them to generate a list of what they thought the subject's strivings were, i.e., what they thought the subject was trying to do. An average of 5.5 peers responded for each subject. From these observer-generated protocols, a consensual list of the subject's strivings was formulated.

Table 2.2 shows the correlations between the NPI factors and the three motives as assessed by the TAT. Need for power is correlated with the total score and with two of the seven factors, and need for intimacy is correlated negatively only with Entitlement. Note that these correlations are uniformly modest. Given that the reliability and validity of these instruments has been established (McClelland, 1985; Raskin & Terry, 1988), these data could be interpreted as supporting McClelland's (1981) contention that operant and respondent measures tap different aspects of personality and, therefore, should not be highly correlated with each other.

TABLE 2.2. Correlations between the TAT motives and NPI.

	nAch	nInt	nPow
Total	.17	−.14	.22*
Authority	.04	−.11	.16
Self-sufficiency	.14	−.21*	.18
Superiority	−.14	.15	.02
Exhibitionism	.34*	−.09	.26*
Exploitativeness	.18	−.11	.20*
Entitlement	.14	−.24*	.07
Vanity	.11	−.05	−.04

Note. N = 60. *$p < .05$.

In order to examine the correlations between the NPI and personal strivings, the strivings were aggregated into content categories to reflect achievement, affiliation, intimacy, and power, as well as other conceptually relevant categories. Correlations between the striving categories and the NPI are shown in Table 2.3. Contrary to predictions, narcissism was unrelated to affiliation strivings and only Entitlement was related to achievement strivings. As predicted, narcissistic individuals are not particularly interested in establishing and maintaining warm interpersonal relations, but they are interested in having impact on and influence over others. It is interesting that Exploitativeness (but not Entitlement) was related to more power strivings, and Entitlement (but not Exploitiveness) was related to fewer intimacy strivings. The fundings support the separation of these two narcissistic components, which had been combined in earlier factor analytic work on the NPI (Emmons, 1984, 1987), and also point to the importance of separating affiliative and intimacy strivings, since the two show different patterns of correlations in these data and correlate with each other only .25.

I have contended that one advantage of the personal strivings approach lies in the idiographic nature of the strivings. What is the relationship between narcissism and the goal strivings of individuals in their everyday lives? In order to examine this, the specific strivings of the two highest and two lowest scorers on the NPI are displayed in Tables 2.4 and 2.5. The themes of domination and exploitation are quite evident throughout "Cat Scratch's" strivings, and possibly the pseudonym chosen by that subject, taken from rock star Ted Nugent, also reflects these concerns. "Crocodile Dundee' admits to a substantially different pattern of strivings, yet they also contain narcissistic overtones. Themes of self-presentation, being overly concerned with appearance, and with being the center of attention are most evident. Contrast these two individuals with the strivings of "Ethel Merman" and "0372", the two lowest scorers on the NPI. "Ethel Merman" is most concerned with minimizing interpersonal conflict, with getting along with and helping others——affiliative concerns. The strivings of subject "0372" contain intimacy themes such

TABLE 2.3. Correlations between striving categories and NPI.

	sAch	sAff	sInt	sPow	sSpr	sPgh
Total	.12	.02	−.30*	.27*	.21*	.09
Authority	.12	−.03	−.28*	.21*	.14	.15
Self-sufficiency	.01	.09	−.17	−.09	.13	.11
Superiority	−.09	.03	−.01	.08	.19	.02
Exhibitionism	.08	.06	−.27*	.41**	.34**	.03
Exploitativeness	.04	−.10	.04	.40**	−.14	−.09
Entitlement	.33**	.11	−.32**	−.03	−.02	.06
Vanity	.01	−.05	−.30*	.20	.37**	.06*

Note. s = striving. Spr = self-presentation. Pgh = personal growth/health

TABLE 2.4. Strivings, high NPI subjects.

(Cat scratch)

1. Dominate people in certain situations.
2. Manipulate people, especially women, to see things from my point of view.
3. Use charm and a smiling face to become friends with someone.
4. Apply my education through my own life and belief.
5. Bring out the best in someone who has been mentally used or abused.
6. Be strong against people who could eventually use me for things.
7. Spend a large amount of money on my friends.
8. Not accept the standard answer in a discussion.
9. Reject authority—church leaders, police, boss.
10. Enjoy my sexuality to the fullest potential, and show my partner the same enjoyment.
11. Be aggressive in team sports.
12. Understand people's problems and not stereotype.
13. Fight for the underdog.
14. Sit next to the most beautiful and physically built woman in class, and then attempt to conquer her attention.
15. Stay active and physically fit.

(Crocodile Dundee)

1. Always appear cool.
2. Not be pessimistic.
3. Keep the peace when conflicts arise in groups.
4. Always amuse others.
5. Always keep physically fit.
6. Always keep socially aware and socially active.
7. Keep myself involved in the peace movement.
8. Not be so defensive with men.
9. Help others with their problems.
10. Avoid the appearance of being aloof.
11. Avoid being anxious.
12. Dress fashionably.
13. Avoid conforming to trends.
14. Wear the other person out.
15. Impress my parents.

as being aware of others' feelings and staying in touch with others. While difficult to quantify, it is clear that these strivings provide us with types of information about these four individuals other than simply knowing their standing on the trait dimension of narcissism. In fact, "Cat Scratch" and "Crocodile Dundee" achieved identical scores, as did "Ethel Merman" and "0372." Yet obviously, the nature of the objectives that these four people are trying to obtain is quite different.

It may be argued that these relationships are a function of the self-report nature of these data. Since "Cat Scratch" is interested in having impact on others, could he not achieve it by boasting about his dramatic strivings? To overcome this possible limitation, ten of the subject's peers were asked to generate a list of what they believed that

TABLE 2.5. Strivings, low NPI subjects.

(0372)

1. Please others.
2. Avoid people that only think of themselves.
3. Tell the truth.
4. Avoid arguments.
5. Be productive in work.
6. Make my parents proud.
7. Be aware of others' feelings.
8. Act mature in times of crisis.
9. Stay in touch with friends and grandparents.
10. Stay in touch with friends from home.
11. Spend as little money as I can on trivial materials.
12. Not interrupt people when talking.
13. Keep a low profile when at a party.
14. Be nice to my fellow man.

(Ethel Merman)

1. Do well in school.
2. Get along with people.
3. Have people I'm around like me.
4. Voice my opinion.
5. Keep an open mind about things.
6. Help other people.
7. Stay thin while doing as little as possible to achieve it.
8. Not get into spats with my mother.
9. Set goals and follow a course to get them.
10. Get out and meet people.
11. Not get in fights with my roomates.
12. Smooth over things so people won't get mad.
13. Only pay attention to what I'm doing at a certain time.
14. Not show people I'm mad.
15. Fit in.

person's strivings to be. Table 2.6 shows the strivings attributed to the target subjects by at least two of their associates. As can be seen, "Cat Scratch's" "friends" were remarkably adept at figuring out what he was up to. "Crocodile Dundee's" associates were able to pinpoint her attention-seeking strivings, and "Ethel Merman's" community of observers were also quite accurate at judging her strivings. Now, undoubtedly, the degree of correspondence between self-reported and peer-attributed strivings are a function of many factors, including the observability of the strivings, familiarity with the target, the target's tendency to self-disclose, etc. Despite ignoring these factors, these fascinating results suggest that people are able to infer what another person is trying to do. Narcissism may be unique in that there is considerable hedonic relevance in knowing what a narcissistic individual is going to try to do to you. In any case, the findings suggest that the relations between narcissism and personal strivings are not solely a function of self-report biases.

TABLE 2.6. Peer attributed strivings, high and low NPI.

(Cat scratch-high NPI)

1. Get ahead by bettering himself.
2. Belittle people who make mistakes.
3. Be liked by others by showing his insights and intelligence.
4. Make himself physically attractive to others.
5. Be liked by everybody.
6. Advance in the social ladder.
7. Act like he is more than he is.
8. Tell others of his strivings and goals in life.
9. Be accepted by others.
10. Please others.

(Crocodile Dundee-high NPI)

1. Give the impression of being a liberal and open-minded person.
2. Look nice—physically by her hair, dress, and make-up.
3. Choose a career that will help build a better world.
4. Be very opinionated.
5. Be independent—not needing a lot from anyone.
6. Keep away from being a burden to others.
7. Make a name for herself.
8. Obtain approval.
9. Accomplish everything/do too much.
10. Stand out in a crowd.

(Ethel Merman-low NPI)

1. Help others with their problems.
2. Listen to other people (she's a good listener).
3. Better her understanding of herself.
4. Understand people's motivations——analyze their actions.
5. Keep private feelings to herself.
6. Seem open, but is typically introverted.
7. Find reasons as to why things happen.
8. Maintain honest and open relationships.

It is clear that several predictable and theoretically meaningful relationships exist between the trait of narcissism and its underlying motivational themes. These themes appeared both in imagery related to TAT cards as well as in self-reported and peer-attributed goal strivings——results that indicate it is feasible to examine the motivational underpinnings of a single trait in a theoretically informed manner. In addition, it would appear that narcissistic individuals possess well-articulated self-representations, which would appear to contradict other findings that narcissists lack insight into their own condition (Kernberg, 1976). Moreover, the current study demonstrated the feasibility of employing different motivational levels of analysis (both idiographic and nomothetic) and the benefits of obtaining multiple data sources (both self- and peer-reports), since considerable convergence was found across these methods.

These findings represent only a beginning. In addition to content, motivational processes such as goal conflict and goal complexity could also be addressed. It has been suggested that narcissistic individuals possess the potentially conflicting goals of self-sufficiency and independence while striving for approval and admiration in order to validate their precarious self-esteem (Kernberg, 1976). Narcissistic individuals ought to be low in self-complexity, or the tendency to differentiate among aspects of the self, since splitting (tendency to see things in all-or-none terms) is a major feature of the narcissistic personality (Emmons, 1987; Raskin & Terry, 1988).

Up to this point, the obvious question has been deliberately sidestepped. Are people narcissistic because of the types of goals they strive after, or do they strive for these goals because they are narcissistic? The answer to this question depends partly on the degree of causal agency one is willing to grant the trait concept. In the absence of a clear physiological substrate (Gottschalk, 1988), as is the case for traits such as extraversion, neuroticism or sensation-seeking, it is difficult to grant narcissism this determining role.

From a different perspective, this question can also be attacked developmentally. There is widespread agreement that narcissistic traits are formed early in childhood (Miller, 1981) and are also highly resistant to change. On the other hand, it has also been argued that certain personal strivings develop early in life (Emmons, 1989). Thus, it is difficult to argue that one temporally precedes the other. Perhaps the most defensible statement that could be made at this time is that both are products of common developmental experiences, and that they are merely correlated, rather than one causing the other.

Arguments concerning causal priority are logical only if one assumes that motives and traits are separable components of personality. As was pointed out earlier, proponents of the motive concept have defended this position, but it is far from a unanimous one. An alternative point of view is represented in the writings of Aronoff & Wilson (1985), Cochran (1984), and Read & Miller (1989). These authors have suggested that traits are megastructures composed of several elements, some of which are motivational in nature. Space does not permit a detailed analysis of all of these positions, however, the framework offered by Read and Miller is especially intriguing and worthy of mention here.

Read and Miller have proposed that stable individual differences (traits) can be viewed as chronic configurations of the individual's *goals, plans* and strategies for achieving those goals, *resources* for acting on the plans, and *beliefs* that affect the choice of plans and strategies. (Note the similarity here with McClelland's tripartite division of personality discussed earlier.) Instead of viewing these as separate constructs, however, their major premise is that central to every trait is a goal. It is not clear where stylistic, temperamental traits fit in here, but, assuming their major premise, I would add that central to most traits is not a single goal but multiple goals, which vary in their relevance to the trait. This would be especially evident in the case of a complex trait like narcissism. Seen in this light, narcissism could be viewed as a chronic configuration of goals regarding exploiting others, seeking attention, appearing confident, etc., coupled with plans and strategies for achieving these goals, beliefs about the efficacy of the plans, strategies for achieving the goals, and resources that constrain or facilitate goal attainment. Perhaps the most notable contribution this framework makes is that it specifies the processes by which trait-structures are translated into action, thus taking a large step toward bridging the much-discussed gap between what personality *is* and what personality *does* (Cantor & Kihlstrom, 1987; Emmons & King, 1989). Goal concepts are ideal units of analysis for bridging this gap as they signify both coherence and discriminativeness, stability and flexibility.

Before judging the heuristic value of this perspective, however, it is first necessary to demonstrate linkages between trait-based and goal-based units of analysis. The present study is significant in that it did demonstrate these linkages between the trait of narcissism and chronic goal concerns in the form of motives and personal strivings. Goals are desirable units for studying such linkages because of their rich hierarchical structure and their access to consciousness. Yet much work remains to be done before we understand 1) the interdependencies between these goals; 2) how these goals become translated into action; 3) situational and biological factors that inhibit or facilitate goal-directed action. Such research will help us to understand the relations between trait-based and motivationally-based structures of personality, and account for the coherence and unity of personality.

References

Akhtar, S. & Thomson, J.A. (1982). Overview: Narcissistic personality disorder. *American Journal of Psychiatry, 139,* 12–20.

Alston, W.P. (1970). Toward a logical geography of personality: Traits and deeper lying personality characteristics. In H.D. Kiefer & M.K. Munitz (Eds.), *Mind, science, and history* (pp. 70–105). Albany, NY: SUNY Press.

Alston, W.P. (1975). Traits, consistency, and conceptual alternatives for personality theory. *Journal for the Theory of Social Behavior, 5,* 17–48.

American Psychiatric Association (1980). *Diagnostic and statistical manual of mental disorders: DSM-III.* Washington, D.C.: Author.

Aronoff, J., & Wilson, J.P. (1985). *Personality in the social process.* Hillsdale, NJ: Erlbaum.

Atkinson, J.W., Heyns, R.W., & Veroff, J. (1954). The effect of experimental arousal of the affiliative motive on thematic apperception. *Journal of Abnormal and Social Psychology, 49,* 405–410.

Buss, D.M., & Craik, K.H. (1983). The act-frequency approach to personality. *Psychological Review, 90,* 105–126.

Cantor, N., & Kihlstrom, J.F. (1987). *Personality and social intelligence.* Englewood Cliffs, NJ: Prentice-Hall.

Cochran, L. (1984). On the categorization of traits. *Journal for the Theory of Social Behavior, 14,* 183–209.

Emmons, R.A. (1981). Relationship between narcissism and sensation seeking. *Psychological Reports, 48,* 247–250.

Emmons, R.A. (1984). Factor analysis and construct validity of the Narcissistic Personality Inventory. *Journal of Personality Assessment, 48,* 291–300.

Emmons, R.A. (1986). Personal strivings: An approach to personality and subjective well-being. *Journal of Personality and Social Psychology, 51,* 1058–1068.

Emmons, R.A. (1987). Narcissism: Theory and measurement. *Journal of Personality and Social Psychology, 52,* 11–17.

Emmons, R.A. (1987, August). *Current status of the motive concept.* In K. Craik & R. Hogan (Chairs), *Fifty Years of Personality Psychology.* Symposium conducted at the 95th Annual Convention of the American Psychological Association, New York.

Emmons, R.A. (1989). The personal striving approach to personality. In L.A. Pervin (Ed.), *Goal concepts in personality and social psychology.* (pp. 87–126). Hillsdale, NJ: Erlbaum.

Emmons, R.A. & King, L.A. (1989). On the personalization of motivation. In T.K. Srull & R.S. Wyer, Jr., *Advances in social cognition. Vol. 2: Social intelligence and the cognitive assessment of personality.* Hillsdale, NJ: Erlbaum.

Gottschalk, L.A. (1988). Narcissism: Its normal evolution and development and the treatment of its disorders. *American Journal of Psychotherapy, 42,* 4–27.

Kernberg, O. (1976). *Borderline conditions and pathological narcissism.* New York: Jason Aronson.

Maddi, S.R. (1989). *Personality theories: A comparative analysis* (5th ed.). Chicago, IL: Dorsey Press.

McAdams, D.P. (1980). A thematic coding system for the intimacy motive. *Journal of Research in Personality, 14,* 413–432.

McAdams, D.P., & Constantian, C.A. (1983). Intimacy and affiliation motives in daily living: An experience sampling analysis. *Journal of Personality and Social Psychology, 45,* 851–861.

McClelland, D.C. (1951). *Personality.* New York: Dryden.

McClelland, D.C. (1961). *The achieving society.* Princeton, NJ: Van Nostrand.

McClelland, D.C. (1981). Is personality consistent? In A. Rabin, J. Aronoff, and R. Zucker (Eds.), *Further explorations in personality* (pp. 87–113). New York: Wiley.

McClelland, D.C. (1985). *Human motivation.* Glenview, IL: Scott, Foresman.

Miller, A. (1981). *Prisoners of childhood.* New York: Basic Books.

Murray, H.A. (1938). *Explorations in personality.* New York: Oxford University Press.

Raskin, R.N., & Hall, C.S. (1981). The Narcissistic Personality Inventory: Alternate form reliability and further evidence of construct validity. *Journal of Personality Assessment, 45,* 159–162.

Raskin, R. N., & Terry, H. (1988). A principal-components analysis of the Narcissistic Personality Inventory and further evidence of its construct validity. *Journal of Personality and Social Psychology, 54,* 890–902.

Read, S.J., & Miller, L.C. (1989). Inter-personalism: Towards a goal-based theory of persons in relationships. In L.A. Pervin (Ed.), *Goal concepts in personality and social psychology*. (pp. 413–472). Hillsdale, NJ: Erlbaum.

Watson, P.J., Grisham, S.O., Trotter, M.V., & Biderman, M.D. (1984). Narcissism and empathy: Validity evidence for the Narcissistic Personality Inventory. *Journal of Personality Assessment, 48,* 301–305.

Winter, D., & Stewart, A.J. (1978). The power motive. In H. London & J.E. Exner, Jr. (Eds.), *Dimensions of personality* (pp. 391–448). New York: Wiley.

CHAPTER 3

Cognitive Strategies as Personality: Effectiveness, Specificity, Flexibility, and Change

Julie K. Norem

As units of personality, *cognitive strategies* describe how individuals use self-knowledge and knowledge about the social world to translate their goals into behavior. The concept of a strategy captures coherent patterns of appraisal, planning, retrospection, and effort (Bruner, Goodnow, & Austin, 1956; Cantor & Kihlstrom, 1987; Norem, 1987; Showers & Cantor, 1985). Strategies focus on *process:* the ways people direct their attention, construct expectations and goals, allocate their time and effort, protect their self-esteem, and react emotionally. Thus, strategies elaborate on the *instantiation* of traits and motives. Analysis of personality and individual differences in terms of strategies shifts emphasis away from general dispositions towards the cognitive links between motives and actions.

This perspective on personality assumes that a general trait, disposition, or motive has many potential manifestations (although some acts may be considered better or more "prototypical" expressions of a disposition, see Buss & Craik, 1984). Need for achievement, for example, may be expressed in cutthroat competition among brokers on Wall Street, or through dedication to improving on a "personal best" in a marathon. Similarly, specific behaviors may represent a number of diverse general characteristics when performed by different individuals in different situations. Organizing departmental colloquia could be an expression of affiliative motives for one person and an expression of power motives for another (Winter, 1988). The contention here is that *personality* is embodied at least as much in the different ways nAch (or introversion or aggression) might be expressed by different individuals, as in differences in those characteristics themselves. Individual differences are expressed in the interpretations of situations and pursuit of specific goals: e.g., beating others vs. improving one's self, or promoting collegial discourse vs. controlling people and resources.

These assumptions, then, locate personality in the specific goals individuals construct for themselves, in the form of "life tasks" (Cantor & Kihlstrom, 1987), "personal projects" (Palys & Little, 1983), "personal strivings" (Emmons, 1986), or even situationally specific expectations; and in the strategies individuals develop to pursue these goals (e.g. Buss, 1987; Cantor, Norem, Niedenthal, Langston & Brower, 1987). There are several important implications of personality conceived of in this way. In this chapter, I plan to discuss these implications, review some recent data that support hypotheses derived from this perspective, and conclude with a consideration of future directions in personality research that build on current data and theory.

Examples of Strategies: Defensive Pessimism and "Illusory Glow" Optimism

Throughout this discussion, research on two particular strategies will serve to illustrate the central tenets of this approach. These strategies are "illusory glow" optimism and defensive pessimism (Norem & Cantor, 1986a). The defensive pessimism strategy involves individuals with acknowledged positive performance histories in a particular domain, who, nevertheless, set unrealistically low expectations when anticipating new situations within that domain. Individuals using the strategy feel anxious and out of control, and play through a "worst-case" analysis—dwelling on possible negative outcomes—even when those outcomes seem improbable.

Data from experimental and field research on defensive pessimism in the achievement domain indicate that these negative expectations do not become self-fulfilling prophecies, or lead to effort withdrawal. Nor do they necessarily have the emotional consequences associated with more generalized pessimistic or depressive attributional style (Peterson & Seligman, 1984; Showers & Ruben, 1988). Instead, individuals using the defensive pessimist strategy invest considerable effort in tasks they see as important (Norem & Cantor, 1986b). Moreover, in the short-run at least, individuals using the strategy perform as well as subjects using an optimistic strategy, and feel just as satisfied with their performance. Unlike optimistic subjects, defensive pessimists do not seem to "revise" their understanding of a performance after the fact in order to protect their self-esteem. For example, in an experimental setting, they did not deny having control when given failure feedback relative to when given success feedback (Norem & Cantor, 1986a).

In contrast, individuals using "illusory glow" optimism do not anticipate negative outcomes; nor do they typically feel anxious or out of control prior to performance situations. Optimists set realistically high expectations, based on their past successes. They then protect or enhance their positive self-image using the battery of positive illusions and biases documented by researchers investigating the differences between depressive and non-depressive cognition (see Taylor & Brown, 1988, for a review). In the study cited in the paragraph above, optimistic subjects showed a typical "illusion of control" for success, while denying control for failure.

It is important to note that individuals using these two different strategies have constructed somewhat different goals for themselves, which follow from their appraisal of relevant situations. Research comparing these groups has focused on situations that both optimists and defensive pessimists see as important, rewarding, and absorbing. The defensive pessimists, however, also see these same situations as more stressful and less within their control than the optimists (Cantor, Norem, Niedenthal, Langston & Brower, 1987). For the defensive pessimist group, therefore, there is an additional crucial dimension to the "problem" presented by these situations: dealing with anxiety and "taking control" of a situation in order to perform well.

For the optimist group, remaining in control and staying "up" is part of the challenge. Indeed, there is some evidence from the studies cited above that their performance may suffer if they confront negative information or do experience anxiety, (ibid). This suggests that their goal may include avoiding negative information and contemplation of the possibility of failure (Miller, 1987).

Another way of understanding the different goals of the two groups is to consider combinations of motives. Both groups resemble, in background, aspiration and cumulative performance, high need for achievement subjects (Atkinson, 1957). Both groups come from families that emphasize achievement-related activities (Norem & Cantor, in press). The high anxiety and low expectations among defensive pessimists, however, resemble that found among high fear of failure subjects in traditional achievement research. (Atkinson & Litwin, 1960). There is some reason to think that individuals using defensive pessimism might be high in nAch and high fear of failure: a motive constellation that Atkinson and his colleagues predict should cause immobilization. Indeed, Self (1988) finds that academic optimists and defensive pessimists do not differ in the satisfaction they expect to derive from success, but that pessimists expect significantly greater unhappiness from failure than the optimists. This fits with the emphasis on "working through" the implications of bad outcomes found in the defensive pessimist group, who, apparently, actively attempt to fight immobilization in order to take control of or "harness" their anxiety so that they may concentrate on the task at hand (Norem & Cantor, 1986b).

The emphasis on these two strategies throughout this chapter is, of course, not meant to suggest that they in anyway exhaust the category of strategies individuals may use, even within the context of performance situations. Various emotional and behavioral self-handicapping strategies come quickly to mind as alternative ways, for example, to approach performance situations, based on somewhat differently constructed goals. There are numerous other strategies individuals may use, especially when one considers different domains of human activity (Folkman & Lazarus,

1985; Frese, Stewart & Hannover, 1987; Kuhl, 1985; Langston & Cantor, in press; Miller, 1987; Paulhus & Martin, 1988; Pyszczynski & Greenberg, 1987; Snyder & Smith, 1986; Zirkel & Cantor, 1988). Aside from the author's convenience, however, there are two reasons why these particular strategies are especially useful examples for the purposes of this chapter. First, research on these strategies includes experimental work, questionnaire studies, and a longitudinal project. There are data from contrived laboratory contexts, and from "messier" real-life situations. There are self-report data, objective-performance data, experience-sampling data, and observer ratings. Although the subjects in these studies have all been college students, they are students drawn from quite different populations, demographically and otherwise. The research reviewed below has been conducted using subjects from the general undergraduate population at the University of Michigan and from a somewhat more select sample of Honors College students. In addition, there are data from undergraduate subjects at Northeastern University, who represent different demographic characteristics, who encounter a different academic environment while attending an urban school known for its cooperative education program, and who arrive at college with a much greater diversity in preparation and aptitude than students at Michigan. The convergence of these different data sources lends substantial support to the argument that strategies provide a powerful tool for exploring personality function.

Second, optimism and defensive pessimism are strategies used by individuals who *do not* appear to differ in other ways, which might suggest that differences in strategy are merely epiphenomena. Among college students, there are no significant demographic or SES differences between those using optimism and those using defensive pessimism. Nor do they differ significantly in high school rank, high school grade point average, SAT scores, or number of family members in college. There is no reason to suspect that the difference in strategies among these individuals is a simple function of intelligence, past performance, scholastic aptitude, preparation for college, or some readily identifiable influence from their social structure. Therefore, they provide a clear opportunity to contrast the expression of personality via different strategies with relatively less "noise" from other variables.

Theoretical Implications of a Strategy-based Approach to Personality

Strategy Effectiveness

One implication of considering personality in terms of strategies is an emphasis on the *effectiveness* of different strategies. Adaptation and coping are thus seen as a function of individual goals, the manner in which individuals pursue their goals, and the probable consequences of various goal-strategy combinations. Strategy effectiveness involves: a) the extent to which a strategy leads to successful outcomes; b) the "costs" of using the strategy, in terms of emotional wear and tear, the response of others, and/or lost opportunities; c) the potential costs of *not* using the strategy (or being without a coherent strategy for pursuing a particular goal). Effectiveness may also be a function of the indirect consequences that using a strategy in one domain has for other domains.

Research on the effectiveness of defensive pessimism and optimism within the academic domain highlights the importance of considering all of the above points when attempting to evaluate the effectiveness of a strategy. Norem and Cantor (1986ab) found that, when left to use their habitual strategy on anagram and puzzle tasks (presented as tests of "different kinds of abilities"), subjects prescreened for self-reported use of defensive pessimism or optimism performed equivalently well.[1] They were also equivalently satisfied with their performances after the fact. This was so even though the defensive pessimism group reported feeling significantly more anxious and out of control prior to the test. When, however, the experimenter interfered with the defensive pessimists' strategy by encouraging them, their performance suffered, relative to optimists in the same condition (whose performance improved) and defensive pessimists in the control condition.

Cantor, Norem, Niedenthal, Langston & Brower (1987), as part of an ongoing longitudinal study of the transition to college life, studied academic optimism and defensive pessimism among freshmen in the Honors College at the University of Michigan. Their results converged with the experimental data in that the students using defensive pessimism appraised their academic tasks significantly more negatively than the students using optimism: they felt less in control, more stressed, found academic tasks more difficult, more important, and more time consuming. They also expected to do more poorly than the optimists expected to do.

---

[1] Prescreening for individuals using defensive pessimism and optimism is done using a nine-item, face valid questionnaire. Subjects indicate the extent to which each item is characteristic of them. The items include questions such as "I generally go into academic situations expecting the worst, even though things usually turn out ok," and "I usually go into academic situations with positive expectations." There are four questions describing aspects of the defensive pessimist strategy and four describing aspects of the optimistic strategy. There is also a question that asks subjects to indicate the extent to which they believe they have done well in the past. The sum of the pessimistic items is subtracted from the sum of the optimistic items. Subjects in the bottom and top thirds of the distribution of answers are selected for use of defensive pessimism and optimism respectively, *providing* that they strongly endorse the item about positive past experience (6 or higher on a 9 point scale). This is done to select for *defensively* pessimistic subjects, as opposed to those whose pessimism is realistic, or based on distortion of past experience.

A similar pattern of emotions and appraisal appeared in data from an experience-sampling study in which a subsample of the Honors students carried electronic pagers that "beeped" on a random schedule several times a day for ten days. At each "beep," the students filled out a report of what they were doing and how they were feeling (Cantor & Norem, in press; Norem, 1987). In these data, defensive pessimist subjects reported feeling significantly less control, less enjoyment, less progress, and more stress than optimists during academic situations, especially in "anticipatory" situations, such as when they were studying for a test. Their reports from other situations, however, were just as positive as the optimists'. As a consequence, their reported feelings of control are significantly more variable across situations than the optimists'.

Just as in the laboratory studies, the negative appraisal and lack of control reported by the defensive pessimists did not impair their performance over the short-run, (although there are suggestions of relatively greater "costs" over the long-run; see below). Defensive pessimists and optimists both performed quite well academically during their first and second years in college (GPAs above 3.30), and there were no differences in average GPA between the two groups. There were also no differences between the two groups in social satisfaction or in an overall measure of perceived stress during their first two years in college.

From these studies, it seems reasonable to conclude that the defensive pessimist and optimist strategies are both *effective* insofar as the individuals using them perform well on academic tasks. It is also important to understand that the characteristic ways in which information about tasks and the self is used by the two strategy groups is not incidental to their performance. Playing through contingency plans is significantly negatively related to GPA for the optimists in the Honors College sample. In contrast, it is significantly positively related for the defensive pessimists, for whom it is an integral part of "dealing with" the problems presented by academic tasks. Negativity about the academic domain and negative beliefs about the self are negatively related to performance for the optimists—a pattern that contrasts markedly with relationships found for the defensive pessimist. Negativity of academic plans is not related to GPA for the latter group (whose plans progress from very negative possible outcomes to successful resolution of those outcomes), and negative beliefs about the academic self are strongly positively related to GPA.

Another way of assessing the effectiveness of optimism and defensive pessimism is to compare the outcomes of those using these strategies with the outcomes of other individuals. Norem and Cantor (in press) looked at the performance of a group of individuals, labelled "aschematics," who, initially, did not seem to have a coherent strategy for the academic domain. These are individuals who are in the middle third of the academic optimism-pessimism prescreening distribution, and who sometimes resemble optimists, sometimes resemble pessimists, but are, characteristically, neither.

The aschematics in the Honors College sample were less absorbed in and anxious about academic tasks than the pessimists, but also felt less in control than the optimists. They were somewhat less reflective than the other two groups, and had significantly fewer mismatches between their actual and ideal self-concepts in the academic domain (Higgins, Klein & Strauman, 1985). Data from the experience-sampling study show that a subgroup of the aschematics spend 29% of their time on academic tasks (relative to 38% and 35% for optimists and defensive pessimists), felt significantly less in control across situations than optimists, and were more lonely, angry, and more in conflict in virtually every situation sampled than the other two strategy groups. For the aschematics, *unlike* the defensive pessimists who seem able to "take control" by using their strategy, feeling out of control is negatively related to GPA performance and academic satisfaction. Finally, the aschematics achieve marginally lower GPAs than the other two groups during their first year in college, and significantly lower GPAs during their second year.

These data show the aschematic group "floundering" in their approach to academic tasks—results interpreted by Norem and Cantor as a consequence of poorly articulated goals within the achievement domain and a resultant lack of a coherent strategy for that domain. Support for that interpretation comes from data gathered in in-depth interviews of subjects during their second year in college (Norem, 1987). The interviews focused on obtaining descriptions from the subjects of their academic and social progress since arriving at the University, their techniques or problems in getting themselves motivated, and difficulties they might be experiencing in academic and interpersonal tasks. The interviews were videotaped: the tapes were coded by trained raters using a Q-sort deck composed of items derived from a number of perspectives on coping and problem-solving strategies and styles, and were sorted for each interview on the basis of how characteristic each item was of the subject being interviewed. Cluster analyses on the observers' ratings of the interview showed that a cluster of items (labelled the "prototype-matching" cluster) was significantly more characteristic of the aschematics than of the other two strategy groups. The items in this cluster included: "refers to standards to check performance"; "judges self with external standards"; "thinks about behavior of prototypical others" "uses information about others as guide in decision making"; "makes tasks similar to others"; "unsure about life tasks". In their first two years of college, then, the aschematics appear somewhat confused and unsure about precisely what they are supposed to do in the academic domain. By the beginning of their third year, they begin to develop a better sense of these tasks by observing and incorporating the interpretations of other students. Indeed, the better they were able to match their understanding of this task domain to that of prototypical or ideal students, the better their academic performance ($r = .67$, $p < .01$ between the characteristicness of the prototype matching cluster for the aschematics and their GPA). As will be seen below, the aschematics were eventually able to develop effective approaches to dealing with their academic tasks, once their goals within that domain crystallized. Initially, however, it seems clear that both the defensive pessimist strategy and the optimistic strategy were considerably more effective than no strategy at all.

The data reviewed so far strongly support the contention that defensive pessimism and optimism can be effective strategies, at least within the academic domain and with respect to performance outcomes. Consideration of strategy effectiveness should, however, also include assessment of the relative "costs" of a strategy to the individual using it. There are no current data showing significant short-term costs to the use of either optimism or defensive pessimism in the academic domain—especially when the use of those strategies is contrasted with the absence of a strategy. Looking in depth at how the strategies of optimism and defensive pessimism unfold over time, however, reveals important differences between the strategies apt to be related to differences in the longer term costs of each. The experience-sampling data reveal much greater variance in emotions—especially in feelings of control—for the pessimists than for the other two groups. Over the course of a few years, the emotional ups and downs of academic defensive pessimism may accumulate and take a heavy toll on well-being. In addition, the pessimists seem to rely heavily on a small group of close friends: they spend more time with a relatively small group of "best friends," while the optimists spend more time with a larger group of "friends." It may be that the pessimists' best friends find themselves wearying of the pessimists' worry and anxiety.

In fact, the costs or "side-effects" of defensive pessimism show up strongly in data from the Honors College sample during their third year in college (Cantor & Norem, in press). A telephone survey assessed reports of physical and psychological symptoms, satisfaction with academic and social performance, and junior year GPA among this sample. Results indicate that the defensive pessimists, although not doing badly in any absolute sense, were suffering somewhat relative to the optimists. They reported experiencing greater frequencies of psychological and physical symptoms, felt less satisfied with their academic and social performances, and had lower GPAs than the optimists. (Again, it is important to note that, although below the optimists' GPA, the pessimists were still performing quite well: Mean GPA = 3.35). In this case, the indirect consequences of using a strategy repeatedly over time are clearly important to assessment of the effectiveness of the strategy. Of course, we do not know from these data what would have happened to the defensive pessimists if they had not been using their strategy. Recall from previous research that defensive pessimists who were "deprived" of their strategy in a performance situation were relatively debilitated (Norem & Cantor, 1986b). The pessimists' appraisal of academic situations focuses on their anxiety and feelings of being out of control. Although it may be stressful to recognize and continually experience those feelings, the pessimists are at least able to "work through" them to some extent by using their strategy. Even though defensive pessimism is apparently not "cost-free" over time, it may be preferable to feeling anxious and out of control, and to having no way of coping with those feelings.

These data about the short- and long-term consequences of different strategies within the academic domain highlight the complexity of the process by which individuals pursue their goals. So far, we have only considered these strategies within one domain——that of academic achievement activities. Another aspect of the effectiveness of strategies, however, concerns the relative fit between strategy and domain. Simply put, some strategies may be better suited to some domains than to others. This raises the question of how domain-specific an individual's strategies are, and the extent to which people can adjust the strategies they use to fit particular contexts.

Domain Specificity, Flexibility and Strategy Change

Strategies stem from appraising a situation and activating relevant goals. One of the reasons that a strategy may not be equally effective in all situations is that all situations do not provide the same opportunities to realize a given goal. Nor, in the absence of monomania, are individuals likely to interpret all situations in the same way. Therefore, there is no a priori reason to assume that individuals will use the same kind of strategy in different kinds of situations.

Moreover, there is no assumption that strategies that characterize an individual at one period in his/her life will continue to do so throughout the passing years. The concept of a strategy explicitly recognizes the potential—indeed, the probability—of change as an individual's goals change. As goals are successfully realized, as cumulative feedback indicates a strategy is unsuccessful or exacts too high a cost, or as tasks in a domain are abandoned or transformed and new goals formulated, one would expect to find corresponding strategy change.

In research to date, the academic and social versions of the defensive pessimism prescreening questionnaire show average correlations of .30 across several samples of University of Michigan students (Norem & Cantor, 1986b, Norem, 1987, Showers, 1986), and .23 for two samples of Northeastern students (Norem, 1988). Both correlations are significant, but modest: it is clear that once categorization into strategy group is made for both domains, not everyone who uses defensive pessimism academically also uses it socially, and that not all academic optimists are social optimists. There is some potential, then, for domain specificity in the application of defensive pessimism. This is also reflected in the academic defensive pessimists' appraisal of the social domain: they do not generalize their negative perspective from the academic to the social domain. Academic pessimists feel just as much control over and have just as high expectations for the social domain as academic optimists, *and* as social optimists (Cantor et al., 1987). Similarly, social defensive pessimists neither set low expectations for their academic performance nor appraise academic tasks negatively (Norem & Illingworth, 1989).

Furthermore, when the self-knowledge of social and academic defensive pessimists and optimists is compared within and across each domain, clear domain specificity appears. Academic defensive pessimists have more negative academic selves than academic optimists, but have equivalently positive social selves. The comparable pattern of domain-specific self-knowledge is found among social optimists and defensive pessimists: the latter have more negative beliefs about their social selves, but not about their academic selves (Cantor et al., 1987; Norem, 1987; Norem & Illingworth, 1989).

In addition to providing support for the idea that use of a given strategy is potentially domain-specific, social defensive pessimism provides an informative look at issues of strategy-situation fit. Recall that defensive pessimism involves setting low expectations, focusing on anxiety, reflecting extensively on negative outcomes, and working very hard on a task. Although academic defensive pessimists experience reasonable success using these procedures, the strategy might be less effective in the social domain.

First, academic situations such as those studied in the research above may differ from many social situations in that, for the most part, there are externally provided, explicit evaluations of performance. Typically, students receive grades, scores, and/or other feedback about their scholastic performance. Even if not entirely "objective," this feedback comes from outside sources and provides easy comparison to past performance and the performance of others. Rarely, in social interactions, are performance outcomes so unequivocal. It may be that in situations where there is relatively less objective positive information about past performance, the defensive pessimist strategy flounders, since it depends on contrasting defensively low expectations with realistically high past performance.

Second, the correlation between the amount of time and effort spent in preparation and eventual performance is probably quite strong and positive within academic situations. In other words, despite what students might say, there is some positive relationship between the amount of time spent studying and final exam grades in most classrooms. The same contingencies, however, may not operate as clearly in the social domain. One can hardly help but think of the prototypical adolescent repeating his/her carefully thought out greeting while waiting for a prospective date to answer the phone—only to find that every word gets jumbled on the way out, and the result is an embarrassing squeak or mumble. It is easy to come up with examples of when "trying too hard" (or being seen that way) can lead to social failure. Indeed, one might even speculate that extensive planning reflection, and effort prior to a social occasion increases the risk of bumbling, stilted interactions, emotional anticlimax, and disappointment.

Data from the Honors College sample do show that social pessimism is less effective than academic pessimism: social pessimists are less satisfied and feel significantly more stressed than social optimists during their first and third years in college (Norem, 1987). Observers of interviews with social pessimists and optimists rate them as less satisfied with their social performance, less interested in trying new things, less apt to try to make new affiliations, more reluctant to think about good social outcomes, more stressed by social tasks, and more apt to ruminate obsessively about problems than are social optimists (see above, and Norem, 1987 for details).

The picture that emerges from these data is not one of individuals *using* defensive pessimism to work through anxiety and motivate themselves; rather, it resembles a picture of unmotivated, mildly depressed subjects, stuck in a repetitive cycle of negativity. It is interesting to note in this context that, among the academic defensive pessimists from the Honors College sample, those who were also defensively pessimistic in the social domain exhibited the most psychological and physical symptoms, the most stress, and the greatest dissatisfaction with their lives (by their junior year) of any group. Indeed, most of the long-term negative consequences found among academic defensive pessimists (relative to optimists) are a function of the low scores of the "pan-domain" pessimists. Defensive pessimism, in other words, may leave a lot to be desired as a social strategy. Those within this sample who use it only within the academic domain seem to fare better than those who overgeneralize or misapply the strategy to tasks in the social domain.

These data have at least two important implications. The first is that the effectiveness of any strategy is apt to vary from situation to situation. One can, therefore, generate a number of testable hypotheses about the relative effectiveness of different strategies in different contexts, which, in turn, have implications for the successful adjustment of people using those strategies in those contexts. Thus, for example, the greater emotional "cost" of defensive pessimism (compared to optimism) would seem to imply that it is relatively inappropriate or ineffective for situations where potential negative outcomes are not strongly influenced by individual effort or not very consequential in and of themselves. Becoming anxious about and planning several different routes for weekly trips to the grocery store is probably not going to result in benefits that compensate for the strain. (It may be that spending time and energy worrying may be more aversive than the actual negative consequences about which one is concerned). When, however, careful reflection, mental rehearsal, and effort do significantly increase the probability of good outcomes, positive outcomes are especially attractive, and/or when negative outcomes are especially disastrous, defensive pessimism may be "worth it"—i.e., highly effective. In contrast, especially to the extent that "illusory glow" optimism involves active avoidance of negative information, there are situations where it may not be a particularly effective strategy. When careful attention to feedback about errors is necessary for learning, when potential negative consequences are extreme, and/or when there are significant risks associated with over-confidence, an optimistic strategy could prove costly. One might hope, for example, that defensive pessimists, as opposed to "illusory glow" optimists, are overrepresented among individuals designing and operating nuclear power plants.[2]

This discussion also suggests that a potentially important aspect of the effectiveness of a given strategy may be the sensitivity with which it is employed from situation to situation. If strategies become overlearned, automatic, or overgeneralized, they may also be relatively less effective. There are corresponding implications: 1) individuals with more strategies available in their repertoire may be better able to adapt to a variety of situations, and may choose to become involved in more different kinds of situations than those with fewer strategies; 2) individuals who are flexible in the way they use the strategies in their repertoire may be better off—especially over time—than those who employ the same strategy over and over.

Recent data provide some support for these hypotheses. A subsample of the Honors College subjects participated in "problem-solving" interviews during their sophomore year, in which they were asked to respond to hypothetical problem situations in different domains, and specific attempts were made by the interviewers to "throw a curve" to each interviewee: i.e., after describing their initial plan, subjects were presented with objections to the plans and asked what they would do if the plans did not work. Among other things, the videotapes of these interviews were coded for "flexibility" of response in each situation (see Norem, 1987, for details). These flexibility ratings correlated positively with sophomore GPA ($r = .39$, $p < .05$), junior year GPA ($r = .24$, $p < .10$), and negatively with physical symptoms ($r = -.37, p < .05$) and psychological symptoms ($r = -.43$, $p < .01$) during the junior year.

In addition, data from the Honors College sample collected during their

---

[2] The word "glow" was not intended—initially—as a pun in this context.

senior year indicate that the academic defensive pessimists have, to a large extent, recovered from their junior year "slump"—*and,* that many of them have begun to use the optimistic strategy within the academic domain (Norem, 1989; see Showers, 1986 for data showing that this change is unlikely to be due to unreliability of the prescreening). The defensive pessimists no longer have lower satisfaction or grade point averages, and they no longer construe the academic domain more negatively than the optimists. Closer analyses of these results reveal that the mean improvement shown by the defensive pessimist group is primarily a function of those academic pessimists who have switched to an optimistic strategy. It is impossible, of course, to tell from these data whether or not this group's improved functioning is a result of their switch to optimism, whether their switch is a function of improved outcomes, or whether some third variable(s) is behind each. Nevertheless, it does seem that individuals have some potential to change their strategies in response to feedback. It is tempting to speculate that the subjects who change strategy do so in response to changes in their primary goals, either within the academic domain, or in other domains which have an impact on their approach to academic tasks.

Analyses in progress on data from these subjects should help to tease out the temporal order in which modification of goals, changes in strategies, feedback about performance and interpretation of feedback occur. This, in turn, should lead to a better understanding of how and when strategy change occurs, and of the extent to which individuals may initiate change in response to satisfaction with the balance of costs and benefits of their original strategies, a switch in emphasis from one task to another, or articulation of new tasks.

The Honors College students who have been the focus of the investigation of these strategies are continuing to participate in this study during their first year after college. As they leave the now familiar and comfortable college environment to make the transition to the working world or graduate/professional school, they will probably work on new life tasks (or old life tasks with substantially new twists). As they pursue new goals in new contexts, one predicts that those whose strategies adjust according to these newly formulated goals will have more success in coping with their new environments. Individuals who try automatically to transfer their college strategies to new contexts, or those who have difficulty articulating new goals, (like the aschematics during their first two years in college) should have a relatively harder time with this new life transition.

Conclusion

A strategy-based approach to the study of personality attempts to illuminate how individuals accomplish (or fail to accomplish) the things that are important to them. Strategies capture the coherence of people's approaches to different domains and highlight important differences between those approaches. A given strategy is part of an individual's personality for as long as he/she is using it to work on current life tasks, or for as long as it remains a viable part of his/her repertoire of strategies. Strategies are, theoretically, among the most malleable units of personality—although, at this point, we know relatively little about the actual limits on flexibility in strategy use, the typical extent of people's strategy repertoires, or how difficult it is to accomplish strategy change. We do, however, have the basis of a model for predicting change. As people move from one set of life tasks to another, we would predict more strategy change than when they remain within the same context over time (Stewart & Healy, 1985). Similarly, consideration of the effectiveness of different strategies in different domains provides the basis for predictions about better and worse coping. Personality adjustment can be considered in terms of the short- and long-term effectiveness of the strategies people employ, and the extent to which they are flexible and sensitive in response to different situations.

From this perspective, personality is the set of goals and strategies that organize an individual's thoughts, feelings and actions, and comprise the tools with which people adapt to their worlds. Personality includes both the tasks that a given group of individuals may have in common (e.g., their desire to get good grades and make new friends during their freshman year in college), and that which distinguishes individuals within that group (e.g., their unique interpretations of those situations in terms of opportunity, challenge, stress, and control). As an instrument of adaptation, personality's potential for change over time is as important as its consistency. Looking at how people articulate their tasks, and the limits and advantages of the strategies they use to work on them should help clarify the conditions under which change is embraced, expected, or resisted.

Acknowledgments. I would like to thank David Buss and Nancy Cantor for the opportunity to participate in the "Emerging Issues" conference in Ann Arbor, as well as for their suggestions and support. I would also like to thank Judy Hall, Stephen Harkins, Shaun Illingworth, Chris Langston, Paula Niedenthal, Carolin Showers and Ellen Veccia for their comments on this work; and Carol Fisher, Dawn Lotter and Denise Marcoux for their help in collecting data. This research was supported in part by NSF grants BNS#84-11778 to Nancy Cantor and Harold Korn, and BNS#87-18467 to Nancy Cantor and Julie K. Norem. Some of the research discussed is from the author's unpublished doctoral dissertation.

References

Atkinson, J.W. (1957). Motivational determinants of risk-taking. *Psychological Review, 64*, 359–372.

Atkinson, J.W. & Litwin, C.H. (1960). Achievement motive and test anxiety conceived as motive to approach success and motive to avoid failure. *Journal of Abnormal and Social Psychology, 60,* 52–63.

Bruner, J.S., Goodnow, J.J., & Austin, G.A. (1956). *A study of thinking.* New York: Wiley.

Buss, D.M. (1987). Selection, evocation, and manipulation. *Journal of Personality and Social Psychology, 53,* 1214–1221.

Buss, D.M. & Craik, K.H. (1983). The act frequency approach to personality. *Psychological Bulletin, 104*(1), 3–22.

Cantor, N. & Kihlstrom, J.F. (1987). *Personality and social intelligence.* New York: Prentice-Hall.

Cantor, N., & Norem, J.K. (in press). Defensive pessimism and stress and coping. *Social Cognition.*

Cantor, N., Norem, J.K., Niedenthal, P.M., Langston, C.A. & Brower, A.M. (1987). Life tasks, self-concept ideals, and cognitive strategies in a life transition. *Journal of Personality and Social Psychology, 53,* 1178–1191.

Emmons, R.A. (1986). Personal strivings: An approach to personality and subjective well-being. *Journal of Personality and Social Psychology. 51,* 1058–1068.

Folkman, S., & Lazarus, D.S. (1985). If it changes it must be a process: Study of emotion and coping during three stages of a college examination. *Journal of Personality and Social Psychology, 48,* 150–170.

Frese, M., Stewart, J., & Hannover, B. (1987). Goal orientation and planfulness: Action styles as personality concepts. *Journal of Personality and Social Psychology, 52,* 1182–1194.

Higgins, E.T., Klein, R., & Strauman, T. (1985). Self-concept discrepancy theory: A psychological model for distinguishing among different aspects of depression and anxiety. *Social Cognition, 3,* 51–76.

Kuhl, J. (1985). From cognition to behavior: Perspectives for future research on action control. In J. Kuhl & J. Beckmann (Eds.), *Action control from cognition to behavior.* New York: Springer.

Langston, C.A., & Cantor, N. (in press). Social anxiety and social constraint: When "making friends" is hard. *Journal of Personality and Social Psychology.*

Miller, S.M. (1987). Monitoring and blunting: Validation of a questionnaire to assess styles of information seeking under threat. *Journal of Personality and Social Psychology, 52*(2), 345–353.

Norem, J.K. (1987) *Strategic realities: Optimism and defensive pessimism.* Unpublished doctoral dissertation. University of Michigan.

Norem, J.K. (1988). *Negativity, specifity and stability of strategies and self-knowledge.* Unpublished manuscript. Northeastern University.

Norem, J.K. (1989) *Changing tasks and changing strategies during adaptation to a life transition.* Manuscript in preparation.

Norem, J.K. & Cantor, N. (1986a). Anticipatory and post hoc cushioning strategies: Optimism and defensive pessimism in "risky" situations. *Cognitive Therapy and Research, 10*(3), 347–362.

Norem, J.K., & Cantor, N. (1986b). Defensive pessimism: "Harnessing" anxiety as motivation. *Journal of Personality and Social Psychology, 51*(6), 1208–1217.

Norem, J.K., & Cantor, N. (in press). Cognitive strategies, coping and perceptions of competence. In R.J. Sternberg & J. Kolligan, Jr. (Eds.), *Perceptions of competence and incompetence across the lifespan.*

Norem, J.K., & Illingworth, S. (1989). *Social vs. academic defensive pessimism: Issues of strategy-situation fit.* Unpublished manuscript. Northeastern University.

Palys, T.S., & Little, B.R. (1983). Perceived life satisfaction and the organization of personal project systems. *Journal of Personality and Social Psychology, 44,* 1221–1230.

Paulhus, D.L., & Martin, C.L. (1987). The structure of personality capabilites. *Journal of Personality and Social Psychology, 52*(2), 345–365.

Peterson, C., & Seligman, M. (1984) Causal explanation as a risk factor for depression: Theory and evidence. *Psychological Review, 91*(3), 347–374.

Pyszczynski, T., & Greenberg, J. (1987). Self-regulatory perseveration and the depressive self-focusing style: A self-awareness theory of reactive depression. *Psychological Bulletin, 102*(1), 122–138.

Self, E.A. (1988) *Defensive pessimism: A strategy for energization?* Unpublished master's thesis. University of Kansas.

Showers, C. (1986). *Anticipatory cognitive strategies: The positive side of negative thinking.* Unpublished doctoral dissertation. University of Michigan.

Showers, C., & Cantor, N. (1985). Social cognition: A look at motivated strategies. In M. Rosenzweig & L.W. Porter (Eds.), *Annual Review of Psychology, 36,* 275–306.

Showers, C., & Ruben, C. (1988). *Distinguishing defensive pessimism from depression: Negative expectations and positive coping mechanisms.* Manuscript under review.

Snyder, C.R. & Smith, T.W. (1986). On being "shy like a fox.": A self-handicapping analysis. In W.H. Jones, J.M. Cheek, & S.R. Briggs (Eds.), *Shyness: Perspectives in research and treatment* (pp. 161–172). New York: Plenum Press.

Stewart, A.J. & Healy, J.M., Jr. (1985). Personality as adaptation to change. In R. Hogan & W. Jones (Eds.). *Perspectives on personality: Theory, measurement, and interpersonal dynamics* (pp. 117–144). Greenwich, CT: JAI Press.

Taylor, S.E. & Brown, J. (1988). Illusion and well being: A social psychological perspective on mental health. *Psychological Bulletin., 103*(2), 193–210.

Winter, D.G. (1988). The power-motive in women—and men. *Journal of Personality and Social Psychology. 54*(3), 510–519.

Zirkel, S. & Cantor, N. (1988). *Independence and identity in the transition to college life.* Paper presented at the Annual Meeting of the American Psychological Association, Atlanta, Georgia.

CHAPTER 4

An Alternative Paradigm for Studying the Accuracy of Person Perception: Simulated Personalities

Jack C. Wright

Introduction

This chapter examines the prospects of the contemporary reprise of person perception accuracy. I identify three components of a paradigm for studying accuracy: a model of social judgment, a model of personality dispositions, and a methodology for examining the relation between social knowledge and behavior. I examine the implications of bounded models of social judgment, then summarize evidence of domain-specific accuracy that supports these models. The role of a conditional model of dispositions in accuracy research is discussed, and criteria for evaluating accuracy are derived from this model. I then describe a "simulated personality" paradigm which combines the strengths of laboratory experiments and observational field studies to permit detailed investigations of the relation between social knowledge and social behavior. Finally, I illustrate how this paradigm has been used to clarify the conditions under which expert clinical judges are more accurate than novices, how the veridical and non-veridical patterning of behaviors across situations influences judgment accuracy, and how observers' interaction goals influence the accuracy of the impressions they form.

The field of person perception has re-discovered long-standing questions about the accuracy of personality impressions. Like its contemporary counterpart, accuracy research during the 50s and 60s focused on the relation between observers' impressions and the actual behavior of the observed. That work revealed that people's impressions of personality often have little predictive utility, and that professional clinicians share many of the layperson's inferential flaws (see Mischel, 1968, for a review). Clinicians, for example, often fail to predict people's behavior in the real world (Mischel, 1965), misdiagnose organic brain damage from test results (Goldberg, 1959), and become increasingly confident in their impressions with greater exposure even when the predictiveness of their impressions is unchanged (Oskamp, 1972).

Interest in accuracy waned for three reasons. Questions about the legitimacy of various criteria for assessing impression accuracy persisted (Cronbach, 1955). Efforts to identify stable individual differences in judgment accuracy proved frustrating (see Oskamp, 1972). And, with the advent of the information-processing paradigm in cognitive psychology, interest shifted from demonstrating poor judgment performance to providing an account of the processes which produced judgment biases and errors (Nisbett & Ross, 1980).

The contemporary reprise of accuracy issues is motivated by several factors. Accuracy research remains high in practical significance, as is evident in recent work demonstrating again the poor performance of clinical judges (Faust & Ziskin, 1988). The renewed interest also stems from improvements in behavior assessment (Patterson, 1982) that allow investigators to assess accuracy using criteria based on extensive direct observations of behavior. Most importantly, the renewed interest in accuracy stems from the conceptual progress made since the earlier phase of accuracy work, as is evident in the recent discussions about the normative status of judgment biases and errors (Funder, 1987; Swann, 1984; McArthur & Baron, 1983; Higgins & Bargh, 1984; Park, 1986; Kenny & Albright, 1987). This theoretical progress now makes it possible to be more explicit about the major components of an accuracy paradigm than was possible thirty years ago.

Components of a Paradigm for Studying Accuracy

Models of Social Judgment

There are three major components of a paradigm for studying person perception accuracy: a model of social judgment; a model of personality dispositions; and methodology for assessing the relation between judgment and behavior. Consider the first component of a paradigm for studying person perception accuracy: a model of the tasks social creatures ought to be able to perform. The accuracy work of the 50s often was not explicit in this regard, so this is an area in which recent efforts, particularly in the literature on decision making under uncertainty, may prove helpful.

For our current purposes, we must distinguish between two approaches to social judgment. The first, which might be characterized as unbounded, defines rational behavior for idealized creatures whose capacities are unlimited and who are assumed to strive for optimal outcomes. Subjective expected utility theory constitutes one example of an unbounded model of rationality in the domains of decision-making under uncertainty (see Raiffa, 1968). Kelley's (1973) covariation model of attribution arguably is an example of an unbounded approach in the domain of person perception.

The second model, which I term bounded, has several variants, each of which has distinctive features, but in this context it is important to appreciate two features they share. One is that they recognize limits on the competencies of observers. The second is that they assume or imply that observers do not strive for optimal outcomes in forming personality impressions and making behavioral predictions. Swann's (1984) pragmatic approach proposes that observers strive for circumscribed accuracy (e.g., in summarizing how the target interacts with them) rather than for global accuracy (e.g., how the target behaves with others). Simon's (1983) bounded rationality posits a limited organism with modest inferential capacities which strives to "satisfice"—that is, to obtain outcomes that are satisfactory given its adaptive needs—rather than to optimize. In their ecological view of social perception, McArthur & Baron (1983) argue that perceivers are selectively attuned to behaviors that are high in adaptive significance, but not to all social behaviors.

The bounded rationality view has major implications for one's concept of rationality in general and one's concept of person perception accuracy in particular. In general, this view emphasizes that the apparent biases and errors people display on person perception tasks can be evaluated only in the context of their adaptive needs. Although it might be reasonable to criticize observers for being insensitive to social behaviors that are adaptively significant for them, it would not be reasonable to criticize observers for being insensitive to social behaviors whose adaptive significance is low.

Bounded rationality and ecological views differ in their assumptions about the role of inference in person perception (see McArthur & Baron, 1983; Wright & Dawson, 1988), but they make similar predictions about the domain-specific accuracy of judgment. For example, if aggression has greater significance than other properties such as conscientiousness, observers are expected to be more sensitive to individual differences in aggression than they are to individual differences in conscientiousness. Wright and Dawson (1988) observe such domain-specific accuracy. Adults' judgments of children's aggressiveness were highly correlated with actual individual differences in children's aggressiveness, whereas their judgments of children's withdrawal correlated poorly with individual differences in withdrawn behavior. These differences in observers' sensitivity in turn were associated with operational measures of the significance of children's aggressive and withdrawn behaviors: Adults assigned higher priorities to attending to aggression than to withdrawal. Moreover, these intervention priorities were not due simply to the greater stimulus intensity of aggressive acts in vivo, as they were observed even when abstract behavioral descriptions were used that controlled for stimulus intensity.

Evidence of domain-specific accuracy raises fundamental questions about the tasks used to study judgment errors. Many experimental tests of judgment errors are convenient, and most are of interest to social, personality, or clinical psychologists, but their adaptive significance to everyday social observers is unknown. What, for instance, is the adaptive significance of assessing one's own variability in conscientiousness (Bem & Allen, 1974)?; of predicting others' self-ratings on questionnaires (Crow, 1957)?; of predicting psychopathology from the results of projective tests (Horowitz, 1962)? In general, the domain-specificity view requires a careful examination of the significance of tasks that have been used to study the accuracy of person perception, and it challenges work that assumes that virtually any behavior can be used to assess the *general* accuracy of person perception.

Models of Personality Dispositions

A second component of a paradigm for studying person perception accuracy is a model of what personality dispositions are and how they should be assessed. Early accuracy work gave a range of answers to this question, so this is a second area in which recent efforts, particularly in the personality assessment literature, may prove helpful. For those who adopted Allportian causal models of dispositions, the implicit research agenda was to assess social observers' intuitions about behavioral consistency—the measure on which causal models of dispositions focused. For example, Bem and Allen (1974) examined the relation between people's assessments of their own variability on certain trait dimensions (e.g., friendliness) and the actual cross-situational consistency of their behavior.

Act frequency views (Buss & Craik, 1983) focus on observers' sensitivity to *act trends*—that is, the overall frequency of a category of behaviors over a period of observation—rather than consistency coefficients. For example, Rushton, Brainerd, and Pressley (1984) examine the relation between adults' judgments of children's honesty and the overall frequency of children's cheating across tests. An important feature of an act frequency model is that it articulates how dispositional judgments may be related to certain aspects of behavior (act tallies), without being related to consistency coefficients used throughout the history of the field (Hartshorne & May, 1929; Newcomb, 1929).

Conditional models of dispositions emphasize different aspects of the relation between judgment and behavior. Briefly, a conditional model represents dispositions as clusters of if-then relations between contexts and behaviors (see Wright & Mischel, 1987). The dispositional construct "aggressive" thus refers not to a general behavioral tendency or act trend, but to clusters of if-then contingencies between categories of situations and categories of behavior (see Mischel, 1973). The conditional model thus implies that neither consistency coefficients nor act tallies are necessarily appropriate for evaluating the relation between impressions and behavior, and instead proposes two alternative criteria for investigating the validity of dispositional judgments. One consists of specific context-behavior contingencies, that is, the probability of dispositionally-relevant behaviors in contexts most likely to elicit individual differences in behavior. For example, Wright and Mischel (1987) observed that people's judgments of children's aggressiveness predicted individual differences in children's aggressive behavior in psychologically demanding situations, but not in non-demanding situations.

The second criterion consists of the *pattern* of contingencies over multiple contexts and behaviors (see Shoda, Mischel, & Wright, 1989). The dispositional construct "aggressive" could constitute a claim about the organization of both aggressive *and* non-aggressive behaviors in both stressful and non-stressful situations. Thus, a child who displays aggression in frustrating situations, but not in non-frustrating ones, could be considered by observers to be a good example of an aggressive child. But a child who displays aggression in both frustrating and non-frustrating conditions could be considered a poorer example of an aggressive child, even though the frequency of aggressive acts is higher. Instead, such a child might be categorized as a member of alternative categories (e.g., emotionally disturbed).

This analysis reveals how the conditional view contrasts with covariation models of attribution. Kelley's (1973) covariation model, for example, asserts that a dispositional attribution (e.g., of aggressiveness) is justified when "distinctiveness" is low (i.e., the person displays aggression toward multiple "entities," or people), "consensus" is low (i.e., the behavior is not expected from most people), and "consistency" is high (i.e., the behavior occurs on multiple occasions). A conditional model shares the requirement for high consistency, but it claims that a dispositional attribution may be justified even when distinctiveness is high—that is, when the target displays dispositionally—relevant behavior only in certain situations. Several lines of research (Dodge, 1982; Patterson, 1982; Wright et al., 1989) indicate that even good examples of aggressive children display aggression in certain situations but not others. In our own work, prototypically aggressive children display verbal and physical aggression primarily when threatened by peers (see Figure 4.1).

The conditional view also contrasts with the "consensus" principle (see Jones & Davis, 1965; Jones, 1977; Kelley, 1973), which states that behaviors that occur when expected are dispositionally uninformative: Observing that a child talks politely when praised by adults and retaliates when threatened by peers does not justify extreme attributions of friendliness or aggressiveness because such behavior is expected from typical children. But in a conditional model, a dispositional attribution may be justified even when the behavior is expected from most people—because certain behavior patterns have relatively high base rates. A child who talks politely when praised by adults and retaliates when threatened by peers is judged a good example of a friendly child, precisely because that patterning of behavior is consistent with the pattern expected of typical—and at the same time, friendly—children (Wright et al., 1989). In sum, the conditional view raises important questions about the conditions under which observers' dispositional judgments will be based on covariation principles, as suggested by attribution theory, or on the patterning of multiple behaviors across contexts, as suggested by a conditional model.

Methodologically, a conditional view requires an explicit treatment of the contexts in which behaviors will be observed, and it requires extensive observations of behavior in a range of contexts. In our own work, we employ two general methods for assessing the organization of behavior across social situations. The bulk of this work is carried out at Wediko Children's Services' 6.5-week residential summer program for children, located in New Hampshire. The program serves a population of about 150 seven to eighteen year-old children and adolescents each summer, a population which includes a range of social adjustment patterns, which allows us to study both aggressive and withdrawn children.

One method decomposes the behavior stream into six-second units, allowing discrete coding of antecedents and responses (see Wright, 1983). A second method focuses on larger temporal units (from several minutes to an hour), but, in exchange, increases the breadth of observation. Using the latter method, we have obtained between 200–300 observations on each of approximately one hundred children for several years. In each observation, an observer identifies the person interacting with the target, particular behaviors that person displays toward the target, and the target's response. Based on independent information about the adult and peer interactants, categories of adults and peers are formed, and the conditional probabilities of the target's response for several behaviors may be computed. Figure 4.1 shows an example of one prototype based on ten aggressive children, using eight antecedent and five response categories. In the following section, I illustrate how such a conditional representation of personality can be used to study the accuracy of person perception.

Methods for Investigating Knowledge-Behavior Relations

A third component of an accuracy paradigm is a methodology that is consistent with one's model of judgment and model of dispositions. Laboratory analogue experiments are appealing in the control they afford, but they are often silent on the ecological significance of the biases people display in them (see Funder, 1987). The stimuli used in such experiments—lists of trait terms or brief descriptions of a hypothetical person's behavior—often bear little relation to the organization of behavior in the environment. Field studies are appealing in their ecologi-

4. Accuracy of Person Perception

			Behavior Category				
Context Category		n	Prosocial Talk	Whine, Cry	Comply	Verbal Aggression	Physical Aggression
Effective Counselor	Praise	710	.66	.01	.33	.00	.00
	Punish	398	.05	.17	.69	.07	.04
Ineffective Counselor	Praise	262	.75	.01	.25	.00	.00
	Punish	351	.07	.26	.58	.01	.08
Aggressive Child	Prosocial	251	.76	.02	.20	.01	.00
	Threat	115	.05	.12	.23	.56	.03
Non-Aggressive Child	Prosocial	276	.79	.02	.18	.02	.00
	Threat	75	.10	.18	.25	.42	.06

FIGURE 4.1. Example of a conditional representation of prototypic aggressive child, based on ~2400 hourly observations of 10 aggressive children. Entries indicate conditional probability of behavior given an antecedent event occurred.

cal representativeness, but the reduced experimental control and flexibility they provide can be problematic (see Wright & Mischel, 1987).

An alternative—a *simulated personality paradigm*—has two desirable features: It allows high experimental control, and it deals meaningfully with the relation between impressions and actual behavior. In a typical simulation (Dawson & Wright, 1988; Wright et al., 1989), we create a computer environment in which the subject can either "interact" with a personality or observe interactions between that personality and other people (see Figure 4.2). In the interactive paradigm, on each trial, subjects select a general situation (e.g., art), select the type of behavior they or another person will display toward the target (e.g., warn), then observe the target's response. Consistent with a conditional model, the probability of a given behavior (e.g., aggression, withdrawal) occurring

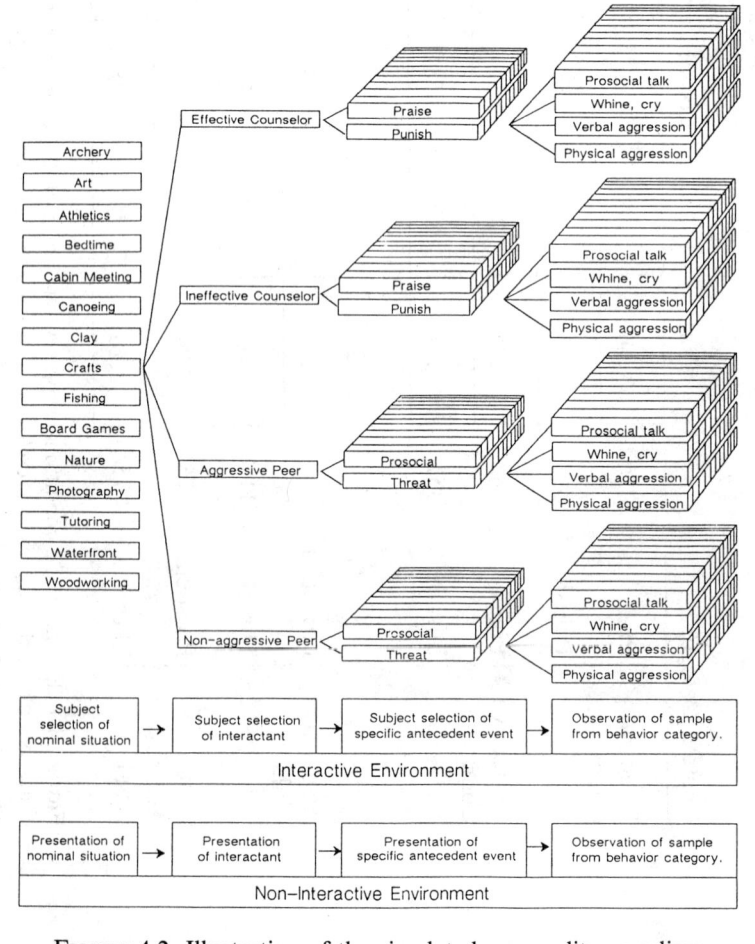

FIGURE 4.2. Illustration of the simulated personality paradigm.

on a given trial in response to a given situation is the conditional probability of that response as defined by the prototype matrix driving the simulated personality. Thus, if the conditional probability of verbal aggression in response to a threat from an aggressive peer is .56 (as shown in Figure 4.1), then there is a 56% chance that the target will respond with verbal aggression to that event on a given trial.

In the non-interactive paradigm, subjects are shown a nominal situation, a particular person with whom the target will interact, a particular behavior that person displays to the target, and the target's response. An important feature of both versions of the paradigm is that the antecedent events and behavioral responses are specific. For example, a typical context-behavior scenario might describe children working on their paintings at art, a counselor warning the target for spilling paint on the table, whereupon the target responds by throwing a paint brush at the counselor. The antecedents and responses are known to be good instances of the relevant antecedent and behavior categories (adult warning and physical aggression in this case), but these categories are never identified for subjects. Thus, subjects must encode their observations into the relevant context and behavior categories.

Applications of the Simulated Personality Paradigm

We have used the simulation paradigm to examine three accuracy issues: (a) experts' and novices' relative accuracy in summarizing and predicting social behavior (Dawson, Zeitz, & Wright, 1988); (b) effects of veridical and non-veridical personalities on the accuracy of observers' dispositional judgments (Shoda et al., 1989; Wright et al., 1989); (c) the effects of observers' interaction goals on implicit theory revision and impression accuracy (Dawson & Wright, 1988). In the following sections, I illustrate briefly how the simulated personality paradigm has been used in each of these areas.

Expert-Novice Differences in the Accuracy of Person Perception

One of the paradoxes of early accuracy research was that expert clinical psychologists performed no better than laypeople on a range of tasks. For example, Horowitz (1962) observed that expert clinicians made predictions from biographic information that were no more accurate than those made by college students with no clinical experience. Crow (1957) observed that observers' accuracy tended to decrease with clinical training. These and related studies led Mischel (1968) to conclude that greater clinical expertise is not associated with increases in person perception accuracy.

In contrast, the expert-novice literature in domains such as physics or chess suggests that these experts have knowledge and judgment strategies that facilitate their performance in their domains (Chase & Simon, 1973; Chi, Feltovich, & Glaser, 1981). Experts' superior performance is, however, highly domain-specific. For example, Chase and Simon (1973) observed that chess experts are better able to reconstruct configurations of chess pieces when those configurations may occur in actual games, but not when those configurations violate the rules of chess.

Dawson et al. (1989) attempted to integrate the two conflicting bodies of evidence on expertise—the evidence of experts' superior performance in "classic" problem-solving literature, and the evidence of experts' modest performance in social domains. Specifically, Dawson et al. (1989) proposed that expertise in person perception involves highly specific knowledge structures and judgment strategies, as specific as those associated with expertise in physics or chess. To explore this, we constructed personalities designed to vary in the degree to which they respected the organization of real children's behavior. We expected that experts' performance would be superior to novices' on tasks with familiar targets that respected the normal organization of behavior (i.e., aggressive targets with whom our experts had extensive experience). We also considered the possibility that experts' performance might be superior to novices' on less familiar problems, provided those problems contained certain important features of social behavior (i.e., covariation between behaviors and the situations in which they occur). Finally, we expected that experts and novices would perform comparably when the simulated personality was neither familiar nor displayed variable behavior across situations.

Three simulated personalities were created. The *prototype aggressive personality* was similar to the one described previously: It was based on the six most aggressive children available in one sample of Wediko children, and its behavioral tendencies (i.e., context-behavior conditional probabilities) were averaged over those aggressive children. The *inverse personality* displayed the same overall frequencies of behaviors and the same magnitude of context-behavior covariation, but certain context-behavior pairings were exchanged so as to violate the organization of veridical aggressive children. For example, the inverse target tended to be aggressive when praised (rather than when punished). Finally, the *random personality* also displayed the same overall frequencies of behavior, but behavioral frequencies were averaged over contexts so that the target's behavior did not vary over situations. For example, the random target was just as likely to be aggressive when praised as it was when punished.

We then created the necessary simulation environment so that experts (consultants at Wediko Children's Services with five to fifteen years of experience) and novices (Brown undergraduates) could observe each target on six occasions responding to each of five antecedent events (peer prosocial, peer tease, adult praise, adult warn, adult punish). A noninteractive environment ensured that both experts and novices observed the same material. On each of thirty trials, subjects observed nominal situation cues (e.g., art, music), the name of the target, a description of the person interacting with him, a specific antecedent event displayed by that person, and a specific response. Subjects performed three tasks: free recall, dispositional judgments, and predictions about behavior in specific situations.

Experts identified the intact target as aggressive, but not the inverse target (see Figure 4.3); novices failed to detect the aggressiveness of the intact target, and instead described the inverse target as more aggressive. No differences occurred between experts and novices for the random

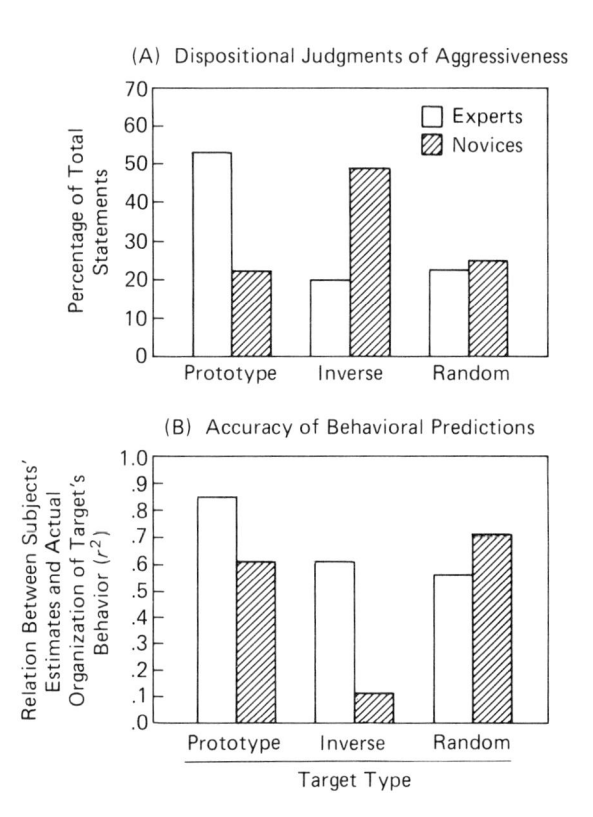

FIGURE 4.3. Expert-novice differences in person perception. (A) Percentage of statements in subjects' descriptions of targets' personality categorized as aggressive, as a function of target type and level of expertise. (B) Correlations between subjects' reconstructed context-behavior conditional probability matrices and the actual organization of targets' behavior, as a function of target type and level of expertise. (From Dawson, Zeitz, & Wright (1989), *Social Cognition*, with permission.)

personality. To assess subjects' performance on the prediction task, in which they were asked to reconstruct the conditional probability matrix driving each of the personalities, each reconstructed matrix was correlated with the actual matrix for that target. For the prototype aggressive and inverse targets, experts' reconstructed matrices corresponded more closely to the actual simulated personalities than did novices'. For the random target, however, there were no significant differences between experts and novices. Despite these expert-novice differences in their sensitivity to the organization of targets' behavior, we obtained no evidence of superior overall recall by experts. That is, there were no differences between experts and novices in the total number of original stimulus units they correctly recalled. If anything, novices performed slightly better than experts.

Clinical experts thus performed better than novices, but this superiority was circumscribed. Experts and novices did not differ in their verbatim recall of stimulus material. Experts displayed superior ability to reconstruct the organization of targets' behaviors, but this superiority occurred only for the intact aggressive target and the inverse target, whose behaviors varied over situations. Experts and novices did not differ in their ability to reconstruct the random target, whose behaviors did not vary over situations. An important task for future research will be to integrate this evidence of expert's superior performance with other evidence of experts' poor performance (Faust & Ziskin, 1988).

Dispositional Inferences and the Effects of Veridical Context-Behavior Relations

The expert-novice experiment took advantage of drastic manipulations of veridical personality organization in order to demonstrate the boundary conditions of expertise in social judgment. Such drastic manipulations of context-behavior linkages leave open questions about the effect of more subtle manipulations of context-behavior linkages on the accuracy of impressions. The expert-novice experiment was also limited in that it focused only on good examples of the selected dispositional category (aggressive). Such conditions are moot concerning observers' sensitivity to a wider range of individual differences in behavior—for instance, moderately aggressive and non-aggressive children.

Shoda et al. (1989) used a modified simulated paradigm to examine the effects of veridical and non-veridical context-behavior relations on the accuracy of dispositional judgments. In this study, the subjects were forty-six counselors who had worked primarily with one of several groups of six to ten children for 6.5 weeks in Wediko's summer program, and were therefore familiar with the children in the living group to which they were assigned. For each of these children with whom the adult subjects were most familiar, we had 200–300 hourly observations similar to those described in Figure 4.1.

For each *individual* child, we created five simulated personalities. One target was "intact" in that the conditional probabilities of his behaviors (e.g., aggression) in several situations (e.g., when praised, when punished) were the conditional probabilities of the actual child on which that simulated personality was based. Three other variants held constant the overall frequencies of all behaviors, but altered the links between contexts and behaviors. For the "low mutation" condition, peer antecedents were exchanged with adults'. For example, this target responded to adult praise the way the intact target responded to peer prosocial talk. For the "medium mutation" target, positive versus aversive events were exchanged. For the "high mutation" condition, both the type of person (peer vs. adult) and the valence of the behavior (positive vs. negative) were exchanged. Thus, this target responded to peer threat the way the intact target responded to adult praise. Finally, in a "context-unspecified" condition, the frequencies of behaviors also were held constant, but behaviors were described without reference to situations. Subjects observed five simulated personalities of the real children with whom they were most familiar. They observed a target (not named) for sixty-four trials, with sixteen occasions in each of four situations, and then provided dispositional judgments before proceeding to the next target.

One way to assess accuracy is to identify the children who were most and least aggressive (e.g., based on the frequency with which the real children displayed physical or verbal aggression), and then examine whether subjects detected the aggressiveness of the simulated personality based on those children. As shown in Figure 4.4, subjects rarely attributed aggressiveness to the least aggressive targets, regardless of the simulated personality they encountered. For aggressive targets, however, the accuracy of subjects' judgments depended on the veridicality of the context-behavior links. When they observed the intact target, subjects attributed high levels of aggressiveness to the target; when veridical context-behavior links were increasingly disrupted, subjects less often detected children's aggressiveness.

Although the mean aggressiveness attributed to intact and context-unspecified targets were comparable, this manipulation affected other measures of accuracy. Consider the correlation between subjects' judgments of aggressiveness and the frequency of aggression displayed by the children on whom the simulated personalities were based. For the context-unspecified targets, the correlation between subjects' judgments and the frequency of children's verbal aggression was significantly lower for the context-unspecified target ($r = .62$, $R^2 = .38$) than for the intact target ($r = .84$, $R^2 = .71$).

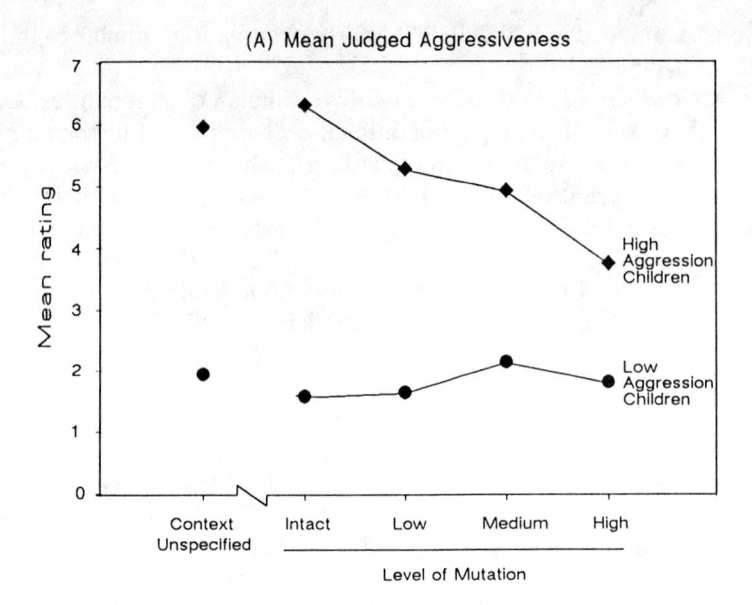

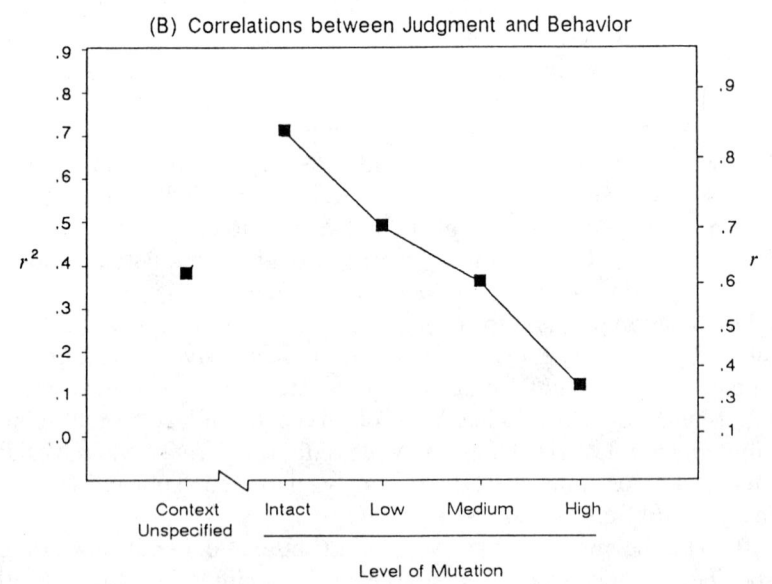

FIGURE 4.4. Effects of context-behavior relations on the accuracy of person perception. (A) Mean judged aggressiveness, as a function of the aggressiveness of the children on which simulated personalities were based and the veridicality of the simulated target. (B) Correlations between subjects' judgments of targets' aggressiveness and actual individual differences in children's verbal aggression, as a function of type of simulated target. (Adapted from Shoda, Mischel, & Wright (1989), *Journal of Personality and Social Psychology,* with permission.)

Like the results of the expert-novice experiment, these results clarify the conditions under which social observers can achieve reasonable levels of accuracy in their personality impressions. When subjects were presented with veridical simulated personalities, observers' judgments were closely related to the children's actual behavioral tendencies. When non-veridical personalities were presented, observers' accuracy was considerably lower, even though the overall frequencies of behaviors were held constant. Similarly, observers' accuracy was impaired simply by removing the context descriptions from the display, again even though the overall frequencies of behaviors were held constant.

These findings qualify conclusions about the inaccuracy of people's personality impressions (see Mischel, 1968, for a review), because those conclusions were based on studies that often did not provide subjects with veridical context-behavior relations. At the same time, it is important not to overgeneralize the present results: Our subjects' accuracy in the intact condition undoubtedly was facilitated by the fact that they were provided with multiple observations of targets' behavior in each situation. Such conditions contrast with tasks in which observers are required to make inferences from a single observation. Future research will be needed to clarify the relation between the phenomena we have observed and previously demonstrated attribution errors (Jones, 1979; Nisbett & Ross, 1980).

Interaction Goals, the Revision of Implicit Personality Theories, and Impression Accuracy

Rationality, as that concept is used in the literature on decision making under uncertainty, concerns the efficiency with which decision makers pursue their goals given their knowledge of the world. Normative models of decision making, such as subjective expected utility theory, thus define the likelihoods of events in terms of decision-makers' subjective probabilities, define the consequences of decision outcomes in terms of decision makers' own subjective values or utilities, and define "rational" decisions to be those which maximize decision-makers' subjective expected utilities.

Accuracy, as that concept is used in the person perception literature, often is less carefully defined. In the early accuracy literature, virtually any divergence from what the researcher considered reasonable might be characterized as an error. One of the most striking features of the judgment literature in this regard is the assumption that forming accurate impressions is important to people. If it were, it would be reasonable to criticize people if they failed to form impressions that were predictive of targets' actual behavioral tendencies. Yet in certain situations, goals other than impression accuracy (e.g., establishing satisfactory social relations) may be equally if not more important, and these goals may conflict with the goal of accuracy (see Higgins & Bargh, 1987; Swann, 1984). Thus, in the interest of maintaining a relationship, an observer may have to avoid embarrassing or difficult questions that might yield diagnostic information. Such a strategy could lead the observer to form impressions that do not correspond to the target's actual personality; nevertheless, it would be impossible to criticize that strategy on normative grounds in the light of the observer's interaction goals.

The interactive version of the simulation paradigm is well-suited to exploring the effects of goals on impression formation: It allows observers to guide the interaction as their impressions form, and it allows us to assess the degree to which observers understand the target's true personality. Indeed, the simulated personality paradigm was first developed by Vicki Dawson to examine how goals drive the impression formation process. In one experiment, we (Dawson & Wright, 1988) employed intact aggressive targets similar to those described earlier. In one condition (personality assessment), we instructed subjects to learn as rapidly as possible about the target's personality. In a second condition (social interaction), we instructed subjects to imagine that they were counselors whose goal was to have enjoyable interactions with the target. All subjects interacted with the target over thirty trials, under conditions that allowed them to control the situations in which they observed the target, then predicted how the target would respond to the full range of context categories built into the target's personality.

We modeled subjects' predictions as a function of two variables: their prior theories of how children behave over contexts and the actual organization of the target's behaviors. To do this, we obtained naive subjects' expectancies about how typical children respond to each context used in the experiment, and then performed multiple linear regressions of experimental subjects' predictions on the naive expectancies and the target's actual behavior. As expected, in the social interaction condition, subjects' predictions of targets' behavior were related both to their prior theories and to the target's actual personality (see Figure 4.5). In the assessment condition, subjects' predictions were very closely related to the behavioral evidence they observed, but were not significantly related to their prior theories. In sum, when the observers' goal was to form accurate impressions, their impressions were correlated with the actual organization of the personality with whom they interacted, but not with their prior theories. When their goal was to engage in enjoyable interactions with another person, their impressions were less closely correlated with the actual organization of the simulated personality with whom they interacted, but were correlated with their prior theories.

Clearly, these results do not imply that all errors occur because

4. Accuracy of Person Perception

Social Interaction Condition

```
Prior Theory ──.33*──┐
                     ▼
.49*            Predictions of      R² = .96
                Future Behavior
                     ▲
Target's    ──.77**──┘
Underlying
Personality
```

Personality Assessment Condition

```
Prior Theory ──.04───┐
                     ▼
.49*            Predictions of      R² = .97
                Future Behavior
                     ▲
Target's    ──.96**──┘
Underlying
Personality
```

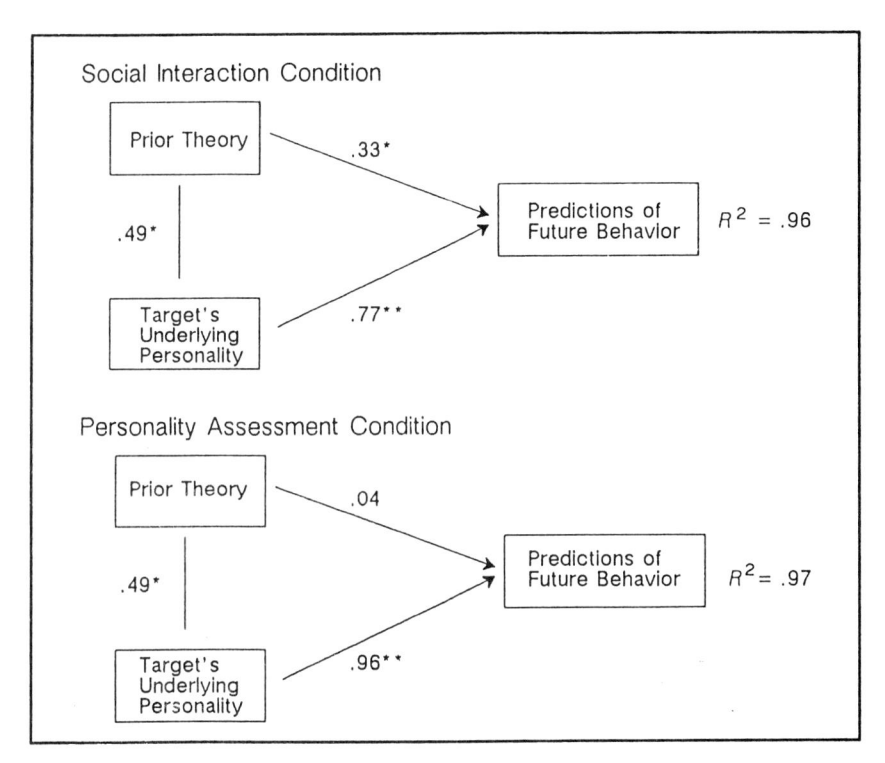

FIGURE 4.5. Effects of interaction goals on the relation between observers' impressions, their prior theories about the organization of social behavior, and the actual organization displayed by simulated targets, as a function of observers' goals. Coefficients are beta-weights from normalized multiple regression of subjects' predictions of targets' future behavior on prior theories about the organization of behavior and targets' behavior during the simulated interaction (* $p < .01$; ** $p < .001$).

subjects are pursuing goals other than accuracy. Clinicians often claim to be striving for accuracy and invest considerable resources in obtaining test information on which to base their predictions. Yet even with experienced clinicians, the predictive utility of their judgments can be quite low, even when their confidence is high (Mischel, 1968; Faust et al., 1988). Moreover, clinicians' interpersonal goals (e.g., smooth interaction) may conflict with the goal of accurate impression formation or behavioral prediction. A challenge for future work will be to clarify experts' and novices' ability to discriminate between tasks in which their accuracy is high (such as ours) and tasks in which their accuracy is low (such as Faust et al., 1988).

Conclusions

I have suggested that this may be a propitious time to bring formal models of social judgment to bear on long-standing questions about the accuracy of person perception. Bounded models of decision-making help to clarify not only the concept of rationality as it is used in the literature on decision-making under uncertainty, but also the concept of accuracy as it is used in the person perception literature. One implication of a bounded view that is worthy of investigation is what might be termed the domain-specific accuracy: If behavioral domains such as aggression and withdrawal differ in their significance, corresponding differences in impression accuracy should be observed over those domains. Future work will be needed to develop converging criteria of behavioral significance and to examine the accuracy of judgment in each domain.

I have illustrated how a conditional model of dispositions may be used to clarify the relation between person perception and behavior. A conditional view contrasts with causal views, which emphasize the relation between trait judgments and cross-situational consistency coefficients, and it contrasts with act frequency models which emphasize the relations between dispositional judgments and overall behavior frequencies. Instead, a conditional approach emphasizes the relation between observers' impressions and patterns of contingencies between multiple behaviors and multiple situations.

The simulated personality paradigm outlined here may be useful in exploring these and related questions about the accuracy of person perception. In this paradigm, observers may either interact with a computer-simulated personality or observe interactions between that personality and other individuals. The paradigm involves a relatively high level of control, which allows the experimenter to manipulate flexibly the behavioral properties of the simulated personality. It also allows the investigator to study the relation between observers' impressions and the organization of real people's behavior in the environment. It makes this study of accuracy possible by driving the simulated interactions with a veridical personality prototype based on extensive observations of people's real-world behavior.

Finally, I have described how such a paradigm can be used to study three issues: expert-novice differences in judgment accuracy; the effects of context-behavior relations on the accuracy of dispositional judgments; the effects of interaction goals on impression accuracy. Taken together, these experiments demonstrate how the domain-specific competencies of social observers may be revealed on familiar person perception problems that respect the organization of behavior in the real world.

As in the debate over the consistency of behavior (see Mischel & Peake, 1982), the renewed interest in accuracy is likely to elicit a sense of déjà vu in those familiar with the earlier literature. Undoubtedly, the accuracy of person perception is not an *emerging* issue for personality and social psychology, but a *re*-emerging one. At this juncture it is critical that this examination of familiar questions not be dismissed as a failure to appreciate the lessons of the past, or with the truism that the debate over accuracy, like all debates, will ultimately end in compromise. Interest in accuracy stems from the fact that the issue is both theoretically rich and high in practical significance. Both those who emphasize judgment shortcomings (Nisbett & Ross, 1980) and those who emphasize people's bounded competencies (Wright & Dawson, 1989; Shoda et al., 1989) have a role to play in resolving the challenges that lie ahead. By identifying the processes that produce inferential flaws *and* the factors that promote impression accuracy, both communities of investigators can help to improve the performance of expert and novice social judges in the real world.

Acknowledgments. This research was supported in part by Biomedical Research Support Grant BS603342 from Brown University to Jack Wright, and by Grants MH39349 and 39263 from the National Institute of Health to Walter Mischel.

I would like to thank the staff and children of Wediko Children's Services, whose cooperation made this work possible. I am especially grateful to Hugh Leichtman and Harry Parad, Wediko's directors, for their support, to Philip Fisher, Mary Powers, Mary Ryan, and Martha Wall for their assistance in conducting the field experiments at Wediko, and to Vicki Dawson for her instrumental role in developing the simulation paradigm. Earlier drafts of this chapter benefited from comments by David Buss, Nancy Cantor, Walter Mischel, and Audrey Zakriski.

Requests for reprints should be addressed to Jack Wright, Hunter Laboratory of Psychology, 89 Waterman Street, Brown University, Providence, Rhode Island, 02912.

References

Bem, D.J., & Allen, A. (1974). On predicting some of the people some of the time: The search for cross-situational consistencies in behavior. *Psychological Review, 81,* 506–520.

Buss, D.M., & Craik, K.H. (1983). The act frequency approach to personality. *Psychological Review, 90,* 105–126.

Chase, W.G., & Simon, H.A. (1973). Perception in chess. *Cognitive Psychology, 4,* 55–81.

Chi, M.T.H., Feltovich, P.J., & Glaser, R. (1981). Categorization and representation of physics problems by experts and novices. *Cognitive Science, 5,* 121–152.

Cronbach, L.J. (1955). Processes affecting scores on "understanding of others" and "assumed similarity." *Psychological Bulletin, 52,* 177–193.

Crow, W.J. (1957). The effect of training upon accuracy and variability in interpersonal perception. *Journal of Abnormal and Social Psychology, 55*, 355–359.

Dawson, V.L., & Wright, J.C. (1988). Forming impressions of simulated people: Goal-driven impressions and the circumscribed accuracy of dispositional judgments. Research in progress.

Dawson, V.L., Zeitz, C., & Wright, J.C. (1989). Expert-novice differences in person perception: Evidence of experts' sensitivities to the organization of social behavior. *Social Cognition, 7*, 1–30.

Faust, D., Hart, K., & Guilamette, T.J. (1988). Pediatric malingering: The capacity of children to fake believable deficits in neuropsychological testing. *Journal of Consulting and Clinical Psychology, 56*, 578–582.

Faust, D., & Ziskin, J. (1988). The expert witness in psychology and psychiatry. *Science, 31*–35.

Funder, D.C. (1987). Errors and mistakes: Evaluating the accuracy of social judgment. *Psychological Bulletin, 101*, 75–90.

Goldberg, L.R. (1959). The effectiveness of clinicians' judgments: the diagnosis of organic brain damage from the Bender-Gestalt test. *Journal of Consulting Psychology, 23*, 25–33.

Hartshorne, H., & May, M.A. (1928). *Studies in the nature of character: Vol. 1. Studies in deceit.* New York: Macmillan.

Higgins, E.T., & Bargh, R. (1987). Social cognition and social perception. *Annual Review of Psychology, 38*, 369–425.

Horowitz, M.J. (1962). A study of clinicians' judgments from projective test protocols. *Journal of Consulting Psychology, 26*, 251–256.

Kelley, H.H. (1971). *Attribution in social interaction.* Morristown, N.J.: General Learning Press.

Kenny, D.A., & Albright, L. (1987). Accuracy in interpersonal perception: A social relations analysis. *Psychological Bulletin, 102*, 390–402.

McArthur, L.Z., & Baron, R.M. (1983). Toward an ecological theory of social perception. *Psychological Review, 90*, 215–238.

Mischel, W. (1965). Predicting the success of Peace Corps Volunteers in Nigeria. *Journal of Personality and Social Psychology, 1*, 510–517.

Mischel, W. (1968). *Personality and assessment.* New York: Wiley.

Mischel, W., & Peake, P. (1982). Beyond deja vu in the search for cross-situational consistency. *Psychological Review, 89*, 730–755.

Mischel, W. (1973). Toward a cognitive social learning reconceptualization of personality. *Psychological Review, 80*, 252–283.

Newcomb, T.M. (1929). The consistency of certain extrovert-introvert behavior patterns in 51 problem boys (No. 382). New York: Columbia University, Contributions to Education.

Nisbett, R., & Ross, L. (1980). *Human inference: Strategies and shortcomings of human judgment.* Englewood Cliffs, N.J.: Prentice-Hall.

Oskamp, S. (1965). Overconfidence in case-study judgments. *Journal of Consulting Psychology, 29*, 261–265.

Park, B. (1986). A method for studying the development of impressions of real people. *Journal of Personality and Social Psychology, 51*, 907–817.

Patterson, G.R. (1982). *Coercive family process.* Eugene, Oregon: Castalia.

Raiffa, H. (1968). *Decision analysis.* Reading, MA: Addson-Wesley.

Rushton, J.P., Brainerd, C.J., & Pressley, M. (1984). Behavior development and construct validity: The principle of aggregation. *Psychological Bulletin, 94,* 18–380.

Shoda, Y., Mischel, W., & Wright, J.C. (1989). Intuitive interactionism and person perception: Effects of context-behavior relations on dispositional judgments. *Journal of Personality and Social Psychology, 56,* 41–530.

Simon, H.A. (1983). *Reason in human affairs.* Stanford, CA.: Stanford University Press.

Swann, W.B. (1984). Quest for accuracy in person perception: A matter of pragmatics. *Psychological Review, 91,* 457–477.

Wright, J.C., & Dawson, V.L. (1988). Person perception and the bounded rationality of social judgment. *Journal of Personality and Social Psychology, 55,* 780–794.

Wright, J.C., Jan, G., Dawson, V.L., & Shoda, Y. (1988). Forming impressions of simulated personalities: Sensitivities to the behavioral organization of "real" and "unreal" people. Manuscript submitted for publication.

Wright, J.C., & Mischel, W. (1988). Conditional hedges and the intuitive psychology of traits. *Journal of Personality and Social Psychology, 55,* 454–469.

Wright, J.C., & Mischel, W. (1987). A conditional approach to dispositional constructs: The local predictability of social behavior. *Journal of Personality and Social Psychology, 53,* 1159–1177.

Wright, J.C., & Murphy, G.L. (1984). The utility of theories and intuitive statistics: The robustness of theory-based judgments. *Journal of Experimental Psychology: General, 113,* 301–322.

Wright, J.C., Shoda, Y., Mischel, W., & Phillips, K. (in press). Domain-specific accuracy of person perception. *Journal of Personality and Social Psychology*

Part II
New Forms of Personality Coherence

CHAPTER 5

On the Continuities and Consequences of Personality: A Life-Course Perspective

Avshalom Caspi

Personality is an organizing force in human behavior. Its functions include the selection and pursuit of goals over extended periods across the life span, as well as the reduction of conflicts between personal desires and social sanctions.

The reemergence of this personological message (Kluckhohn & Murray, 1953; Murray, 1938) has oriented contemporary personality research towards the study of the effects of personal dispositions on choices and goals, on social and familial relationships, as well as on interactions with social institutions (Maddi, 1984). Current research concerns have also shifted from debates about cross-situational consistency and temporal stability to the coherence of behavior across time and circumstance (Block, 1981, pp. 40–41):

What is contended is that how experience registers, how environments are selected and modified, and how the stages of life are negotiated depends, importantly and coherently, on what the individual brings to these new encounters—the resources, the premises, the intentions, the awareness, the fears and the hopes, the forethoughts and afterthoughts that are subsumed by what we call personality.

Longitudinal studies are an integral part of these (re)emerging directions. In this essay, I shall consider some of the problems and promises entailed in "exploring personality the long way" (White, 1981) with specific reference to a conceptual framework for the analysis of personality in the life course.

The Search for Developmental Continuities

Most longitudinal research focuses on regularities over time in the same characteristics (Moss & Susman, 1980). The search for phenotypic persistence has exerted a strong influence on how longitudinal researchers analyze their data and, in turn, on how their critics evaluate the results. Indeed, Livson and Peskin (1980) have suggested that longitudinal research has been fundamentally handicapped by an exclusive focus on the individual-difference stability of personality characteristics over time.

There does, of course, exist a convincing body of evidence pointing to regularities in the persistence of specific traits (McCrae & Costa, 1984). Not surprisingly, these are primarily characteristics in the sphere of temperament, for which biological underpinnings have been assumed and increasingly confirmed: introversion-extraversion is a prime example. The difficulty with this approach, however, is that phenotypic regularities provide only a select view of connectedness across the life span (Hinde & Bateston, 1984).

A formulation of psychological structures that is isomorphic with behavior is misleading, because the phenotypic display of a given disposition may change with age as a result of maturation and learning (Kagan, 1969). Livson and Peskin (1980) argue that personality dispositions can be shown to be predictive of meaningful social outcomes only if we abandon the search for the simple persistence of specific characteristics and seek genotypic continuities—relationships across time and circumstance between phenotypically dissimilar manifestations of an underlying disposition.

To identify genotypic continuities, we need to view development in terms of the organizations and reorganizations of behavior that take place in response to a series of salient developmental issues presented in the social environment. Consider the case of children's friendships. Gottman & Mettetal (1987) have argued that the significant contexts for social interaction change according to the salient developmental goals of the age period. In early childhood, coordinated dyadic play offers the most opportunities for emotional and cognitive growth. In middle childhood, these opportunities are provided in the context of interaction within the larger same-sex peer group. In preadolescence, the salient developmental task is achieving intimate relations with others, particularly with youth of the same sex. The onset of puberty adds sexual desires to the need to achieve interpersonal intimacy, and creates difficulties for achieving relationships with persons of the opposite sex in which both needs are met.

Developmental considerations about the changing goals and opportunities in children's social worlds imply that we should tailor measures toward the assessment of how individuals respond to salient developmental tasks. Thus, Parker and Asher (1987), in their review of research on children's peer relations and later adjustment problems, note that measures of honesty in early childhood may not predict later outcomes because issues of trustworthiness do not become salient until the preadolescent years. Similarly, solitary activity is quite normal in the early years, and children who exhibit such behavior cannot be considered deviant from age-group play norms. In the middle years of childhood, however, children who continue to remain alone despite a strong press for social interaction may be deviating from social play norms, and thus establishing the grounds for negative peer reputations as well as possibly peer rejection.

Accordingly, consistent individual differences are to be found in the ways that individuals organize their behavior to meet environmental demands and new developmental challenges. Moreover, an appreciation of contextual and developmental factors suggests that longitudinal studies must attend to qualitative similarities in behavior patterns rather than simply to behavioral constancies. The way forward may not lie in aggregating more measures across more settings, but in seeking to understand the dynamics of personality in different contexts at different ages. Thus, an important step in developing a predictive framework for the study of personality is to provide information about the nature of developmental challenges that are likely to be encountered by the developing person in diverse settings.

Sroufe (1979, 1989) has been an eloquent advocate of this approach, arguing that continuity across development can best be discerned by assessing children's functioning with respect to the challenges they face at each developmental phase. This approach has informed the Minnesota Longitudinal Studies on pathways to adaptation and maladaptation in childhood. With assessments of behavior conceptualized in terms of age-appropriate developmental issues, these studies have shown that children who are securely attached as infants are more likely than children with histories of anxious attachments to explore their environments as toddlers (Matas, Arend, & Sroufe, 1978), are less dependent on their teachers in the preschool years (Sroufe, Fox, & Pancake, 1983), and attain higher sociometric status in late childhood (Sroufe, 1989).

Beyond childhood, the search for developmental continuities becomes somewhat more complicated. In particular, a purely psychological approach is inadequate for the analysis of personality in the life course, since most psychological formulations lack a satisfactory concept of the life course itself. How are life trajectories structured? How are lifelong adaptational processes patterned? To answer these questions, a sociological framework is needed; a framework that not only takes account of the person, but also of the person's engagement in society.

A Sociological Conception of the Life Course

In our own work, we have found it useful to adopt a sociological perspective and to conceive of the life course as a sequence of culturally defined, age-graded roles that the individual enacts over time (Caspi, 1987). This conception of the life course is borrowed from the sociology of age-stratification, which emphasizes the social meaning of age in referring to the ordering of life transitions and roles by age-linked expectations, sanctions, and options (Elder, 1975, 1985).

Two concepts are central to this formulation: age-stratified social roles and the age-grading of life events. Both concepts refer to the same phenomenon, but at different levels of analysis (Parsons & Shils, 1951). The stratification of social roles by age refers to phases of the life course that are differentiated by unique clusters of roles and statuses, such as student, worker, and parent. The age-grading of life events, implied in the aforementioned definition, refers to the time dependence (vs. random occurrence) of these roles (Featherman, 1986). Age strata thus describe a sociological reality that is partly rooted in biological processes, whereas age-grades describe a social psychological reality parallel to the age-stratification structure.

Almost every society has a way of allocating, defining, and conferring social membership on individuals as they progress through the life course (Riley, Johnson, & Foner, 1972). Moreover, studies that have explored regularities in age expectations among adults suggest that there exists a shared system of social age definitions that provides a frame of reference for evaluating life experiences (Foner & Kertzer, 1978). Shared social judgments about age expectations define a normative timing of role transitions, such as leaving home, getting married, and childbearing (Neugarten, Moore, & Lowe, 1965), and, as people move through the age structure, being "offtime" can have negative consequences for both the individual and society. For example, the woman who becomes pregnant as a teenager is off-time, and she risks negotiating the demands of this role without the benefit of those social and institutional structures that support and smooth the way for women who are "on-time" (Furstenberg, Brooks-Gunn, & Morgan, 1987). In addition, concepts about the proper phasing of the life course may be registered as cognitive descriptions or predictions of what will happen. Ethnographic accounts of the life course have shown that self-evaluations drawn vis-à-vis collective standards—shared expectancies about how lives are lived—play a central role in regulating a person's sense of personal worth throughout life (LeVine, 1980).

Age strata and age norms thus represent important dimensions of the social context of lives. Moreover, these concepts suggest profitable directions to follow in constructing life-span developmental models. Specifically, if age strata emerge in most societies, and if the system of age expectations is normative, it should be possible to identify and delineate a social time clock that, superimposed upon a biological clock, is more or less compelling for all people.

The concept of a social clock focuses attention on the age-related life schedules of individuals in particular societies and cohorts, and it organizes the study of lives in terms of patterned movements into, along, and out of multiple role-paths such as education, work, marriage, and parenthood (Helson, Mitchell, & Moane, 1984). In this fashion, the life course can be charted as a sequence of social roles that are enacted over time.

According to this framework, successful transitions and adjustments to age-graded roles are the core developmental tasks faced by the individual across the life course. The corresponding research agenda for personality psychology is to examine *how* individuals confront, adapt, and make adjustments to age-graded roles and social transitions.

Dispositions and Situations in the Life Course: When Does Personality Matter?

Individual differences interact with situational demands at numerous points. Research has demonstrated, however, that the influence of dispositional factors on behavior is most pronounced in settings that are unstructured—when individuals are forced to rely primarily on their own internal traits to guide their behavior—and in settings that require them to master and negotiate new demands and tasks (Monson, Hesley, & Chernick, 1982; Snyder & Ickes, 1985).

This conclusion emerges most clearly from research in social psychology. For example, Ickes (1982) developed the Unstructured Interaction Paradigm to elicit, in dyadic social episodes, spontaneous behaviors that are relatively free of the constraints characteristic of more traditional experimental paradigms. Findings from this research program reveal clear-cut and strong dispositional influences on social behavior in situations where the interpersonal and role requirements are new and ambiguous.

Convergent evidence for this conclusion is provided by research in the field of behavior genetics. Thus, twin studies suggest that genetic effects are most pronounced in relation to novel social encounters and in unstructured settings. For example, Plomin and Rowe (1979) have argued that heredity affects individual differences in social responding more to unfamiliar persons than to familiar persons. Specifically, Plomin and Rowe imported the Strange Situation paradigm, a popular procedure for assessing infants' attachment with their mothers, to the homes of twins. Here they found significant differences between monozygotic and dizygotic pairs for social behaviors directed towards the stranger, but not for behaviors directed towards the mother. A similar finding is contained in a report from the Louisville Twin Study. In their longitudinal study of twins from nine-to-thirty-months of age, Matheny and Dolan (1975) have shown that identical twin pairs behave more similarly than fraternal twin pairs in both playroom and test room settings. Importantly, the difference between identical and fraternal twin pairs was consistently weaker in the test room setting, where the range of reactions was potentially more restricted, than that permitted in the less structured playroom setting.

In combination, these findings suggest a more general life-course process. Dispositional factors should be most pronounced when people enter new relationships and assume new roles. Thus, the central strategy for research on personality in the life course is to trace personality variables through a succession of social events while tracking their emergent manifestations. We have done this by tracing the continuities and consequences of interactional styles from late childhood to midlife. Specifically, our longitudinal research has sought to explore the coherence of interactional styles across social transformations in the age-graded life course, to discern how individuals meet developmental challenges and adapt to new roles and settings, and to combine the longitudinal assessment of persons with the longitudinal assessment of situations in order to discover how childhood interactional styles shape the life course itself (Caspi, Bem, & Elder, 1989).

Childhood Dispositions and the Prediction of Life-Course Patterns

Data for our research were obtained from the archives of the Institute of Human Development at the University of California, Berkeley. The subjects are members of the Berkeley Guidance Study (Eichorn, 1981)—an ongoing study, initiated in 1928, of every third birth in the city of Berkeley over a period of eighteen months. The original sample contained 102 males and 112 females of which a maximum of eighty-seven and ninety-five participants, respectively, have been followed up into adulthood.

Childhood data on the Berkeley subjects were obtained from yearly clinical interviews with their mothers, which were subsequently organized into ratings on five-point behavior scales by Macfarlane (1938; Macfarlane, Allen, & Honzik, 1954). On the basis of these materials, we identified three distinctive interactional styles in late childhood: ill-temperedness ("moving against the world"), shyness ("moving away from the world"), and dependency ("moving toward the world") (Horney, 1945). Ill-temperedness refers to an interactional style characterized by explosive temper tantrums in reaction to frustration and authority. Shyness refers to an interactional style characterized by emotional inhibition and discomfort in social settings. Dependency refers to an interactional style characterized by the tendency to seek attention, company, approval, and help.

Our exploration begins in late childhood (ages eight to ten), partly because longitudinal research has shown that individual-difference stability in behavioral profiles like aggression, dominance, dependency, sociability, and shyness emerges most clearly during this period (Kagan & Moss, 1962). Clinical observations similarly suggest that if children persist in problem behavior by age ten it is more difficult to alter behavior patterns thereafter (Patterson, 1982). The appearance of stable individual differences in late childhood may be due to the emergence of belief systems and expectations that find continuous affirmation in an expanding social environment (Kagan, 1984). It is also possible that the degree to which experiences and environments are influenced by personality dispositions increases with development (Scarr & McCartney, 1983). From infancy to late childhood, children become increasingly effective in creating environments that are compatible with their motivations and needs. As self-regulatory capacities and competencies increase, individuals begin to make choices, display preferences, and take actions that preserve their social relations and maintain their social networks (Lerner, 1982).

To examine these choices, preferences, and actions, we have organized the analysis of life-course patterns around two themes: the transition to adulthood and subsequent aspects of work and family life. In our exploration, we obtained measures of adjustment to age-graded events and roles by sampling behavior from the life-record domain—actual records of a person's behavior in society (Cattell, 1957). Childhood dispositions should relate importantly to L-data, to observations made in situ that are embedded in the group culture pattern. There are sound methodological grounds for this claim. Rather than measuring behavior at a given moment, L-observation is usually spread over longer periods of time, thus rendering the data relatively free of unreliability (e.g., Block, 1977). In addition, Cattell suggested equally compelling theoretical reasons for emphasizing L-data. Insofar as life-span development involves interaction with institutions, mores, and the general culture pattern, the natural history mapping of behavior as expressed in L-data is most promising because L-data are ultimately concerned with inclination and volition—with how, whether, and when a person chooses to perform. There are, of course, limitations to this approach (cf. Moskowitz, 1986). What one sacrifices by not directly observing the immediate settings in which people are embedded is, however, compensated for by an increased understanding of the cultural and structural conditions that shape those settings.

Indeed, our analysis of ill-temperedness pointed to the discriminativeness of this childhood interactional style across many of life's tasks, from patterns of early adult achievement to family relations (Caspi, Elder, & Bem, 1987). Thus, men who reacted with temper tantrums to frustration and adult authority as children encountered difficulties when they again faced frustration and controlling authority—in school, the armed services, and low-level jobs—or were immersed in life situations requiring the frequent management of interpersonal conflicts—as in marriage.

For example, these men achieved less in formal education; in the military, they attained a lower rank; in the workplace, they experienced greater instability; and their marriages were more likely to end in divorce or separation.

Women's performance in the world of work did not show the significant correlates with childhood ill-temperedness that we found for the men. Although a large majority of the Berkeley women were employed at some point in their lives, there was insufficient comparable variation in their occupational roles. Historically, however, a woman's socioeconomic status has derived from her husband's status, and it is here that we can discern the socioeconomic consequences of childhood ill-temperedness for the female subjects. Women with a history of childhood ill-temperedness fared less well than their even-tempered peers in the marriage market and married men who were significantly less well-positioned in their occupational careers. A history of childhood ill-temperedness also had clear implications for their family life. These women were more likely to divorce and were described by their husbands and children as less adequate, more ill-tempered mothers.

Our analysis of shyness showed that individuals who experienced acute discomfort in meeting new acquaintances and in entering social settings as children became adults who tended to delay or avoid action and were, generally, more reluctant to enter new and unfamiliar situations (Caspi, Elder, & Bem, 1988). In particular, a shy interactional style affected men's transition to adulthood and proved somewhat problematic in their efforts to negotiate traditional masculine roles involving mate selection and vocational decision making. A large percentage of men who were shy and reserved as children were normatively off-time in their transitions to these age-graded roles; they married, became fathers, and assumed a stable career line at a significantly older age than their more outgoing counterparts. Moreover, the findings showed that by entering an occupational career at an older age, men with a childhood history of shyness may have forgone investments in skills and benefits, thus increasing their vulnerability to career disruptions and sacrificing higher achievements.

Unlike their male counterparts, women with a childhood history of shyness were not delayed or off-time in entering marriage, or in starting families. Instead, they were more likely than other women in their cohort to follow a conventional pattern of marriage, childbearing, and homemaking, and, in general, were dispositionally suited to adhere to the female social clock (cf. Helson, Mitchell, & Moane, 1984). Again, it is pertinent to recall that the men and women in this study reached the age of majority during the late 1940s, a time of relatively traditional sex roles, and the results suggest that shyness was much more compatible with the traditional female role than with the traditional male role in our society.

Finally, our analysis of dependency also implicated this childhood interactional style in the formation and maintenance of work and family roles (Caspi, Elder, & Bem, 1989). Men with this childhood history adhered to conventional roles across the life course. In particular, they were on-time in their transition to adulthood and adhered to an orderly sequence of age-graded events. For example, they were more likely than the other men in the sample to follow the normative sequence of finishing school and launching a career before getting married. A history of childhood dependency also had implications for the stability and quality of their marriages. Men with such a history were significantly more likely to have an intact first marriage; their wives were more satisfied with their marriages than wives of other men; and they and their wives agreed more with one another on childrearing practices.

Among women, expressions of childhood dependency were also observed in events surrounding family formation and in parenting investments. Two findings stand out for women with a history of childhood dependency; their relatively early entry into marriage and parenthood, and their extended investment in parenting. In their transition to adulthood, these women were more likely to leave the parental home earlier, to marry, and to have children more quickly. Although women with this childhood history did not, on average, bear more children, their child-bearing period was significantly longer. It would appear that women who tended to seek help, approval, and attention as children became adults who submerged their individuality in family ties, creating for themselves a life locally focused on attachments to their spouses and children.

In general, then, it appears that life-course patterns are related, importantly and coherently, to interactional styles observed in late childhood. Invariant behavior patterns do not emerge in the findings, but a predictable way of approaching and responding to the environment in different social settings is clearly indicated by the results.

Of course, these specific results must be viewed in cultural and historical perspective. Particular life-course patterns depend not only on the individual's distinctive interactional style, but also on the structure of the environment in any given historical period. How, then, shall we treat the results briefly summarized here if we are to remain steadfast in our mission to identify generalizable principles that govern personality functioning?

I suspect that longitudinal researchers have erred in asking whether *specific* findings will generalize across historical epochs and have fretted unnecessarily about whether historical relativity poses a danger to a nomothetic science of personality. The fact that all samples and behaviors are bound by history should not discourage the personologist. In fact, the use of historically and culturally specific data places no constraints on the specificity or universality of the inferences drawn, or the theories constructed therefrom. The obverse argument, however, is not equally valid: when personality research is carried out without a sense of history, without recognition that phenotypic expressions represent a point of articulation between historical, social, and ontogenetic processes, specific findings may be difficult to apprehend. The changing environmental context of development must be thoroughly understood and analyzed before an adequate account of the role of dispositional factors in social behavior is possible.

This point is illustrated by a comparison of findings on personality and substance use obtained in two separate research projects carried out with normal samples, whose members were born four decades apart.

Jones (1981), using the Oakland Growth and Berkeley Guidance studies, asked whether midlife drinking problems among men born in the 1920s could be predicted on the basis of their earlier personality characteristics. The answer is yes. In adulthood, men with drinking problems could be differentiated by a constellation of items from the California Q-set in adolescence. Similarly, Block, Block, and Keyes (1988), in their sample of children born in the late 1960s, asked if drug use could be predicted on the basis of early personality characteristics. Again, the answer is yes. Marijuana use at age fourteen is foretold by a constellation of items from the California Child Q-set at ages three to four.

The overall conceptual and measurement similarity between the two studies is striking. In both instances, a constellation of personality characteristics encompassed by the concept of ego undercontrol (e.g., inability to delay gratification, rapid tempo) predicts the use of cohort-specific substances. The behavioral connections observed in these two longitudinal investigations suggest that certain life outcomes (e.g., drug use) depend on the structure of the environment (e.g., the availability and popularity of particular drugs), as well as on a transhistorically coherent set of personality attributes that implicate undercontrolled behavior.

An even more striking illustration is provided by longitudinal research on adult correlates of adolescent intellectual competence. Livson and Day (1977), working with a sample of women from the Oakland Growth and Berkeley Guidance studies, found that intellectual competence, a dimension derived from California Q-sort data in adolescence, significantly predicted, for those born in the early and late 1920s, their completed family size during the post-war baby boom. The relationship is positive and linear: intellectually competent girls grew up to have larger families.

It is unlikely that this correlation will be replicated with contemporary cohorts, because historical forces have created opportunities for women that will reverse the sign of this correlation. Indeed, in a provocative essay, Herrnstein (1989) has recently argued that the positive correlation between IQ and fertility was probably restricted to a unique historical period. For earlier, and more recent times, the correlation between tested intelligence and fertility is negative (cf. Retherford & Sewell, 1988).

Under what conditions do claims for generalizability apply? Studies have shown that individual differences in adolescent competencies can and do predict those socially-valued life outcomes prescribed by changing social conditions in different historical settings. Thus, Livson and Day (1977, p. 321), appropriately cautious, note that their results are useful for understanding and predicting such outcomes

. . . only if they are interpreted not as direct if-then relationships, but as providing an understanding of the intrapsychic and interpersonal characteristics that mediate one's child-bearing response to a social context prevailing during the period in which fertility decisions are made.

Similarly, it has not been my aim to claim cross-cohort generality from the single-cohort longitudinal findings summarized here. On the contrary, the analysis has been undertaken with explicit reference to the social climate experienced during the lifetime of the sample studied. Instead of seeking information about life-course patterns that transcend this sociohistorical context, I sought to provide a longitudinal survey of the environmental landscape as it is influenced by dispositional factors, and to document the manifestations of childhood interactional styles in the timing, sequence, and content of social roles across the life course as they are grounded in historically-bound circumstances. Social changes may well alter these circumstances and produce changes in particular manifestations of a disposition. We can, however, still hope to abstract the general principles of personality that produce these manifestations by investigating how individuals bring their unique characteristics to bear on the interpretation and enactment of the roles they are required to play in the course of their lives.

Acknowledgments. This research was supported in part by a grant from the National Institute of Mental Health to G. H. Elder, Jr., and A. Caspi (MH-41827). I am indebted to the Institute of Human Development, University of California-Berkeley, for permission to use archival data from the Berkeley Guidance Study.

References

Block, J. (1971). *Lives through time.* Berkeley: Bancroft.
Block, J. (1977). Advancing the psychology of personality: Paradigmatic shift or improving the quality of research. In D. Magnusson & N.S. Endler (Eds.), *Personality at the crossroads: Current issues in interactional psychology* (pp. 37–63). Hillsdale, NJ: Erlbaum.
Block, J. (1981). Some enduring and consequential structures of personality. In A.I. Rabin, J. Aronoff, A.M. Barclay, & R.A. Zucker (Eds.), *Further explorations in personality* (pp. 27–43). New York: Wiley.

Block, J., Block, J.H., & Keyes, S. (1988). Longitudinally foretelling drug usage in adolescence: Early childhood personality and environmental precursors. *Child Development, 59,* 336–355.

Caspi, A. (1987). Personality in the life course. *Journal of Personality and Social Psychology, 53,* 1203–1213.

Caspi, A., Bem, D.J., & Elder, G.H., Jr. (in press). Continuities and consequences of interactional styles across the life course. *Journal of Personality.*

Caspi, A., Elder, G.H., Jr., & Bem, D.J. (1987). Moving against the world: Life-course patterns of explosive children. *Developmental Psychology, 23,* 303–308.

Caspi, A., Elder, G.H., Jr., & Bem, D.J. (1988). Moving away from the world: Life-course patterns of shy children. *Developmental Psychology, 24,* 824–831.

Caspi, A. Elder, G.H., Jr., & Bem, D.J. (1989). Moving toward the world: Life-course patterns of dependent children. Unpublished manuscript, Harvard University.

Cattell, R.B. (1957). *Personality and motivation structure and measurement.* New York: World Book.

Eichorn, D. (1981). Samples and procedures. In D. Eichorn, J. A. Clausen, N. Haan, M.P. Honzik, & P. Mussen (Eds.), *Present and past in middle life* (pp. 33–51). New York: Academic Press.

Elder, G.H., Jr. (1975). Age differentiation and the life course. *Annual Review of Sociology, 1,* 165–190.

Elder, G.H., Jr. (1985). Perspectives on the life course. In G. H. Elder, Jr. (Ed.), *Life course dynamics: Trajectories and transitions, 1968–1980* (pp. 23–49). Ithaca, NY: Cornell University Press.

Featherman, D.L. (1986). Biography, society, and history: Individual development as a population process. In A.B. Sorensen, F.E. Weinert, & L.R. Sherrod (Eds.), *Human development and the life course: Multidisciplinary perspectives* (pp. 99–149). Hillsdale, NJ: Erlbaum.

Foner, A., & Kertzer, D.I. (1978). Transitions over the life course: Lessons from age-set societies. *American Journal of Sociology, 83,* 1081–1104.

Furstenberg, F.F., Jr., Brooks-Gunn, J., & Morgan, S.P. (1987). *Adolescent mothers in later life.* New York: Cambridge University Press.

Gottman, J.M., & Mettetal, G. (1987). Speculations about social and affective development: Friendship and acquaintanceship through adolescence. In J.M. Gottman & J.G. Parker (Eds.), *Conversations of friends: Speculations on affective development* (pp. 192–237). New York: Cambridge University Press.

Helson, R., Mitchell, V., & Moane, G. (1984). Personality and patterns of adherence and nonadherence to the social clock. *Journal of Personality and Social Psychology, 46,* 1079–1096.

Herrnstein, R.J. (1989). IQ and falling birth rates. *Atlantic Monthly,* May, 72–79.

Hinde, R.A., & Bateston, P.P.G. (1984). Continuities versus discontinuities in behavioral development and the neglect of process. *International Journal of Behavioral Development, 7,* 129–143.

Horney, K. (1945). *Our inner conflicts.* New York: Norton.

Ickes, W. (1982). A basic paradigm for the study of personality, roles and social behavior. In W. Ickes & E. Knowles (Eds.), *Personality, roles and social behavior.* New York: Springer.

Jones, M. C. (1981). Midlife drinking patterns: Correlates and antecedents. In D. Eichorn, J.A. Clausen, N. Haan, M.P. Honzik, & P. Mussen (Eds.), *Present and past in middle life* (pp. 223–242). New York: Academic Press.

Kagan, J. (1969). The three faces of continuity in human development. In D.A. Goslin (Ed.), *Handbook of socialization theory and research* (pp. 983–1002). Chicago: Rand McNally.

Kagan, J. (1984). Continuity and change in the opening years of life. In R.N. Emde & R.J. Harmon (Eds.), *Continuities and discontinuities in development* (pp. 15–39). New York: Plenum.

Kagan, J., & Moss, H.A. (1962). *Birth to maturity.* New York: Wiley.

Kluckhohn, C., & Murray, H.A. (1953). Personality formation: The determinants. In H.A. Murray, C. Kluckhohn, & D.M. Schneider (Eds.), *Personality in nature, society, and culture* (pp. 53–67). New York: Alfred A. Knopf.

Lerner, R.M. (1982). Children and adolescents as producers of their own development. *Developmental Review, 2,* 342–370.

LeVine, R.A. (1980). Adulthood among the Gusii of Kenya. In N. J. Smelser & E. Erikson (Eds.), *Themes of work and love in adulthood* (pp. 77–104). Cambridge, MA: Harvard University Press.

Livson, N., & Day, D. (1977). Adolescent personality antecedents of completed family size: A longitudinal study. *Journal of Youth and Adolescence, 6,* 311–324.

Livson, N., & Peskin, H. (1980). Perspectives on adolescence from longitudinal research. In J. Adelson (Ed.), *Handbook of adolescent psychology* (pp. 47–98). New York: Wiley.

Macfarlane, J.W. (1938). Studies in child guidance I: Methodology of data collection and organization. *Monographs of the Society for Research in Child Development, 3,* Serial No. 6.

Macfarlane, J.W., Allen, L., & Honzik, M.P. (1954). *A developmental study of the behavioral problems of children between twenty-one months and fourteen years.* Berkeley: University of California Press.

Maddi, S. (1984). Personology for the 1980s. In R.A. Zucker, J. Aronoff, & A.I. Rabin (Eds.), *Personality and the prediction of behavior* (pp. 7–41). New York: Academic Press.

Matas, L., Arend, R., & Sroufe, L.A. (1978). Continuity of adaptation in the second year: The relationship between quality of attachment and later competence. *Child Development, 49,* 547–556.

Matheny, A.P., Jr., & Dolan, A.B. (1975). Persons, situations, and time: A genetic view of behavioral change in children. *Journal of Personality and Social Psychology, 32,* 1106–1110.

McCrae, R.R., & Costa, P.C., Jr. (1984). *Emerging lives, enduring dispositions.* Boston: Little, Brown.

Monson, T.C., Hesley, J.W., & Chernick, L. (1982). Specifying when personality traits can and cannot predict behavior: An alternative to abandoning the attempt to predict single-act criteria. *Journal of Personality and Social Psychology, 43,* 385–399.

Moskowitz, D.S. (1986). Comparison of self-reports, reports by knowledgeable informants, and behavioral observational data. *Journal of Personality, 54,* 294–317.

Moss, H.A., & Susman, E. J. (1980). Longitudinal study of personality development. In O.G. Brim, Jr., & J. Kagan (Eds.), *Constancy and change in human development* (pp. 530–595). Cambridge, MA: Harvard University Press.

Murray, H.A. (1938). *Explorations in personality.* New York: Oxford University Press.

Neugarten, B., Moore, J., & Lowe, J.W. (1965). Age norms, age constraints, and adult socialization. *American Journal of Sociology, 70,* 710–717.

Parker, J.G., & Asher, S.R. (1987). Peer relations and later personal adjustment: Are low-accepted children at risk? *Psychological Bulletin, 102,* 357–389.

Parsons, T., & Shils, E.A. (Eds.). (1951). *Toward a general theory of action.* Cambridge, MA: Harvard University Press.

Patterson, G.R. (1982). *Coercive family process.* Eugene, OR: Castalia.

Plomin, R., & Rowe, D.C. (1979). Genetic and environmental etiology of social behavior in infancy. *Developmental Psychology, 15,* 56–63.

Retherford, R.D., & Sewell, W.H. (1988). Intelligence and family size. *Social Biology, 35*(1&2), pp. 1–40.

Riley, M.W., Johnson, M., & Foner, A. (1972). *Aging and society: A sociology of age-stratification.* New York: Russell Sage Foundation.

Scarr, S., & McCartney, K. (1983). How people make their own environments: A theory of genotype-environment correlations. *Child Development, 54,* 424–435.

Snyder, M., & Ickes, W. (1985). Personality and social behavior. In G. Lindzey & E. Aronson (Eds.), *Handbook of social psychology* (Vol. 2, pp. 883–947). New York: Random House.

Sroufe, L.A. (1979). The coherence of individual development. *American Psychologist, 34,* 834–841.

Sroufe, L.A. (in press). Pathways to adaptation and maladaptation: Psychopathology as developmental deviation. In D. Cicchetti (Ed.), *First Rochester symposium on developmental psychopathology.* Hillsdale, NJ: Erlbaum.

Sroufe, L.A., Fox, N., & Pancake, V. (1983). Attachment and dependency in developmental perspective. *Child Development, 54,* 1615–1627.

White, R.W. (1981). Exploring personality the long way: The study of lives. In A.I. Rabin, J. Aronoff, A.M. Barclay, & R.A. Zucker (Eds.), *Further explorations in personality* (pp. 3–19). New York: Wiley.

CHAPTER 6

Life Paths of Aggressive and Withdrawn Children

Debbie S. Moskowitz and Alex E. Schwartzman

Introduction

Aggression and social withdrawal are two major dimensions of individual differences in behavior during childhood. The present paper introduces a longitudinal study of the development of children selected from a general school population who were high on aggression and withdrawal and describes results relating aggression and withdrawal to outcomes during adolescence. High aggressiveness was predictive of low intelligence, poor school achievement, and psychiatric problems. For females, high aggressiveness was also predictive of general health problems. High social withdrawal appeared to be predictive of inaccurate, negative self-perceptions. In addition, females who were high on withdrawal were more likely than the others to have had an abortion. Individuals who were high on both aggression and withdrawal had relatively poor social competence, general problems with behavior, low intelligence, and were performing poorly in school. Expectations for the future development of these individuals are considered, and plans for the incorporation of contextual variables in future studies are described.

Life Paths of Aggressive and Withdrawn Children

There is a well-established tradition in the personality literature of using longitudinal methods to describe the course and texture of people's lives. The purpose of the present report is to highlight results from a longitudinal study of children selected in childhood for aggressiveness and social withdrawal. The present report describes their functioning during adolescence, speculates on their functioning in the future, and considers contextual issues that may affect their future development.

Aggression and social withdrawal have been used by several personality researchers to study dispositional patterns in children's behavior (e.g.,

Wiggins & Winder, 1961; Wright & Mischel, 1987). Aggression has frequently been defined as behaviors whose intent is to hurt the person or property of others. Referent behaviors include bullying, fighting, and teasing. Social withdrawal refers to behaviors which isolate the individual from others. Factor analytic studies suggest that withdrawn behaviors closely cluster with fear, anxiety, and sadness (Quay, 1986). Referent behaviors include shyness, sadness, and staying alone.

The most developed literature on the relation between these childhood characteristics and subsequent patterns of adaptation concerns aggressive behavior in boys. Numerous studies indicate that aggression in males is highly stable (Olweus, 1979). There is also evidence that aggression by boys is predictive of antisocial activity (e.g., Huessman, Eron, Lefkowitz, & Walder, 1984; Loeber & Dishion, 1983; Magnusson, 1988; Robins, 1966, 1986). There are few studies of outcomes for aggressive females, but those available indicate moderate stability for aggression, at a somewhat lower level than for males, and some reports indicate fewer negative outcomes for aggressive girls than for aggressive boys (Huesmann, et al., 1984; Moskowitz, Schwartzman, & Ledingham, 1985; Olweus, 1981). It is possible, though, that reports of fewer negative outcomes for aggressive girls may not have examined a sufficient variety of aspects of life adaptation to detect the outcomes that may occur for aggressive girls (Robins, 1986).

The literature on the stability and consequences of social withdrawal in children is less developed and less consistent than the literature on aggression. One view is that childhood withdrawal is neither stable nor a predictor of later outcomes (see Kohlberg, et al., 1984). The negative conclusions concerning the relevance of childhood withdrawal to later adjustment may, however, be misleading or restricted in their genralizability, because they are based largely on the findings of a limited number of follow-up studies of relatively small samples of clinic-referred withdrawn children (see Parker & Asher, 1987). In several studies using children sampled from the community and schools, there is evidence that social withdrawal is stable and that, by ten years of age, the level of stability is similar to that found for aggression (Bronson, 1966; Moskowitz, et al., 1985; Wiggins & Winder, 1961).

Research on the prediction of behavior suggests that, when using global variables such as aggression and withdrawal as predictors, replicable predictions are most likely to be obtained using global outcome variables that reflect multiple occasions and situations (e.g., Block, 1977; Epstein, 1980; Moskowitz, 1982, 1986, 1988). The variables in the two studies to be described reflect characteristics aggregated across many occasions and situations. The global variables assessed a range of possible outcomes, including measures of behavior problems, social activities, cognitive ability, academic achievement, and health.

In one study, individuals were assessed in the laboratory approximately six years after identification. The measures included an intelligence test and self-reports about behavior, school achievement, and social relationships. In the second study, archival records were obtained concerning individuals' physical and mental health for a four-year period beginning approximately four years after identification.

Several of the predicted variables reflected dispositions (e.g., behavior problems and participation in school activities). Others were acts that were not primarily caused by dispositions (e.g., seeing a physician), and sometimes the acts reflected events initiated by others (e.g., seeing a psychiatrist). So rather than purely representing aspects of personality, the variables to be described represent diverse aspects of functioning along a life path during adolescence.

General Method

Identification of the sample. Initially, assessments of aggression and withdrawal were collected for 4,109 students in Grades 1, 4, and 7. Students in these grades were seven, ten, and thirteen-years-old. The number of boys and girls screened was approximately equal, as was the number of children in each of the three grades.

Children from the screening population were assigned to the aggressive group ($n = 198$) if they had scores in the 95th percentile or greater on aggression, and scores below the 75th percentile on withdrawal. Children selected for the withdrawal group ($n = 220$) had scores equal to or greater than the 95th percentile on withdrawal, and scores below the 75th percentile on aggression. The aggressive-withdrawn group ($n = 238$) consisted of those whose scores exceeded the 75th percentile on both aggression and withdrawal. This group was included because it was expected that individuals who were high on both aggression and withdrawal might be at risk for schizophrenia (see Schwartzman, Ledingham, & Serbin, 1985). The control group ($n = 1114$) contained children who scored below the 75th percentile and above the 25th percentile on both aggression and withdrawal.

Selection instrument. A modified version of the Pupil Evaluation Inventory (PEI), a peer nomination assessment technique developed by Pekarik, Prinz, Liebert, Weintraub, and Neale (1976), was used to measure aggression and withdrawal. The withdrawal scale included items such as "those who are too shy to make friends easily" and "those who often don't want to play." Among the items on the aggression scale were: "those who are mean and cruel to others" and "those who pick fights." Details about the administration of the modified PEI can be found in Moskowitz, et al., 1985.

Study 1: Intelligence, Behavior Problems, and Social Competence

Method

Five to seven years after identification, individuals from the four peer classification groups were invited to participate in laboratory testing. The percentage of each group that agreed to participate was approximately equal: aggressive group = 21%, withdrawn group = 23%, aggressive-withdrawn group = 29%, and control group = 22%.

Intelligence. To assess intelligence, six subtests from the WISCR or the WAISR (for individuals seventeen years and older) were administered, and the scaled scores were summed. The subtests were Information, Vocabulary, Comprehension, Similarities, Block Design, and Picture Arrangement.

Behavior problems and social competence. Individuals completed the Youth Self-Report (YSR, Achenbach & Edelbrock, 1983). This measure has two components, one examining behavior problems and the other examining social competence. From this measure, the following scores were analyzed: the total scores for behavior problems and social competence and the subscale scores for internalizing, externalizing, activities, school competence, and interpersonal aspects of social competence.

Results

Intelligence. Total intelligence was analyzed using a hierarchical stepwise multiple regression. Two covariates were entered first: age at time of testing and socioeconomic status (Nock & Rossi, 1979). The predictor vectors were entered in steps in the following fixed order: sex, age group, classification group, sex by age group interaction, sex by classification group interaction, and age group by classification group interaction. Results involving classification group are presented. A difference between an extreme group and the control group is described when the post hoc test (Scheffé procedure, alpha = .05) was significant.

Classification group accounted for a significant increment in the proportion of explained variance for total intelligence ($F(3,390) = 9.9$, $p < .001$). The aggressive and the aggressive-withdrawn individuals scored significantly below the control individuals on total intelligence (see Table 6.1).

Behavior problems. The analysis of total behavior problems and the externalizing and internalizing subscales followed the same hierarchical regression procedure as the analysis of intelligence with the addition of one covariate, social desirability (Crowne & Marlowe, 1964).

TABLE 6.1. Classification group effects on intelligence, behavior problems and social competence.

	\multicolumn{8}{c}{Classification group}							
Variables	Aggressive		Withdrawn		Aggressive-Withdrawn		Control	
	M	SD	M	SD	M	SD	M	SD
Intelligence	53.4	11.9	61.3	15.8	56.5	11.4	61.4	11.1
Externalizing	62.9	9.6	60.3	4.8	63.6	7.7	60.8	6.2
Behavior problems	74.1	8.7	72.5	7.1	75.4	7.7	72.7	6.3
School competence	39.0	14.6	41.4	14.5	38.6	15.5	48.1	15.5
Total social competence	42.4	10.6	42.2	9.3	39.7	8.9	44.2	9.6

Note. Cell sizes varied slightly because of missing data. Cell sizes were: aggressive group, $n = 36$-42; withdrawn group, $n = 49$-51; aggressive-withdrawn group, $n = 66$-69; control group, $n = 222$-239.

On the measure of total behavior problems, there was a classification group effect ($F(3,375) = 3.1$, $p < .05$). The aggressive-withdrawn individuals had more behavior problems than the control individuals (see Table 6.1).

On the externalizing subscale, there was a main effect for classification group ($F(3,375) = 5.9$, $p < .001$). The aggressive-withdrawn group had an elevated externalizing score relative to the control group (see Table 6.1).
Social competence. The total and subscale scores for social competence were analyzed using the same procedure followed for the behavior problem scales.

There was a main effect for classification group on total social competence ($F(3,364) = 4.1$, $p < .01$). The aggressive-withdrawn individuals were depressed on total social competence relative to the control individuals (see Table 6.1).

There was a main effect due to classification group on the school competence subscale ($F(3,367) = 10.4$, $p < .001$). Aggressive, withdrawn, and aggressive-withdrawn individuals were lower on school competence than the control individuals (see Table 6.1).
Summary. Intelligence, social competence, and behavior problems were affected by classification group. The aggressive and the aggressive-withdrawn individuals scored below the control individuals on intelligence, while the withdrawn individuals were not different from the control individuals. The aggressive-withdrawn individuals reported problems in the areas of behavior and social competence, including poor competence in school. The aggressive individuals and the withdrawn individuals reported problems in school, but not in other areas of competence.

Study 2: Medical and Psychiatric Treatment

Method

Virtually all medical care in the province in which the subjects reside is paid for by the provincial government. Medical records were obtained from a centralized provincial office for a four-year period beginning approximately four years after identification. These records were provided without individuals' names but with information about each individual's sex, age group, and classification group. Records were obtained for more than 95% of the original sample, that is, 1,677 individuals.

Measures. The following measures were generated from the records for all individuals: (1) whether the person received medical treatment for a nongynecological and nonpsychiatric problem; (2) frequency of medical treatment; (3) whether the person received treatment for a psychiatric problem; (4) frequency of psychiatric treatment. Additional measures extracted for the females were: (1) whether the individual was treated for a gynecological problem; (2) frequency of gynecological problems; (3) whether the individual had received treatment related to pregnancy; (4) whether the individual had had an abortion.

Results

The dichotomous variables were analyzed using a logistic regression procedure with a fixed order of entry for the independent variables. Frequency variables were analyzed using a hierarchical multiple regression procedure. For both kinds of analyses, the order of entry of the independent variables was: sex, age group, classification group, sex by age group, sex by classification group, age group by classification group, and sex by age group by classification group. For variables collected for females only, the sex main effect and interactions were omitted. Results involving classification group are reported. Differences between each extreme group and the control group were examined using the Scheffé procedure (alpha = .05).

Medical treatment. More than 97% of the sample had received medical care during the four-year period. On frequency of medical treatment, there was a significant main effect for classification group ($F(3,1670) = 6.5$, $p < .001$) and a significant interaction effect for sex by classification group ($F(3,1665) = 2.6$, $p = .05$). The aggressive group had an elevated frequency of medical treatment (see Table 6.2). The aggressive females had a particularly elevated frequency of treatment (see Table 6.3 and Figure 6.1). The aggressive males were not elevated relative to the control males.

Psychiatric treatment. There was a significant main effect for classification group for whether psychiatric treatment had been received (improvement in chi-square, log linear ratio (3) = 11.9, $p < .01$). Aggressive

TABLE 6.2. Classification group effects on frequency of medical and psychiatric treatments.

	Classification group							
Variables	Aggressive		Withdrawn		Aggressive-Withdrawn		Control	
	M	SD	M	SD	M	SD	M	SD
General medical	25.7	22.3	22.5	22.9	21.6	22.2	19.3	18.3
Psychiatric	1.1	5.9	.3	1.0	.3	1.2	.2	1.9

Note. Cell sizes were: aggressive group $n = 194$; withdrawn group $n = 207$; aggressive-withdrawn group $n = 224$; control group $n = 1052$.

TABLE 6.3. Sex by classification group effect on frequency of medical treatment.

Classification Group	Sex					
	Males			Females		
	M	SD	n	M	SD	n
Aggressive	17.7	17.7	95	35.7	25.3	99
Withdrawn	18.9	20.8	99	26.5	24.9	108
Aggressive-withdrawn	20.9	21.8	104	22.6	23.4	120
Control	15.9	15.0	519	23.2	21.0	533

individuals were more than twice as likely as control individuals to have received psychiatric treatment (aggressive group = 18%; withdrawn group = 12.6%; aggressive-withdrawn group = 7.6%; control group = 7.8%).

There was also a classification group effect for frequency of psychiatric treatments ($F(3,1670) = 6.7$, $p < .001$). The aggressive group received more frequent psychiatric treatments than all other classification groups (see Table 6.2).

Gynecological problems. There was a classification group effect on whether a female had been treated for a gynecological problem (improvement in chi-square, log linear ratio (3) = 21.1, $p < .001$). The aggressive group was most likely to have received treatment (aggressive group = 20.2%; withdrawn group = 16.7%; aggressive-withdrawn group = 6.7%; and control group = 11.8%).

Pregnancy. There were no classification group differences related to pregnancy.

Abortions. Given the nature of the data, we could not determine whether a pregnancy was planned. There might, however, be differences in whether the pregnancy was allowed to go to term. There was a significant effect due to classification group on having had an abortion (improvement in chi-square, log linear ratio (3) = 12.5, $p < .01$). The withdrawn group had a higher probability than the other groups of having had an abor-

Sex by Classification Subgroup Effects on Medical Treatment

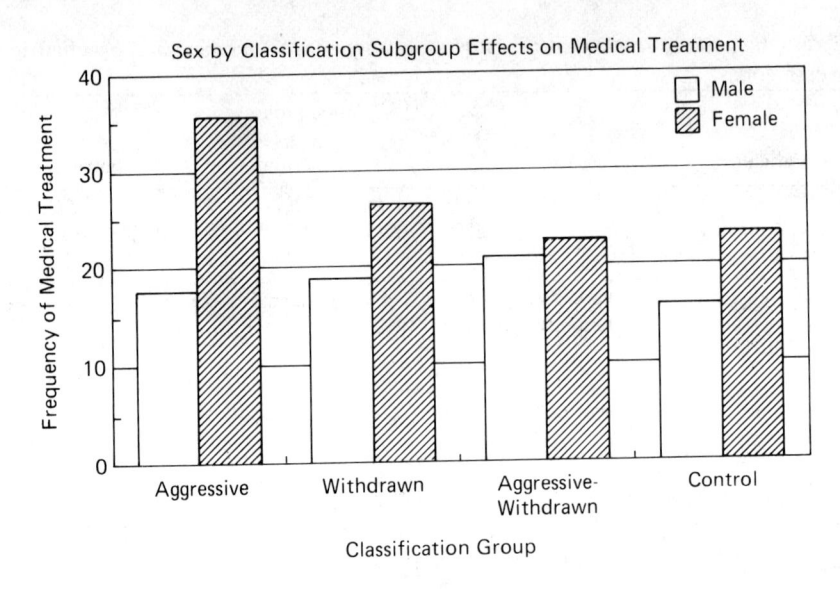

FIGURE 6.1. Classification Group

tion (aggressive group = 5.1%; withdrawn group = 7.4%; aggressive-withdrawn group = 2.5%; control group = 2.8%).

Summary. The aggressive individuals were more likely than control individuals to have received psychiatric treatment, and they received more frequent psychiatric treatment than the other groups. The aggressive females received the highest rate of medical treatment, more than the other groups of females and more than the aggressive males. The aggressive females also were more likely to have been treated for a gynecological problem. There were no differences among the classification groups in the probability of pregnancy, but the withdrawn females had a higher proportion of terminated pregnancies than the other females.

Discussion

Aggressives

At the time of first assessment, the aggressive individuals were not different from control subjects on intelligence, but they were achieving poorly on standardized tests of language and mathematics (Moskowitz & Schwartzman, 1988). The present results indicate that the pattern of poor academic achievement continued into adolescence. In contrast to findings at the time of first assessment, six years after first assessment the aggressive individuals were relatively low on intelligence. These results are consistent with a pattern described by Huesmann, Eron, and Yarmel

(1987) that aggression in childhood is predictive of lowered intelligence in adolescence and adulthood. The aggressive behavior and the poor academic achievement may be interfering with the development of intellectual skills. It is also possible that both the aggression and the problems with school achievement may be stemming from common underlying deficits that eventually interfere with the development of intelligence.

A relatively high proportion (almost 20%) of the aggressive individuals had received psychiatric treatment, and they received more frequent psychiatric treatments than the others. It appears then that these individuals, who were initially identified by their peers, were sufficiently deviant to be brought to the attention of mental health service providers.

The females who were high on aggressiveness had more frequent treatments for health problems. These treatments were for general physical health, for gynecological problems, and for abortions. There is considerable evidence that women seek more medical treatment than men (see Weissman & Klerman, 1977), so it is not surprising that the aggressive females received more health treatment than the aggressive males. It is notable, however, that the aggressive females were seeking more health treatment than other females, a fact about which, at this point, it is only possible to speculate. There is evidence from adoption studies that women who have frequent sick leaves are more likely to have biological fathers who fight and commit other violent crimes than women who do not have frequent sick leaves (Bohman, Cloninger, von Knorring, & Sigvardsson, 1984), suggesting the possibility that sex moderates the expression of a genetic tendency that can lead either to aggression in males or to physical complaints in women. A possible mechanism for this pattern is suggested by the work of McClelland and his associates on the relation between immune function, illness, and inhibition of the power motive (McClelland, Davidson, Floor, & Saron, 1980). Aggressiveness towards others is one way in which the power motive can be manifested. Given social norms about sex-appropriate behavior, females may inhibit aggression more, and consequently experience depressed immune function and more disease.

Withdrawns

The individuals who were high on social withdrawal reported that they were low on school competence. Their self-reports suggested that their school achievement was comparable to the aggressive individuals. There was some evidence, though, that the withdrawn individuals were exaggerating their poor achievement. They were not low on intelligence either at the time of first assessment or in the period overlapping with their reports of poor achievement (Moskowitz & Schwartzman, 1988). Moreover, shortly after individuals were interviewed, the parents of a subsample were interviewed (Schwartzman & Moskowitz, 1987). The parents of withdrawn individuals did not perceive their children to be doing poorly in school. In contrast, the parents of the aggressive and the aggressive-withdrawn individuals agreed with their offspring that they were performing poorly in school. Some of the withdrawn individuals may have been performing poorly in some areas, but poor achievement was probably not as low or as pervasive as for the aggressive and the aggressive-withdrawn individuals. Thus, it seems likely that the withdrawn individuals' self-perceptions of their poor school achievement were inaccurate.

The withdrawn females had a relatively high proportion of abortions, the reasons for which are unclear. As with the health data for the aggressive females, this is an area that needs to be explored further.

Aggressive-withdrawns

When originally assessed, individuals who were high on both aggression and withdrawal were achieving poorly on standardized tests of achievement (Moskowitz & Schwartzman, 1988). The finding that approximately six years after first identification they were low on intelligence and academic achievement continued a pattern that began when they were first identified. In addition to performing poorly in school, the combination of aggressiveness and withdrawal predicted problems in social relationships: individuals who were high on both characteristics got along less well with others and participated less in organizations, sports, hobbies, and jobs.

There was evidence of psychopathology and antisocial behavior among the aggressive-withdrawn individuals. The aggressive-withdrawn individuals had elevated scores on the externalizing scale. This scale included some items that were similar to the items originally used to identify subjects as aggressive, such as fighting and cruelty to others, but the scale was broader than aggression and also included items involving delinquency and hyperactivity, such as stealing, vandalism, and difficulties with concentration. The elevated externalizing scores suggested that the aggressive-withdrawn individuals were continuing in the aggressive-hostile behaviors that originally led their peers to perceive them as aggressive, and they may have had additional problems with impulsivity.

Future Directions

In current studies of these groups, information is being collected about a diverse set of variables. Several of these variables are similar to ones that have been previously assessed—for example, treatments for health and psychiatric problems. Other variables, such as academic achievement and social relationships, are closely related to previously assessed variables, but have been modified in order to be appropriate to events in the lives of young adults. Other variables are new additions that reflect age-appropriate changes, specifically, occupational status and financial independence.

Achievement. A continuation of results already found is expected for academic achievement. Achievement is expected to be quite poor among individuals who, in childhood, had been aggressive and aggressive and withdrawn. The achievement of individuals who had been withdrawn is of particular interest. As previously explained, their belief in their poor achievement is exaggerated compared to other available evidence, so, the accuracy of their self-perceptions will be clarified by obtaining objective information about whether they fare poorly in school.

The poor academic achievement of the individuals who had been high on aggression is likely to lead to lower social status in their later employment. If a pattern of generally poor academic achievement is found for the individuals who had been high on withdrawal, their occupational status should be affected. Even without depressed school achievement, individuals who are high on withdrawal may have low occupational status if these individuals consistently underestimate their own achievement, and if their low expectancies for achievement inhibits their pursuit of opportunities.

Social relationships. In social relationships, a pattern of instability is expected among the individuals who had been aggressive. They may have serious relationships, but these relationships will be of briefer duration than those of the control individuals. This result would be similar to another study (Caspi, Elder, & Bem, 1987), which found instability in the marital relationships of men and women who had explosive temper tantrums during middle childhood. The individuals who had been withdrawn may have good friends of the same sex, but dating and marriage may be delayed. If their early, anxious, inhibited, fearful behavior continues, they may have more difficulty in becoming involved with the opposite sex. Men who had been withdrawn may have particular problems initiating dating (also see, Caspi, Elder, & Bem, 1988). Individuals who were high on both aggression and withdrawal may be least likely to have friendships or long-term relationships. At the time of the first assessment, they were perceived by their peers as both anxious and withdrawn and hostile and aggressive. By their own report during adolescence, they were low on social competence. Thus, they should have problems beginning and sustaining social relationships.

Financial independence. Another issue to be pursued is whether these individuals, who are now in late adolescence and young adulthood, are establishing financial independence. Females are less likely to be financially independent than males, but, among the females, there should be individual differences. The women who were high on aggression may make greater use of social welfare because they are likely to leave home earlier, but then have more trouble supporting themselves.

Adult social competence. The variables academic achievement, occupational status, and financial independence are interrelated. It is possible to combine them into a composite that has been referred to as adult social competence (Cannon-Spoor, Potkin, & Wyatt, 1982; Zigler & Phillips, 1960; Zigler & Levine, 1981). The individuals who were high on aggression are expected to have poor academic achievement, poor occupational achievement, and unstable relationships; so, they are likely to have poor social competence scores. The individuals who were high on withdrawal are not expected to be achieving as poorly as the individuals who were aggressive, but their social relationships are expected to be delayed. They should have higher social competence scores than the individuals who were aggressive, but lower social competence scores than the control individuals. Since a pattern of delay with subsequent progress is expected, the difference between individuals who were withdrawn and the controls may decrease with age, while the difference between those who were aggressive and those who were withdrawn may increase with age.

Sex differences. Crime and health are two areas of life data in which strong sex differences are expected. Men are more likely to commit crimes than women, and males who were high on aggression are expected to have elevated rates of crimes. Women receive more health care than men, and the women in this sample who were high on aggression as children have particularly high rates of medical treatment. This pattern needs to be examined in more detail.

Contexts

Personality psychologists have frequently noted that behavior occurs in meaningful contexts. In the present research, outcome variables have thus far been conceptualized as aggregating across occasions and situations and referring to particular spans of time in much the way the act frequency approach does (Buss & Craik, 1983). Contextual variables, though, may be important determinants of outcomes for these individuals. For example, what contextual variables are associated with the decision to terminate a pregnancy?

An issue underlying the inclusion of information about situations and contexts in longitudinal studies is how to conceptualize contexts for global variables that span periods of time. One approach would be to examine situational events that are associated with particular outcome events and abstract important recurring environmental events. Social roles, such as marriage and parenthood, may be useful ways to refer to context (see Caspi, 1987), because these roles refer to repetitive sets of social interactions. Status in a social role may well affect the probability of certain acts. For example, marriage is probably an excellent predictor of whether a pregnancy is allowed to go to term.

Another approach to the definition of contexts may be the specification of interpersonal processes that recur across numerous social interactions. From this perspective, level of social support (e.g., Cohen & Wills, 1985; Thoits, 1986; Turner, 1983) becomes a contextual variable. The person's dispositional acts occur within a context of the level of social support received in the past and expected in the future. A pregnancy may be allowed to go to term not because of marriage per se, but because of the level of social support associated with the marriage. When a comparable level of social support is available outside of marriage (i.e., from the boyfriend, from family, from friends), the pregnancy may also be allowed to go to term.

Another possibility for defining contexts may consist of identifying significant events in the environment that are neither necessarily repetitive nor specifically associated with the individual's actions. Macro-stressful events such as the death of a loved one (e.g., Sarason, Siegal, & Johnson, 1978) may well provide context affecting many actions. Micro-stressful events, such as hassles at work, (Dohrenwend & Shrout, 1985), may lead to particular actions by an individual at work and become important when aggregated over occasions. The existence of chronic stress may also provide contextual effects on behaviors and feelings outside of work, such as in interpersonal relationships.

The analysis of contextual variables in longitudinal research will be difficult, because at times there will be confusion about whether a context is an independent or a dependent variable. Individuals have influence over the selection and creation of specific situations in which they find themselves (Snyder & Ickes, 1985; Wachtel, 1973). In longitudinal research, sometimes a context will be a consequence of an individual's actions; the context that has been created may then subsequently affect future acts. For example, socially withdrawn individuals may have a relatively low level of social support as a consequence of their socially inhibited behavior. The absence of social support may then mediate other decisions, such as the decision to terminate a pregnancy.

Conclusions

Aggressiveness during childhood was predictive of future adaptational problems for an individual, including low levels of academic achievement and high rates of psychiatric treatment. While it has sometimes been thought that aggressiveness is only an important predictor for males, the consequences described were found for both males and females. Moreover, the aggressive females had additional problems with poor health. Social withdrawal appeared to be a predictor of negative self-perceptions. Withdrawn individuals seemed to exaggerate their poor school achievement. An unexpected result was that withdrawn females were more likely than other females to have had an abortion during adolescence. When individuals were high on both aggression and social withdrawal, they had multiple problems, including low intelligence, poor academic achievement, poor social competence, and behavior problems.

Physics separates the description of moving objects into two parts, kinematics and dynamics: kinematics describes the paths of moving bodies (e.g., the trajectory of a bullet); dynamics describes the forces causing bodies to behave as they do. The present research is analogous to kinematics in generating data points to trace the life paths of individuals with specific characteristics. We have speculated about some reasons for these outcomes. An integrated theory awaits future developments incorporating dynamics–the processes which cause individuals to follow these life paths.

Acknowledgments. This research has been supported by grants from Health and Welfare Canada, the Quebec Ministry of Social Affairs, the Conseil Québécois de la Recherche Sociale, and the National Institute of Mental Health. Concordia University provided resources and facilities to support this project.

We acknowledge the contributions of Jane Ledingham to the identification of the subjects, of Joseph Beltempo and Claude Senneville to the collection of data, and of Punam Bhargava to the computer programming. David Zuroff, H. Gerry Taylor, Richard Koestner, and Avshalom Caspi provided helpful comments on earlier drafts of this chapter.

References

Achenbach, T.M., & Edelbrock, C. (1983). *Manual for the Child Behavior Checklist and Revised Child Behavior Profile.* Burlington, VT: Department of Psychiatry, University of Vermont.

Bohman, M., Cloninger, C.R., von Knorring, A.L., & Sigvardsson, S. (1984). An adoption study of somatoform disorders. III. Cross-fostering analysis and genetic relationship to alcoholism and criminality. *Archives of General Psychiatry, 41,* 872–878.

Block, J. (1977). Advancing the psychology of personality: Paradigmatic shift or improving the quality of research. In D. Magnusson & N.D. Endler (Eds.), *Personality at the crossroads: Current issues in interactional psychology* (pp. 37–63). Hillsdale, N. J.: Erlbaum.

Buss, D.M., & Craik, K.H. (1983). The act frequency approach to personality. *Psychological Review, 90,* 105–126.

Bronson, W.C. (1966). Central orientations: A study of behaviour organization from childhood to adolescence. *Child Development, 37,* 125–155.

Caspi, A. (1987). Personality in the life course. *Journal of Personality and Social Psychology, 53,* 1203–1213.

Caspi, A., Elder, G.K., Jr., & Bem, D.D. (1987). Moving against the world: Life course patterns of explosive children. *Developmental Psychology, 23,* 308–313.

Caspi, A., Elder, G.K., Jr., & Bem, D.D. (1988). Moving away from the world: Life course patterns of shy children. *Developmental Psychology, 24,* 824–831.

Cannon-Spoor, W.E., Potkin, S.G., & Wyatt, R.J. (1982). Measurement of premorbid adjustment in chronic schizophrenia. *Schizophrenia Bulletin, 8,* 470–484.

Cohen, S., & Wills, T. A. (1985). Stress, social support, and the buffering hypothesis. *Psychological Bulletin, 98,* 310–357.

Crowne, D.P., & Marlowe, D. (1964). *The approval motive: Studies in evaluative dependence.* New York: Wiley.

Dohrenwend, B., & Shrout, P.E. (1985). "Hassles" in the conceptualization and measurement of life stress variables. *American Psychologist, 40,* 780–785.

Epstein, S. (1980). The stability of behavior: II. Implications for psychological research. *American Psychologist, 35,* 790–806.

Huesmann, L.R., Eron, L.D., Lefkowitz, M.M., & Walder, L.O. (1984). The stability of aggression over time and generations. *Developmental Psychology, 20,* 1120–1134.

Huesmann, L.R., Eron, L.D., & Yarmel, P.W. (1987). Intellectual functioning and aggression. *Journal of Personality and Social Psychology, 52,* 232–240.

Kohlberg, L., Ricks, D., & Snarey, J. (1984). Childhood development as a predictor of adaptation in adulthood. *Genetic Psychology Monographs, 110,* 94–162.

Loeber, R., & Dishion, T. (1983). Early predictors of male delinquency: A review. *Psychological Bulletin, 94,* 68–99.

McClelland, D.C., Floor, E., Davidson, R.J., & Saron, C. (1980). Stressed power motivation, sympathetic activation, immune function, and illness. *Journal of Human Stress, 6,* 11–18.

Magnusson, D. (1988). *Individual development from an interactional perspective: A longitudinal study.* New York: Wiley.

Moskowitz, D.S. (1982). Coherence and cross-situational generality in personality: A new analysis of old problems. *Journal of Personality and Social Psychology, 43,* 754–768.

Moskowitz, D.S. (1986). Comparison of self-reports, reports by knowledgeable informants, and behavioural observation data. *Journal of Personality, 54,* 294–317.

Moskowitz, D.S. (1988). Cross-situational generality in the laboratory: Dominance and friendliness. *Journal of Personality and Social Psychology, 54,* 829–839.

Moskowitz, D.S., & Schwartzman, A.E. (1988). Intellectual characteristics of aggressive and withdrawn children. Unpublished manuscript, McGill University.

Moskowitz, D., Schwartzman, A.E., & Ledingham, J. (1985). Stability and change in aggression and withdrawal in middle childhood and adolescence. *Journal of Abnormal Psychology, 94,* 30–41.

Nock, S.L., & Rossi, P.H. (1979). Household types and social standing. *Social Forces, 57,* 1325–1345.

Olweus, D. (1979). Stability of aggressive reaction patterns in males: A review. *Psychological Bulletin, 86,* 825–875.

Olweus, D. (1981). Continuity in aggressive and withdrawn, inhibited behavior patterns. *Psychiatry and Social Sciences, 1,* 141–159.

Parker, J.G. & Asher, S.R. (1987). Peer relationships and later personal adjustment: Are low-accepted children at risk? *Psychological Bulletin, 102,* 357–389.

Pekarik, E.G., Prinz, A.J., Liebert, D.E., Weintraub, S. & Neale, J.M. (1976). The Pupil Evaluation Inventory: A sociometric technique for assessing children's social behavior. *Journal of Abnormal Child Psychology, 4,* 83–97.

Quay, H.C. (1986). Classification. In H.C. Quay & J.S. Werry (Eds.), *Psychopathological disorders of childhood,* (3rd ed, pp. 1–34). New York: Wiley.

Robins, L.N. (1966). *Deviant children grown up.* Baltimore: Williams & Wilkins.

Robins, L., (1986). The consequences of conduct disorder in girls. In D. Olweus, J. Block & M. Radke–Yarrow (Eds.), *Development of antisocial and prosocial behavior: Research, theories, and issues* (pp. 385–414). New York: Academic Press.

Sarason, I.G., Johnson, J.H., & Siegal, J.M. (1978). Development of the Life Experiences Survey. *Journal of Consulting and Clinical Psychology, 46,* 932–946.

Schwartzman, A.E., Ledingham, J., & Serbin, L. (1985). Identification of children at risk for adult schizophrenia. *International Review of Applied Psychology, 34,* 363–380.

Schwartzman, A.E., & Moskowitz, D.S. (1987). Aggressive, withdrawn, and aggressive-withdrawn children: Social competence and health status. Paper presented at the meeting of the Society for Research in Child Development, Baltimore, MD.

Snyder, M., & Ickes, W. (1985). Personality and social behavior. In G. Lindsay and E. Aronson (Eds.), *Handbook of social psychology* (pp. 883–947). New York: Random House.

Thoits, P.A. (1986). Social support as coping assistance. *Journal of Consulting and Clinical Psychology, 54,* 416–423.

Turner, R.J., Frankel, G., & Levine, D.M. (1983). Social support: Conceptualization, measurement, and implications for mental health. In J.R. Greenley (Ed.), *Research in community and mental health,* (Vol 3, pp. 67–111). Greenwich: JAI Press.

Wachtel, P. (1973). Psychodynamics, behavior therapy, and the implacable experimenter: An inquiry into the consistency of personality. *Journal of Abnormal Psychology, 83,* 324-334.

Weissman, M.M., & Klerman, G.L. (1977). Sex differences and the epidemiology of depression. *Archives of General Psychiatry, 34,* 98–111.

Wiggins, J.S., & Winder, C.L. (1961). The Peer Nomination Inventory: An empirically derived sociometric measure of adjustment in preadolescent boys. *Psychological Reports, 9,* 643–677.

Wright, J.C., & Mischel, W. (1987). A conditional approach to dispositional constructs: The local predictability of social behavior. *Journal of Personality and Social Psychology, 53,* 1159–1177.

Zigler, E., & Levine, L. (1981). Age on first hospitalization of schizophrenics: A developmental approach. *Journal of Abnormal Psychology, 90,* 458–467.

Zigler, E., & Phillips, L. (1960). Social competence and symptomatic behaviors. *Journal of Abnormal and Social Psychology, 62,* 231–238.

CHAPTER 7

Emotional Adaptation to Life Transitions: Early Impact on Integrative Cognitive Processes

Joseph M. Healy, Jr.

For almost everyone, the life course is marked by a series of life transitions—major, relatively permanent changes in our physical or psychological environment that demand the establishment of new behavior patterns and/or ways of conceptualizing the world and the life tasks that confront us. Studies of individuals coping with specific life changes have often pointed to the disorganizing, and sometimes permanently debilitating, effects of life transitions (e.g., Gleser, Green, and Winget, 1981; Lindemann, 1944, 1979). From one perspective, major life changes represent just those instances when our cognitive schemas fail us: by definition, the novelty and importance of major life changes provide demands for new coping patterns and a wealth of new information which, at least initially, exceeds our ability to assimilate it (Block, 1983; Mandler, 1975, 1982). The result is, at least, temporary cognitive disequilibrium and emotional distress until schemas can be revised and new modes of coping can be developed.

Folkman and Lazarus have suggested recently (1988) that the bi-directional relationship between coping and emotion processes must be more carefully conceptualized to take into account the complexity of emotional experience before we can develop a more accurate understanding of how people negotiate stressful life events. Primarily, explorations of the effects of affect on cognition have focused on mood or arousal, and have demonstrated that mood clearly influences our expectations of success or failure (Wright & Mischel, 1982), evaluations of risk (Pietromonaco & Rook, 1987), speed of information processing (Isen et al., 1982; Clark, 1982) and memory recall (Bower, 1981; Bower, Gilligan, & Monteiro, 1981). Yet, with the increasing focus on the cognitive basis of personality processes (Cantor, in press; Cantor & Kihlstrom, 1987) and their implications for how individuals contend with the life tasks they encounter, it is perhaps time to begin to examine emotion processes more closely tied to major life tasks.

One goal is to begin to clarify some of the confusion about what appear to be the disorganizing effects of some of the emotional components of major life changes. In particular, this chapter focuses on the consequences of a process of emotional adaptation to major life changes for cognitive processes. Although there may be long-term benefits (both cognitive and emotional) that result from successful adaptation to a major life change, the focus here is on the relationship between emotional adaptation and cognitive processes in the period immediately following a major life change.

The Process of Emotional Adaptation to Life Changes

The present research grows out of a framework for studying the emotional commonalities in individuals' responses to life transitions over the life course. In particular, it is based on a recursive sequence of four emotional stances that occur in response to any major life change, regardless of when it is experienced in the life course (Stewart, 1982). To date, Stewart and her colleagues have provided evidence for a return to the start of the sequence of stances shortly after a transition, and for progress through the sequence over time in a new situation. These data have been obtained from studies of children, adolescents, and adults experiencing major life changes that include positive and negative, chosen and imposed, and expected and unexpected changes (see, e.g., Healy & Stewart, 1984; Stewart et al., 1982, 1986; Stewart & Healy, 1985). Thus, following any major, permanent life change, whether positive or negative, individuals return to the beginning and renegotiate the sequence of emotional stances.

The first stance, *Receptivity,* involves feelings of helplessness, sadness and loss; others are seen as benevolent sources of aid, and a predominantly passive orientation is adopted. This gradually gives way to *Autonomy,* in which others are viewed as less helpful, feelings of incompetence and indecision dominate, and limited initiatives are attempted. *Assertion,* the third stance, includes feelings of hostility; others are seen as objects to be manipulated for one's own purposes, and often there is a rebellious attitude toward authority figures. Finally, the fourth stance, *Integration,* is characterized by a realistic, reciprocal, and differentiated view of others, complex and ambivalent affect is possible, and there is emotional involvement in and commitment to work (see Stewart, 1982, for a more detailed discussion of the stances and a description of the measure).

Two aspects of the recursive sequence of emotional stances may have specific implications for the cognitive processes we use in thinking about others and in solving life's problems. First, life changes precipitate a shift in the balance of power between the self and the environment. The novelty of a new situation demands a heightened awareness of the external circumstances and a correspondingly reduced sense of the power of the self over that external environment (Stewart & Healy, 1985). Thus, for individuals in the receptive stance, the salience of the environment is magnified and, as a result, reactivity to the environment is increased. Secondly, although a hypervigilant stance toward the environment is adopted after a major life change, that stance is characterized by a lack of differentiation between self and environment. In a sense, the individual confronted by a drastically altered life situation is embedded in, hyper-aware of, and extremely reactive to his or her new situation. The new situation is unfamiliar, and the individual's reactivity to the environment precludes any "non-subjective" perspective on the new situation. An individual's perspective on the environment becomes narrowed, perhaps to facilitate coping with the immediate demands of living in a changed world.

Evidence of this kind of shift in stance toward the environment can be found in several different studies of individuals experiencing life changes. Gleser, Green and Winget (1981) and Titchener and Kapp (1976) describe heightened sensitivity to the environment, in the form of increased concern and vigilance, and a perceived lack of control over their lives in victims of a devastating flood at Buffalo Creek. This is understandable given the nature of their particular crisis. Other studies of less traumatic changes, however, describe findings consistent with these general principles. In studies of the transition to college and immigration to other nations, Wapner and his colleagues (Grosslight, Grosslight, Reed, & Wapner, 1977; Wapner, 1978; Wapner, Kaplan, & Cohen, 1973) examined the development of people's "cognitive maps" of their new environment. Early in the new situation, individuals display increased sensitivity to the most salient features of their environment by overrepresenting them in maps they draw depicting their environment: other features are completely omitted. As time progresses, their maps become increasingly differentiated and much less distorted. One might argue that the increasing differentiation of the "cognitive map" over time is the result of increased knowledge of the environment. Nevertheless, it also seems plausible to suggest that the early exaggeration of some aspects of the environment is the result of the restricted "egocentric" stance that an individual may adopt in response to a life transition; as the individual's emotional stance becomes less restricted, and more realistic and differentiated, he or she gains knowledge about the new environment. Thus, emotional stances act as a lens through which we view and interpret the novel world around us. Receptivity, the first stance in the sequence, can be said to impose a "functional egocentrism" on individuals beginning to adapt to major life changes; their perspective is both narrowed and distorted, but, as emotional adaptation proceeds, the focus becomes broader and less distorted.

On the basis of this argument, I would like to suggest that those cognitive processes dependent upon an open, differentiated, and realistic perspective on the environment should be impaired by the "functional egocentrism" imposed by the process of emotional adaptation. The crucial link between emotional adaptation and cognitive processes depends upon the organized emotional orientation inherent in each stance. That is, during the course of adaptation, each stance organizes and structures the way we attend to and perceive the external environment and our position in it. In the early stances in the sequence, our perspective is both narrowed and distorted. Thus, social cognitive processes like *perspective-taking* and *complexity of person concepts,* and information-processing skills such as the *ability to structure an argument,* marshalling evidence under a central organizing principle, and *isolating elements in causal relationships* from confusing multivariate contexts, should be impaired in individuals adapting to a major life change. Each of these skills requires an individual simultaneously to process and coordinate information from different sources and/or to view the world in a detached "non-subjective" manner. This kind of cognitive activity should become difficult for those laboring under the "functional egocentrism" imposed by the process of emotional adaptation. Other cognitive skills that do not require the simultaneous coordination and processing of information from multiple sources should not be impaired by the process of emotional adaptation.

An important distinction should be maintained between the process of emotional adaptation and general arousal or mood disturbance. The process of emotional adaptation from which this work derives has been observed in individuals adapting to positive, relatively happy life changes, such as marriage, as well as individuals negotiating less happy life crises, such as marital separation. Moreover, in studies including measures of both emotional adaptation and mood disturbance, these measures have been found to be statistically unrelated (see, e.g., Stewart, 1984). Thus, both theoretically and empirically, general mood disturbance and emotional adaptation are independent. Moreover, the emotion-cognition link I have articulated depends on the effect of the organized perceptual qualities of the emotional stances on specific cognitive processes.

Emotional Adaptation and Cognition: Empirical Evidence

To date, three studies have directly examined the relationship between the process of emotional adaptation and cognitive processes. Each of these studies examines the relationship between emotional stance and cognitive processes in individuals who have recently experienced a major life change. In general, the early stances in the process of emotional adaptation should be associated with impaired performance on the cognitive tasks used in these studies.

Study One: Children of Recently Separated Parents

In the first study, 108 six- to twelve-year-old children whose parents had recently separated completed questionnaires and participated in interviews within six months of the separation. Among the data collected were measures of emotional stance (Stewart, 1982), perspective-taking (White et al., 1986), and complexity of person concepts (Peevers and Secord, 1973). The sample was divided at the median on modal emotional stance for the purpose of analysis (modal emotional stance scores are assigned on the basis of the most dominant stance—1 for receptivity, 2 for autonomy, 3 for assertion, and 4 for integration). Since we might expect age differences in these kinds of cognitive skills, as well as differences attributable to emotional adaptation, I conducted age by adaptation group ANOVAs on each of the cognitive skills. As you can see from Table 7.1, the predicted differences in complexity of person concepts between advanced and less advanced adaptation groups did appear. There was a main effect for adaptation group ($F=3.79, p=.05$) on complexity of person concepts, and a main effect for age ($F=3.79, p=.06$) and an age by adaptation group interaction ($F=5.94, p<.05$) on perspective-taking. In the case of perspective-taking, the results were slightly different although still in keeping with the linkage proposed here. For young children, who are less adept at perspective-taking, emotional adaptation does not seem to interfere with performance. For the older children, however, those who were still in the early stances did have lower scores on perspective-taking than those who had progressed further in the course of adaptation.

Alternative explanations could, of course, be offered for these results. Children of recently separated parents are likely to be suffering from generally increased levels of emotional distress, and the process of successful emotional adaptation may be characterized by gradually

TABLE 7.1. Age by adaptation group ANOVAs on perspective-taking and complexity of person concepts in children of recently separated parents

	Less advanced adaptation	Advanced adaptation	Significant effects
Perspective-taking			
6–8 year olds (n = 49)	4.13	3.78	$F = 5.94, p < .05$ Age X Adaptation
9–12 year olds (n = 55)	4.03	4.65	$F = 3.79, p = .06$ Age
Total	4.08	4.22	
Complexity of person concepts			
6–8 year olds (n = 53)	.21	.25	$F = 3.79, p = .05$ Adaptation Group
9–12 year olds (n = 55)	.24	.27	
Total	.22	.26	

decreasing emotional distress. A measure of the children's emotional distress about their parents' separation was available, however, and covarying emotional distress did not affect the results. Similarly, performance might be a function of intelligence. Covarying WISC vocabulary subscale scores also left the results unaffected. Thus, the results provide some support for a link between the process of emotional adaptation and the kinds of cognitive skills that, I have argued, should be at least temporarily impaired by the process of emotional adaptation.

Study Two: Adaptation to College and Structured Argument

In the second study, fifty-nine freshmen from a private mid-western college provided questionnaire data shortly after they began college. Included in their packets were measures of emotional stance and structured argument—the ability to form a coherent argument against some issue by marshalling evidence and presenting it under a central organizing principle (Winter, McClelland, and Stewart, 1981). In this study, those students who had not progressed beyond the early emotional stances were expected to perform less well at structuring arguments than those who were further along in the adaptation process. The sample was divided at the median on emotional adaptation in order to perform a sex by adaptation group ANOVA on structured argument scores. As you can see in Table 7.2, the results supported the prediction. Those who were further along in the course of adaptation scored higher in structuring arguments than those who were less advanced (F=8.60, $p<.01$). Total covarying Scholastic Achievement Test scores to control for intelligence did not alter these results.

Study Three: Marital Separation

The third study is more complicated than the previous two and includes a variety of cognitive measures given to two samples. Forty-five recently separated parents were recruited from a larger, ongoing study of the

TABLE 7.2. Sex by adaptation group ANOVA on structured argument in college freshmen

	Less advanced adaptation	Advanced adaptation	Significant effects
Males (n = 26)	41.39	51.86	F = 8.60, $p < .01$ Adaptation Group
Females (n = 33)	48.45	52.46	
Total	44.92	52.16	

effects of marital separation on parents and children. In addition, a comparison sample of married parents was recruited and matched to the separated parents on age, education, SES of job, number of children, age ranges of children, and number of past change experiences (see Healy, 1985, for a more detailed explanation of the recruitment procedures). In addition, since the purpose of the comparison sample was to enable a comparison of individuals in transition with those not in transition, the married parents were screened for other life changes. Only those married parents who had not had any major life changes in the preceding two years were included. Each sample consisted of twenty-six women and nineteen men.

In addition to a measure of emotional stance, the participants completed measures of perspective-taking (Sommers, 1978, 1981; Feffer, 1959), structured argument (Winter, Stewart, & McClelland, 1981), isolating elements or the ability to isolate causal relationships in a multivariate context (Kuhn & Angelev, 1976; Kuhn & Brannock, 1977; Kuhn & Ho, 1977), and generative fertility or the ability to generate large numbers of discrete solutions to real life problems (adapted from Guilford, 1962, and DeBono, 1968). The first three cognitive processes were included because they represent exactly those kinds of processes that are expected to be impaired, at least temporarily, by the early stances of emotional adaptation. The measure of generative fertility was included in order to determine whether cognitive skills that do not depend on the simultaneous coordination and processing of different sources of information might also be impaired by the process of adaptation. Finally, each participant completed a measure of mood disturbance (McNair, Lorr, and Droppleman, 1971), which was included for the purpose of verifying that observed differences in cognitive performance are a function of emotional stance rather than merely a reflection of increased emotional arousal.

Because of the combined cross-sectional design, two kinds of comparisons were possible: (1) comparisons of the separated and married samples on both emotional stance and the cognitive processes; (2) comparisons within the separated sample between those who are less advanced in the course of emotional adaptation and those who are further along in the adaptation process on the cognitive measures.

Comparison of Married and Separated Parents

In order to examine the general prediction that the kinds of cognitive processes included here would be impaired by the early stances in the process of emotional adaptation, I created an aggregate measure of cognitive performance by t-scoring and averaging across all cognitive measures. Sex by sample ANOVAs on the average cognitive performance measure indicated that there was an overall sample difference on this measure (See Table 7.3, $F=6.91$, $p<.01$). In order to intrepret this finding

TABLE 7.3. Sex by sample ANOVA on average cognitive performance in separated and married men and women

	Separated sample	Married sample	Significant effects
Males (n = 38)	48.62	51.56	$F = 6.91, p = .01$ Sample
Females (n = 52)	48.68	51.21	
Total	48.64	51.38	

as support for a connection between emotional stance and cognitive processes, however, we need to be confident that the differences are attributable to emotional stance differences between the two samples rather than some other sample differences. Because of the matching process, the samples do not differ on any of the demographic variables mentioned above. A sex by sample ANOVA on emotional adaptation revealed a sex by sample interaction (See Table 7.4, F=3.15, P<.08), indicating that only the men differed in the predicted direction. The women in the two samples did not differ at all. This result is not inconsistent with findings in other studies suggesting that there is not much support for autonomy and assertion in the female sex role, perhaps especially in the context of marriage (see, e.g., Stewart et al., 1986; Guttman, 1975). Thus, although they are not in the process of adapting to a life change, the women in the married sample seem to have formed a stable adaptation at one of the early stances. One possible implication of this finding is that the connection established here between emotional stances and cognitive processes holds while individuals are adapting to changed circumstances, but not when they have become habituated to their environment (as the married women presumably have).

An alternative explanation for the cognitive performance differences between the married and separated samples could be that the separated

TABLE 7.4. Sex by sample ANOVA on emotional adaptation in separated and married men and women

	Separated sample	Married sample	Significant effects
Males (n = 34)	2.06[a]	2.94[a]	$F = 3.15, p < .08$ Sex by Sample
Females (n = 54)	2.26	2.26	
Total	2.16	2.60	

Note: Means identified by the same superscript are significantly different from each other ($p < .05$) according to Newman-Keuls post-hoc comparisons.

TABLE 7.5. Sample differences on individual cognitive skills

	Separated sample	Married sample	Significance
Cognitive skills			
Perspective-taking	47.42	52.10	$F = 6.39$, $p = .02$
Structured Argument	.16	.46	$F = 11.06$, $p < .01$
Isolating Elements	2.51	3.18	$F = 6.99$, $p = .01$
Generative Fertility	6.28	6.07	n.s.

parents are experiencing more emotional distress. It is clearly the case that they are: a sex by sample ANOVA revealed a significant sample difference (M=46.97 for separated parents, M=21.12 for married parents, F=11.86, $p<.001$). Covarying mood disturbance in the analysis of cognitive performance did not, however, alter the result. Thus, the most apparent difference between the two samples is that one is in the process of adapting to a major life change and one is not.

In order to assess whether the specific cognitive skills proposed would be affected by emotional adaptation, separate sex by sample ANOVAs were conducted on each cognitive skill. Table 7.5 summarizes the sample differences in those analyses (there were no main or interaction effects involving sex) and reveals that, as predicted, perspective-taking, structured argument, and isolating elements scores are lower in the separated sample than in the married sample, and that the only unaffected skill is generative fertility. The lack of differences in generative fertility is consistent with expectations, since cognitive skills that are not dependent on simultaneous coordination and processing of information should not be affected by emotional stance. Again, for each of these analyses, covarying mood disturbance did not alter the results.

Emotional Adaptation and Cognition in Separated Parents

Comparison of advanced and less advanced adaptation groups within the sample of recently separated adults also provided support for the emotional stance-cognition link proposed here. Table 7.6 shows the results of a sex by adaptation group ANOVA on the average cognitive performance measure. Overall, those who were further along in the course of adaptation performed better than those who were less advanced (F=7.78, $p<.01$). Covarying mood disturbance did not change the results. Moreover, it is possible that those with more education or more resources might adapt more quickly and perform better on the cognitive measures. After covarying education and SES, the significant difference remained.

Individual analyses of the various cognitive processes within the

TABLE 7.6. Sex by adaptation group ANOVA on average cognitive performance in separated men and women

	Less advanced adaptation	Advanced adaptation	Significant effects
Transitional adults			
Males (n = 17)	48.39	53.60	$F = 7.78, p < .01$ Adaptation Group
Females (n = 27)	49.42	51.92	
Total	48.96	52.67	

separated sample failed to provide any significant differences, although all of the differences in the means were in the predicted direction. Perhaps the lack of results in these analyses is due to restricted variance (since all of the participants were, in fact, in the process of adaptation) or to the reduced power of analysis with a smaller sample.

Conclusions and Future Directions

Clearly, the overall results provide encouraging support for the idea that there is a specific link between the process of emotional adaptation to major life changes and certain cognitive skills. The data presented above support this notion in studies of children, adolescents, and adults experiencing three different life transitions. In each case, the evidence indicated that the process of emotional adaptation seems to interfere, at least in the short term, with cognitive processes dependent upon a detached, differentiated, and realistic perspective on the environment. This affective process entails a shift in the perceived relationship between oneself and one's environment that drastically alters how we attend to and construe the world around us. As a result, we are temporarily limited in our ability to attend to and process the wealth of novel information available to us. Moreover, although receptivity may actually facilitate (through passive vigilance) efforts to take in as much novel information as we can about our new situation, we are not yet able to integrate this information because we are also in the process of revising our schemas (see Stewart, 1988 for more discussion of this issue).

Although the relationship portrayed here between the process of emotional adaptation and cognition appears to be primarily detrimental, this research program is based on the assumption that life changes are an opportunity for growth as well as a threat to current modes of coping. In fact, evidence from a longitudinal study of college students has shown that while freshman receptivity interferes with integrative cognitive skills in the short-term, it actually facilitates increases in information-processing skills from freshman to senior year (Stewart and Healy, 1985).

On the basis of these results, we may tentatively conclude that life transitions, and the attendant process of emotional adaptation, result first in temporary deficits in certain cognitive processes (perhaps as extant cognitive schemas are broken down) and then in a cognitive restructuring as novel experiences are integrated with revised schemas. Thus, the connection between the course of emotional adaptation and cognition examined here represents only part of the process—the immediate impact of a return to the beginning of the emotional stance sequence after a major life change on specific kinds of cognition. The other side of the model focuses on elaborating the role of emotional adaptation in promoting long-term beneficial changes in cognitive processing.

Finally, if we extend this argument further, the process of renegotiating the sequence of emotional stances after a major transition would seem to have implications for a variety of processes that depend on how we view others, how we view ourselves in relation to them, and how we conceptualize the tasks we undertake. For example, in the case of life tasks, personal projects or personal strivings (see, e.g., Cantor et al., 1987; Emmons, 1986; Little, 1983; Palys & Little, 1983), we might predict that individuals who have adopted a passive-receptive stance would lower their estimates of the probability of success in life tasks, and would feel either unable to take the initiative in pursuing them or unclear about what needs to be done to succeed. Individuals in the autonomous stance may experience more conflict about personal projects and doubt their ability to succeed, or waiver in their commitment to them. Assertive individuals may overestimate the likelihood of their success and experience an inflated sense of control over the outcome. Progress toward one's goals may be inconsistent in predictable ways during the course of emotional adaptation, and changes in the ways people conceive of their plans and goals may be influenced by emotional stances after a major life change. Similarly, conceptions of ourselves (i.e., self-schemas) may also undergo at least temporary modification as we redefine both who we are and who we might become in a new situation. Presumably, our possible selves (Markus & Nurius, 1986) will change as we experience ourselves as helpless and overwhelmed at first, then active but timid and lacking confidence, then overconfident and omnipotent, and, finally, committed and realistic. Thus, the process of emotional adaptation offers one possibility for increasing our understanding of change and growth in cognition-based personality processes, at least in the context of major life change.

References

Block, J. (1983) Assimilation, accomodation, and the dynamics of personality development. *Child Development, 53,* 181–195.

Bower, G. (1981) Mood and memory. *American Psychologist, 36,* 129–148.

Bower, G., Gilligan, S., & Monteiro, K. (1981) Selectivity of learning caused by affective states. *Journal of Experimental Psychology, 110,* 451–473.

Cantor, N. (in press) From thought to behavior: "Having" and "doing" in the study of personality and cognition. *American Psychologist.*

Cantor, N. & Kihlstrom, J.F. (1987) *Personality and social intelligence.* Englewood Cliffs, NJ: Prentice-Hall.

Cantor, N., Norem, J.K., Niedenthal, P.M., Langston, C. & Brower, A.M. (1987) Life tasks, self-concept ideals, and cognitive strategies in a life transition. *Journal of Personality and Social Psychology, 53,* 1178–1191.

Clark, M.S. (1982) A role for arousal in the link between feeling states, judgment, and behavior. In M.S. Clark & S.T. Fiske (Eds.) *Affect and cognition* (pp. 263–290). Hillsdale, NJ: Erlbaum.

DeBono, E. (1968). *New think.* New York: Basic.

Feffer, M. (1959) The cognitive implications of role taking. *Journal of Personality, 27,* 152–158.

Folkman, S., & Lazarus, R. S. (1988) Coping as a mediator of emotion. *Journal of Personality and Social Psychology, 54,* 466–475.

Gleser, G., Green, B. & Winget, C. (1981) *Prolonged psychosocial effects of a disaster: A study of Buffalo Creek.* New York: Academic.

Grosslight, J.H., Grosslight, J., Reed, R. & Wapner, S. (1977) Cognitive maps of London during a five-month sojourn. Presented at Southeastern Psychological Association, Hollywood, CA.

Guilford, J. (1962) Creativity: Its measurement and development. In S. Parnes & H. Harding (Eds). *A sourcebook for creative thinking.* New York: Scribner's.

Guttman, D. (1975) Parenthood: A key to the comparative study of the life cycle. In N. Datan & L.H. Ginsburg (Eds.) *Life-span developmental psychology: Normative life crises.* New York: Academic.

Healy, J.M., Jr. & Stewart, A.J. (1984) Adaptation to life changes in adolescence. In P. Karoly & J.J. Steffen (Eds). *Adolescent behavior disorders: Foundations and concerns.* Lexington, MA: D.C. Heath.

Healy, J.M., Jr. (1985) Emotional adaptation to life transitions and cognitive performance. Unpublished doctoral dissertation, Boston University.

Isen, A.M., Means, B., Patrick, R., & Nowicki, G. (1982). Some factors influencing decision-making strategy and risk-taking. In M.S. Clark & S.T. Fiske (Eds.), *Affect and cognition,* (pp. 243–262). Hillsdale, NJ: Erlbaum.

Kuhn, D. & Angelev, J. (1976) An experimental study of the development of formal operational thought. *Child Development, 47,* 697–706.

Kuhn, D. & Brannock, J. (1977) Development of the isolation of variables scheme in experimental and 'natural experiment' contexts. *Developmental Psychology, 13,* 9–14.

Kuhn, D., & Ho, V. (1977) The development of schemes for recognizing additive and alternative effects in a 'natural experiment' context. *Developmental Psychology, 13,* 515–516.

Lindemann, E. (1944) Symptomatology and management of acute grief. *American Journal of Psychiatry, 101,* 141–149.

Lindemann, E. (1979) *Beyond grief: Studies on crisis intervention.* New York: Jason Aronson.

Little, B. (1983) Personal projects: A rationale and method for investigation. *Environment and Behavior, 15,* 273–309.

Mandler, G. (1975) *Mind and emotion.* New York: Wiley.

Mandler, G. (1982) The structure of value: Accounting for taste. In M.S. Clark & S.T. Fiske (Eds.) *Affect and Cognition* (pp. 3–36). Hillsdale, NJ: Erlbaum.

Markus, H. & Nurius, P. (1986) Possible selves. *American Psychologist, 41,* 954–969.

Palys, T.S. & Little, B. (1983) Perceived life satisfaction and the organization of personal project systems. *Journal of Personality and Social Psychology, 44,* 1221–1230.

Peevers, B.H. & Secord, P.F. (1973) Developmental changes in attribution of descriptive concepts to persons. *Journal of Personality and Social Psychology, 52,* 399–408.

Pietromonac, P. R. & Rook, K. S. (1987) Decision style in depression: The contribution of perceived risks versus benefits. *Journal of Personality and Social Psychology, 52,* 399–408.

Sommers, S. (1978) The undivided mind: The relationship between affect and social cognition. Unpublished doctoral dissertation, Boston University.

Sommers, S. (1981) Emotionality reconsidered: The role of cognition in emotional responsiveness. *Journal of Personality and Social Psychology, 3,* 553–561.

Stewart, A. J. (1982) The course of individual adaptation. *Journal of Personality and Social Psychology, 42,* 1100–1113.

Stewart, A. J. (1984) Family changes and children's affective development. Unpublished manuscript, Boston University.

Stewart, A. J. (in press) Social intelligence and adaptation to life change. In R. S. Wyer & T.K. Srull (Eds.) *Advances in social cognition: Vol. 2.* Hillsdale, NJ: Erlbaum.

Stewart, A.J. & Healy, J.M., Jr. (1985) Personality and adaptation to change. In R. Hogan & W. Jones (Eds.) *Perspectives on personality.* Greenwich, CT: JAI Press.

Stewart, A.J., Sokol, M., Healy, J.M., Jr., Chester, N.L., & Weinstock-Savoy, D. (1982) Adaptation to life changes in children and adults: Cross-sectional studies. *Journal of Personality and Social Psychology, 43,* 1270–1281.

Stewart, A. J., Sokol, M., Healy, J. M., Jr. & Chester, N. L. (1986) Longitudinal studies of psychological consequences of life changes in children and adults. *Journal of Personality and Social Psychology, 50,* 143–151.

Titchener, J. L. & Kapp, F. T. (1976) Family and character change at Buffalo Creek. *American Journal of Psychiatry, 133,* 295–299.

Wapner, S. (1978) Environmental transition: A research paradigm deriving from the organismic-development systems approach. In L. Van Ryzin (Ed.) *Proceedings of the Wisconsin conference on research methods in behavior-environment studies.* Madison, WI.

Wapner, S., Kaplan, B. & Cohen, S.B. (1973) An organismic-developmental perspective for understanding transactions of men and environments. *Environment and Behavior, 5,* 255–289.

White, K.M., Speisman, J.C., Jackson, D., Bartis, S. & Costos, D. (1986) Intimacy maturity and its correlates in young married couples. *Journal of Personality and Social Psychology, 50,* 152–162.

Winter, D.G., McClelland, D.C. & Stewart, A.J. (1981) *A new case for the liberal arts.* San Fransisco: Jossey-Bass.

Wright, J. & Mischel, W. (1982). Influence of affect on cognitive social learning person variables. *Journal of Personality and Social Psychology, 43,* 901–914.

CHAPTER 8

Performance Evaluation and Intrinsic Motivation Processes: The Effects of Achievement Orientation and Rewards

Judith M. Harackiewicz

When individuals freely engage in an activity for its own sake, their behavior is considered intrinsically motivated. In reality, however, very few behaviors occur in a social vacuum. Most people eventually encounter external constraints on their behavior, and these constraints can interfere with intrinsic motivation (Lepper, Greene, & Nisbett, 1973). A common constraint is the external evaluation of performance at an activity—task performance is constantly evaluated in educational, athletic, and professional domains. When teachers, coaches, and supervisors evaluate performance on an interesting and involving activity, their evaluation represents an extrinsic intrusion into what had been an intrinsically motivated activity, and may undermine subsequent intrinsic motivation. The effects of performance evaluation on intrinsic motivation depend on the properties of the evaluative situation, and on characteristics of the individual whose performance is evaluated.

The Effects of Performance Evaluation and Reward

Evaluative situations have their effects on performance and motivation over the course of time, and it is important to consider the *process* of performance evaluation. Before beginning a task, individuals anticipate that their performance will be evaluated, and they are aware of external evaluation while they perform. They may attribute their behavior to the external constraint (Amabile, 1979), or experience performance pressure (Deci & Ryan, 1985), thus reducing their intrinsic interest in the task. While engaged in the task, individuals may worry about their performance, become distracted from the task (Harackiewicz, Manderlink, & Sansone, 1984), and may not have a clear sense of how they are doing. Performance feedback is not usually available during task performance, but external feedback may ultimately provide positive information about competence at an activity. When evaluative outcomes are positive, they should enhance subsequent intrinsic motivation (Deci, 1975; White,

1959). Thus, performance evaluation has both positive and negative implications for subsequent interest. It could have negative effects due to the experience of evaluation during task performance, and positive effects due to the resultant (positive) evaluative outcomes.

Rewards often accompany positive evaluative outcomes, and when their attainment is contingent upon achieving a certain level of performance, they are considered performance-contingent (Harackiewicz, 1979; Ryan, Mims, & Koestner, 1983). When rewards are associated with competence, they can enhance interest independently of the competence feedback communicated in the evaluative situation (Harackiewicz & Manderlink, 1984). A reward can have *cue value* because it makes the potential evaluative outcome more salient, and it symbolizes a meaningful performance accomplishment (Boggiano, Harackiewicz, Bessette, & Main, 1985; Harackiewicz et al., 1984). It can magnify the emotional significance of competence and make people more concerned about doing well in an evaluative situation. The effects of cue value may occur at the outset of performance, when individuals are motivated to achieve competence and earn the reward, and at task conclusion, when the receipt of performance-contingent rewards makes the positive evaluative outcome more salient.

In summary, evaluative situations possess three critical properties: the promise of performance evaluation, the competence feedback provided by evaluative outcomes, and the cue value of performance-contingent rewards. Harackiewicz et al (1984) examined the effects of evaluation anticipation and cue value on intrinsic motivation in two comparisons. Evaluation groups expected their performance on a pinball game to be evaluated against an 80th percentile criterion, and then learned that they had surpassed it. Performance-contingent reward subjects were promised a movie pass if their performance exceeded the same criterion; they, too, learned that their performance was in the top 20th percentile, and received the promised reward. Feedback control subjects were not promised rewards and did not expect evaluation, but they did receive unanticipated feedback that they had scored above the 80th percentile. Thus all subjects received positive competence feedback.

Evaluation subjects subsequently played significantly less pinball in a free choice situation than did feedback control subjects, thus revealing the negative effect of evaluation anticipation on intrinsic motivation. Reward subjects played significantly more pinball than did subjects exposed to the same performance evaluation and feedback, thus revealing the positive effect of cue value. This comparison, therefore, controls for both the performance evaluation and competence feedback inherent in performance-contingent rewards and isolates the effect of receiving a reward as a consequence of positive evaluative outcomes. The results demonstrate that symbolic rewards can enhance interest independently of the competence feedback they convey.

A Process Model of Intrinsic Motivation

Carol Sansone and I have begun to develop a model of the motivational processes that mediate these effects (Harackiewicz & Sansone, 1989). Figure 8.1 presents a schematic version of our process model. The model accounts for the effects of evaluative contingencies and individual differences on subsequent intrinsic motivation in terms of the motivational processes initiated during task engagement. Our emphasis is on how individuals approach and experience a task during the performance period. Three processes are critical: competence valuation, task involvement, and perceived competence. All three processes can be initiated during the course of task performance, but competence valuation and task involvement are the motivational states most likely to affect task engagement during the performance. Perceived competence is typically more important later, after people have received performance feedback. Because we often control for evaluative outcomes by providing all subjects with positive performance feedback in our research (thereby minimizing variance in perceptions of competence), we have devoted less attention to the perceived competence process (however, see Boggiano & Ruble, 1979; Harackiewicz & Larson, 1986; Sansone, 1986).

Competence Valuation

Competence valuation reflects the degree to which individuals care about doing well and is a motivational process that mediates the effects of cue value on intrinsic motivation. The promise of a performance-contingent reward can make competence at an activity more salient and can promote competence valuation (Harackiewicz & Manderlink, 1984). A person starting a task may care more about doing well because of a reward offer, and, the more they value competence, the more they will enjoy a task after they receive positive feedback. This process represents an active, positive orientation towards achieving competence at the task and can offset the negative effects of performance evaluation. We typically measure competence valuation at the outset of performance by asking subjects how concerned they are about doing well in the upcoming session, and how important it is for them to do well.

Of course, some individuals are characteristically more oriented towards competence across situations: these are people who approach *all* tasks with a greater interest in doing well. Competence valuation is also influenced by stable individual differences in achievement motivation, which we measure with the Achievement Orientation Scale from the Personality Research Form (Jackson, 1974). This scale was developed according to Murray's (1938) theory of needs, and represents a well-constructed and validated measure (Anastasi, 1982). People scoring high on this 16-point scale are described as maintaining high standards, challenge-seeking, purposeful, and competitive. Depending on the experi-

```
┌─────────────────────┐  ┌─────────────────────┐
│    EVALUATIVE       │  │    INDIVIDUAL       │
│   CONTINGENCIES     │  │   DIFFERENCES       │
│   Reward offered    │  │                     │
│  Evaluation promised│  │ Achievement orientation│
│Performance goals assigned│                     │
└──────────┬──────────┘  └──────────┬──────────┘
           │                        │
           └───────────┬────────────┘
                      ▼
         ┌─────────────────────────┐
         │     MOTIVATIONAL        │
         │      PROCESSES          │
         │  Competence Valuation   │
         │    Task Involvement     │
         │  Perceived Competence   │
         └───────────┬─────────────┘
                     ▼
         ┌─────────────────────────┐
         │      EVALUATIVE         │
         │       OUTCOMES          │
         │  Performance feedback   │
         │ Performance-contingent  │
         │        Reward           │
         └───────────┬─────────────┘
                     ▼
         ┌─────────────────────────┐
         │       INTRINSIC         │
         │                         │
         │      MOTIVATION         │
         └─────────────────────────┘
```

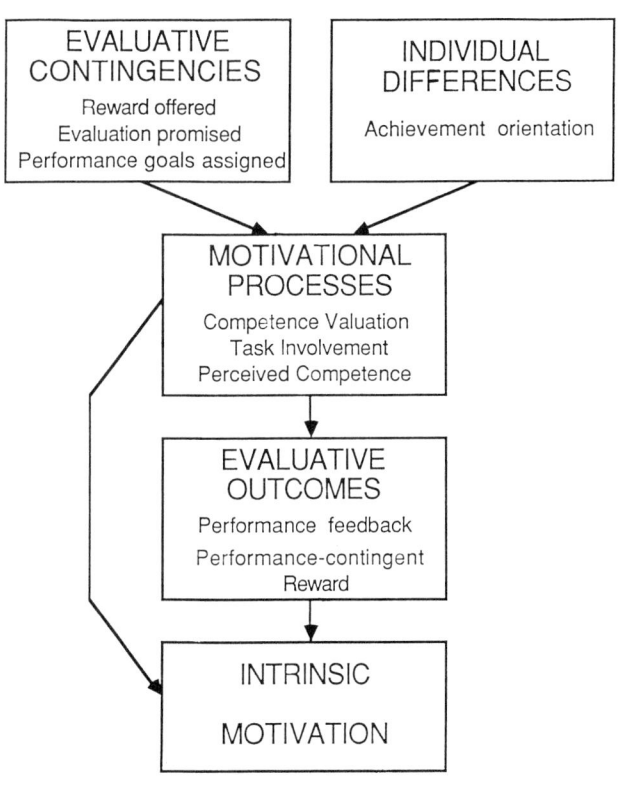

FIGURE 8.1

mental conditions we run, we see the effects of achievement orientation on competence valuation either as a main effect (Harackiewicz, Abrahams, & Wageman, 1987), or in interaction with situational cues (Harackiewicz, et al, in press; Sansone, 1989). For example, we have found that high achievers particularly value competence when given a positive expectancy about their future performance (Harackiewicz, Sansone, & Manderlink, 1985). In competitive situations, high achievers especially value competence when they receive information about their opponent's prior performance (Epstein & Harackiewicz, 1989).

Competence valuation is, therefore, influenced by both situational factors (e.g., performance-contingent rewards, performance expectancies, opponent information in competitions) and personality factors (e.g., achievement orientation). Moreover, we have documented that competence valuation *mediates* the direct effects of these variables on subsequent intrinsic interest (Harackiewicz & Manderlink, 1984). The logic of mediation analysis (Judd & Kenny, 1987) requires that we first demonstrate the direct effects on interest, then, that situational and person factors significantly influence competence valuation, and finally, that competence valuation significantly affects intrinsic interest, controlling for the effects of the situational and personality factors. We have conducted several studies in which these requirements were satisfied and found that, in evaluative situations resulting in positive feedback, competence valuation enhanced subsequent interest (Harackiewicz & Manderlink, 1984; Harackiewicz et al, 1985, 1987). In other words, the more that individuals value competence going into a task, the more they enjoy it following positive evaluative outcomes. Competence valuation has, therefore, been shown to be a motivational process that mediates the positive effects of performance-contingent reward and achievement orientation on intrinsic interest.

Task Involvement

The second process we have studied in some detail is task involvement, which we hypothesize to mediate the negative effects of evaluation. When anticipating evaluation, people may worry about their performance and become distracted from a task (Wine, 1971); this cognitive interference may reduce task enjoyment. In one study, we collected a cognitive measure of task involvement during the process of playing pinball, loosely based on Sarason's (1980) measure of cognitive interference. We asked subjects how frequently they thought about the ongoing game (e.g., manipulating the flippers, keeping the ball in play). The results on this measure paralleled those on intrinsic motivation: evaluation-condition subjects were significantly less involved in the game than feedback control or reward-condition subjects (Harackiewicz et al, 1984). Performance evaluation, therefore, seemed to distract subjects from the pinball game.

In another study, we found that low achievers were the ones most likely to show this effect, which suggests that they may be particularly vulnerable to the distracting effects of performance evaluation (Harackiewicz et al, 1987). In general, however, task involvement is less sensitive to individual differences in achievement orientation. Task involvement concerns attention and immersion in the activity at hand, and is less responsive to an individual's characteristic orientation towards competence. It is a more situationally constrained process that reflects task-specific factors such as task structure or complexity. Competence valuation is the process more likely to pick up a general orientation towards success, as well as situationally determined effects.

The Focus of Performance Evaluation: A Contextual Factor

One reason that performance evaluation might be so distracting and detrimental for intrinsic interest is that it often involves normative comparisons with peers. When people expect evaluation relative to others, not only do they worry about their own performance, they also worry about how other people are doing, and this cognitive activity may be particularly likely to distract them from the task at hand. In the intrinsic motivation literature, external evaluation and performance feedback have almost always been based on normative definitions of competence (cf, Sansone, 1986 for an exception), and we hypothesized that this emphasis on normative competence might be responsible for the negative effects of evaluation. If we could deemphasize the social comparison element and focus external evaluation more on the task itself, we might be able to boost task involvement in evaluative situations and so maintain, or even enhance, intrinsic motivation.

To test this, we performed an experiment with three conditions: performance-contingent reward, evaluation anticipation, and feedback controls crossed by a manipulation of evaluative focus (Harackiewicz et al, 1987). High school students played an enjoyable word game, and all received positive feedback about their performance on the game. The evaluation manipulation and performance feedback were couched in terms of attaining a task-specific criterion score on the activity—the "New Jersey Standard Score" (task focus), or performing better than 50% of their peers (normative focus). Students in task-focus conditions were informed that the New Jersey Standard Score was based on normative testing (insuring that the level of competence feedback was comparable across focus conditions), but this information was downplayed. Instead, the evaluation, reward, and feedback manipulations all emphasized surpassing a particular score on the task at hand. In contrast, the manipulations in the normative focus conditions stressed outperforming other high school students, and emphasized comparisons with peers. We measured students' thoughts while playing the word game, and found that the task focus manipulation was successful in enhancing task involvement across conditions, relative to the normative focus.

The results on a measure of task enjoyment were striking. Under a normative focus, we found that evaluation reduced interest relative to both the reward group and feedback controls, thus replicating earlier findings. Under a task focus, however, evaluation enhanced interest relative to feedback control conditions. These results indicate that the focus of evaluation is an important moderator of evaluation effects. When competence was defined in terms of a task-focused criterion score, evaluation anticipation did not reduce interest. The significant enhancement of interest relative to the feedback control group was unanticipated, but may have been due to the facilitative effect of the task-focused evaluation manipulation; it may have helped subjects to concentrate on their performance without worrying about how it compared to that of other students. These results suggest that performance evaluation is most distracting and debilitating for intrinsic interest when competence is defined with respect to normative criteria.

In our model, the focus of evaluation is a contextual factor—evaluation takes place in a context where competence is defined in terms of the task, or in terms of social norms. The model predicts that the processes that influence intrinsic motivation will vary according to the context of evaluation (cf., Harackiewicz et al, 1987; Sansone, Sachau, & Weir, 1989). Our measure of competence valuation does not specify how competence is defined; rather, we ask subjects how much they care about "doing well." Since, however, adolescents and adults usually define competence in terms of normative comparisons (Boggiano & Ruble, 1986; Jagacinski & Nicholls, 1984; Nicholls, 1984), competence valuation is more likely to reflect attitudes and feelings about normatively-based competence, as opposed to task mastery. We would, therefore, expect that competence valuation would be a more critical mediator of interest in an evaluative context that emphasizes social comparisons.

Harackiewicz et al (1987) found that subjects in reward conditions were more concerned about doing well than subjects in evaluation and feedback control conditions, thus replicating earlier findings (Harackiewicz, et al, 1984), and that high achievers cared most about doing well across all conditions. The mediating effect of competence valuation varied dramatically, however, according to the focus of evaluation. It was very strong in normative focus conditions (beta = +.71), but much weaker under a task focus (beta = +.15). Thus competence valuation was a more important process in contexts emphasizing normatively based performance evaluation. When normative comparisons were deemphasized, an individual's competence valuation was not significantly related to his or her subsequent interest.

Under a normative focus then, evaluation anticipation had the negative effects observed in earlier studies, but performance-contingent rewards could counteract this negative effect through the competence valuation process (by making people care about doing well). Achievement-oriented individuals maintained interest through the same process: they came into the situation concerned about doing well and showed higher levels of interest following positive normative feedback.

Under a task focus, however, different motivational processs were relevant. Task-focused evaluation minimized the negative effects of cognitive interference and promoted task involvement. By defining competence in terms of a task criterion, however, we sapped rewards of their affective power. Rewards for surpassing a task criterion enhanced competence valuation, but this process did not mediate interest under these conditions. For the same reason, achievement orientation was not related to subsequent interest in task focus conditions. Although achievement-oriented individuals were more concerned about doing well, competence valuation was unrelated to intrinsic interest in these conditions.

Personality and Motivational Processes in Context

Considered together, these studies underscore the importance of examining context and mediating processes in intrinsic motivation. We have identified two very different ways of enhancing interest in evaluative situations, depending on context. We can emphasize the importance of doing well by offering performance-contingent rewards that will make competence salient and valued, or by appealing to achievement-oriented individuals' characteristic orientation towards normatively defined competence. Alternatively, we can deemphasize the normative component of evaluation and focus people on the task as much as possible. The competence valuation and task involvement processes represent two very different ways of becoming involved in a task—people can become involved in ongoing performance and the pursuit of competence, or they can become immersed in the more task-intrinsic aspects of the activity itself. The good news here is that, in a field plagued by factors that detract from interest, our research points to two different kinds of involvement that can promote intrinsic motivation.

Another advantage of this process approach is that it allows us to consider situational and personality variables in one theoretical context. Process analysis can reveal the situational contexts in which individual differences will be particularly relevant in predicting behavior, and it allows us to explore person by situation interactions in greater detail. We can study the specific mechanisms by which some individuals respond differently to performance evaluation. The mediating mechanisms identified in our model give equal weight to situational and personality determinants, and translate them into a common unit of analysis——the motivational processes that operate in evaluative situations.

Acknowledgments The research described in this chapter was supported by grants from the Spencer Foundation. The author was supported by a Spencer Fellowship awarded by the National Institute of Education. I thank John Kihlstrom and Carol Sansone for helpful comments on earlier versions of this chapter.

References

Amabile, T.M. (1979). Effects of external evaluation on artistic creativity. *Journal of Personality and Social Psychology, 37,* 221–223.

Anastasi, A. (1982). *Psychological testing* (5th ed.). New York: Macmillan.

Boggiano, A.K., Harackiewicz, J.M., Bessette, J.M., & Main, D.S. (1985). Increasing children's interest through performance-contingent reward. *Social Cognition, 3,* 400–411.

Boggiano, A.K., & Ruble, D.N. (1979). Competence and the overjustification effect: a developmental study. *Journal of Personality and Social Psychology, 53,* 450–467.

Boggiano, A.K., & Ruble, D.N. (1986). Children's responses to evaluative feedback. In R. Schwarzer (Ed.), *Self-related cognitions in anxiety and motivation* (pp. 195–227). Hillsdale, NJ: Erlbaum.

Deci, E.L. (1975). *Intrisic motivation.* New York: Plenum.

Deci, E.L., & Ryan, R.M. (1985). The general causality orientations scale: Self-determination in personality. *Journal of Research in Personality, 19,* 109–134.

Epstein, J.A., & Harackiewicz, J.M. (1989). Winning is not enough: The effects of competition and opponent information on intrinsic motivation. Under editorial review.

Harackiewicz, J.M. (1979). The effects of reward contingency and performance feedback on intrinsic motivation. *Journal of Personality and Social Psychology, 37,* 1352–1363.

Harackiewicz, J.M., Abrahams, S., & Wageman, R. (1987). Performance evaluation and intrinsic motivation: The effects of evaluative focus, rewards, and achievement orientation. *Journal of Personality and Social Psychology, 53,* 1015–1023.

Harackiewicz, J.M. & Larson, J.R., Jr. (1986). Managing motivation: The impact of supervisor feedback on subordinate task interest. *Journal of Personality and Social Psychology, 51,* 547–556.

Harackiewicz, J.M., & Manderlink, G. (1984). A process analysis of the effects of performance-contingent rewards on intrinsic motivation. *Journal of Experimental Social Psychology, 20,* 531–551.

Harackiewicz, J.M., Manderlink, G., & Sansone, C. (1984). Rewarding pinball wizadry: Effects of evaluation and cue value on intrinsic interest. *Journal of Personality and Social Psychology, 47,* 287–300.

Harackiewicz, J.M., Manderlink, G., & Sansone, C. (in press). Competence processes and achievement orientation: Implications for intrinsic motivation. In A.K. Boggiano & T.S. Pittman (Eds.), *Achievement and motivation: A social-developmental analysis.* New York: Cambridge University Press.

Harackiewicz, J.M., & Sansone, C. (1989). A process model of intrinsic motivation: The case of performance-contingent rewards. Manuscript in preparation.

Harackiewicz, J.M., Sansone, C., & Manderlink, G. (1985). Competence, achievement orientation, and intrinsic motivation: A process analysis. *Journal of Personality and Social Psychology, 48,* 493–508.

Jackson, D.N. (1974). *Personality Research Form Manual.* Goshen, NY: Research Psychologists Press.

Jagacinski, C.M., & Nicholls, J.G. (1984). Conception of ability and related affects in task involvement and ego involvement. *Journal of Educational Psychology, 76,* 909–919.

Judd, C.M., & Kenny, D.A. (1981). Process analysis: Estimating mediation in treatment evaluations. *Evaluation Review, 5,* 602–619.

Lepper, M.R., Green, D., & Nisbet, R.E. (1973). Undermining children's intrinsic interest with extrinsic reward: A test of the overjustification hypothesis. *Journal of Personality and Social Psychology, 28,* 129–137.

Murray, H.A. (1938). *Explorations in personality*. New York: Oxford University Press.

Nicholls, J.G. (1984). Conceptions of ability and achievement motivation. In R. Ames & C. Ames (Eds). *Research on motivation in education: Vol I* (pp. 39–73). New York: Academic Press.

Ryan, R.M., Mims, V., & Koestner, R. (1983). Relation of reward contingency and interpersonal context to intrinsic motivation: A review and test using cognitive evaluation theory. *Journal of Personality and Social Psychology, 45,* 736–750.

Sansone, C. (1986). A question of competence: The effects of competence and task feedback on intrinsic interest. *Journal of Personality and Social Psychology, 51,* 918–931.

Sansone, C. (1989, in press). Competence feedback, task feedback, and intrinsic interest: An examination of process and context. *Journal of Experimental Social Psychology*.

Sansone, C., Sachau, D.A., & Weir, C. (1989). The effects of instruction on intrinsic interest: The importance of context. *Journal of Personality and Social Psychology*.

Sarason, I.G. (1980). Introduction to the study of test anxiety. In I.G. Sarason (Ed.), *Test anxiety: Theory, research, and applications* (pp. 3–14). Hillsdale, NJ: Erlbaum.

CHAPTER 9

The Problem of Life's Meaning

Roy F. Baumeister

Some years ago I became interested in understanding the modern dilemma of identity: identity crisis, finding oneself, knowing oneself, being all that you can be—these phrases are so familiar that they have become clichés. I wanted to understand why our whole society, in general, and our social sciences, in particular, had become so concerned with the self.

I thought that the answer must be that the self had somehow become increasingly problematic. To understand how the self had changed, I surveyed historical and literary trends relevant to self, and found that the self had indeed become more complex, overgrown, and problematic (Baumeister, 1986, 1987). That is, over the centuries, our society had come to expect more of the self, to conceptualize it in more complex and elaborate ways, and to increase the assumptions about what the self could and should do.

Toward the end of this project, however, I realized that the fascination and concern with self are often merely manifestations of a deeper problem with life's meaning. When people say they are struggling to find themselves or having an identity crisis, the issue is not always a problem of knowing the self so much as finding a meaningful life. There are important reasons (to which I shall return) underlying the confusion of identity problems with meaning problems. The key point is, however, that understanding the modern dilemma requires not only seeing the difficulties in how the self is defined, but also understanding what is happening to life's meaning. My recent efforts have, therefore, been devoted to understanding the problems of life's meaning.

Life and Meaning

To treat the problem of life's meaning as a psychological issue, it is necessary to have some understanding of the respective natures of life and meaning. A related issue is the nature of motivation, and here one may distinguish natural and cultural motivations.

Life. Life is a biological process. Living things are made of atoms and molecules, are physically real, are characterized by ongoing biochemical reactions, and so forth. Living things act as unities; thus, digging up the roots of a plant will affect its leaves, or stepping on a person's toe will usually cause the head and shoulders to move.

Life encounters the problems of dealing with the environment and with its own needs and wants. Living things are vulnerable to discomfort and damage caused by external events. They also come endowed with natural motivations, which typically include the desires for air, food, water, sex, sleep, and warmth. It also appears that living things have certain avoidance motivations that are, if not innate, at least innately prepared, such as fears of darkness, falling, and snakes. Human beings may also be predisposed to fear exclusion from social groups and may feel anxious when inclusion is threatened (Baumeister, in press; see also Bowlby, 1969, 1973).

Meaning. Meaning does not have physical existence or follow the laws of physics. Meaning begins with the animal's capacity to learn associations and distinctions, but human language, of which sharedness is a vital aspect, goes far beyond this capacity. Language is social, i.e., members of a community have it in common. The meaning of a dollar bill does not reside in one individual's associations to it but rather in the empirical fact that all members of the community understand and use it in similar ways.

Most social scientists focus on symbols when discussing meaning. Symbolism is important, to be sure, but it is only one part of meaning—even dogs and cats can learn, and use, symbols. The special power of human culture arose from the capacity of speech and intelligence to *combine* symbols. The meanings that pervade, enable, and complicate human social life are combinations of symbols; much more can be expressed with sentences than with single words.

Meaning also comes in clusters rather than in isolated doses. For example, the number 29 does not exist in isolation, and it would be useless and meaningless if there were no other numbers. A given number only makes sense in connection with other numbers, i.e., in the context of a system of numbers and, perhaps, of mathematical relationships in general.

Life encounters the immediate physical environment and events. Meaning is essentially relational: it relates stimuli and events across time and space. The concept of *tree,* for example, links together a large number of particular wooden plants. Using meaning, therefore, is a matter of *interpretation,* which means relating the particular event or stimulus to other events or stimuli. For example, the meaning of an act of giving advice, threatening harm, or sexual intercourse is probably established by placing it in the context of past and future events (e.g., an ongoing relationship); inferring intentions, implications, traits, and consequences; and evaluating it against general attitudes and expectations.

Thus, most of human cognitive activity is a matter of superimposing meaning on events: Things that occur are related to others and to broad, general meanings (principles, inferences, attitudes). Social intelligence is centrally concerned with learning to use the meanings provided by the culture in the ways the culture stipulates as appropriate (Cantor & Kihlstrom, in press).

Occasionally people want to escape from meanings—when, for example, these become painful. The process of *cognitive deconstruction* is the effort to avoid meaningful thought and is typically accomplished by returning awareness to the immediate physical present—sensations, movements, stimuli (Baumeister, in press). Masochism, for example, can be understood as a set of techniques for deconstructing the self, that is, reducing awareness of self from identity to body (Baumeister, 1988a, 1988b, 1989a).

One important class of meanings is standards. Standards are abstract representations of the way things could be, and they include norms, values, and expectations, as well as criteria for evaluating performances. Cultures provide individuals with standards, and cultural change often appears to involve changing standards. Standards are, therefore, an important aspect of *cultural motivations,* that is, motivations that are based on meaning. People feel motivated to live up to positive standards.

In many cases, cultural motivations are simply superimposed on natural motivations: The culture takes some natural pattern of behavior and elaborates it with meanings and contexts that transform behavior and experience. Thus, sexual desire is apparently universal and natural, but certain patterns of sexual activity and culturally relative (again, masochism is a good example; see Baumeister, 1988a, 1989a). Often, the transformation includes surrounding the behavior with standards. Thus, cultural patterns of etiquette and culinary values are superimposed on the natural desire for food; cultural rules and restrictions are superimposed on the natural desire for sex; cultural rules about private ownership, status symbolism, and monetary exchange are superimposed on the natural desires for territory and shelter.

False Constancy

Two further consequences of the analysis of life and meaning are important. The first is what I call *false constancy*. False constancy is the tendency for ideas and concepts to overestimate the stability of the phenomena to which they occur, thus producing highly pervasive psychological errors (often including disappointment). To understand the causes of false constancy, it is necessary to consider one more fact about the differences between life and meaning.

9. Life's Meaning

Life, as a physical and social process, is inherently a matter of change: Biologically, the organism is in a constant state of flux. Life consists of breathing, eating food, eliminating wastes, growth, movement, learning, desire and satisfaction, sleep and waking, illness and recovery, aging, and death. All of these involve change. Similarly, human social life consists of relentless change: Relationships begin, evolve, and end, family roles gradually change, new groups are joined, old groups disintegrate, conflicts arise and are resolved, and so forth.

Meaning, in contrast to life, is based on stability. Some meanings do gradually change, but this is a necessary and often problematic concession to the changes in social life—meanings may change to keep up. For the most part, however, meanings have to be constant in order to be useful. It would be impossible to talk if words changed their meanings overnight. The number 6 means very much the same thing it did thousands of years ago, and this consistency is necessary for the system of mathematics to operate.

To apply meaning to life, therefore, is to apply something inherently stable and constant to something that is inherently a relentless process of change. This incongruity will result in false constancy, that is, the tendency for ideas and concepts to be more stable than the phenomena to which they refer. This pattern appears to occur whenever meaning is applied to life. It is apparent in person perception, for example, in the suggestion that a perceiver's impression of someone will overestimate the stability and consistency of that person's behavior (e.g., Jones & Nisbett, 1971; Ross, 1977). It is also apparent in the cultural construct of marriage, which defines marriage as a stable, unchanging state from the wedding day "till death do us part," contrary to the multiple processes of evolution and change that actually characterize mating relationships. It is also apparent in ideas about fulfillment, which tend to be thought of as stable, enduring states of positive feelings, whereas all evidence indicates that these states of fulfillment tend to be ephemeral and subject to alteration even if repeated (for example, consider the various cultural ideals of love, fame, and religious enlightenment).

False constancy is not simply an accidental result of an odd incongruity between life and meaning. The nature of life includes relentless change, but also a recurrent *desire* for stability that is apparent in the body's homeostatic mechanisms, the endless efforts to achieve a stable, secure environment, and the quest for stable social bonds. Life is a process of change that yearns for stability, and, among human beings, meaning is one of the principal tools in the quest for stability. So it is not surprising that meaning is inherently stable, and that the application of meaning to some phenomena will tend toward distorting them in the direction of greater constancy. That is a large part of what meaning is *for*.

Shortfall Denial

The second consequence of the analyses of life and meaning can be called *shortfall denial*. Indeed, false constancy can be considered as a special case of shortfall denial.

As already stated, an important class of meanings is *standards,* that is, abstract generalizations against which actual events can be evaluated. Culture regulates individual behavior by attaching positive and negative affect to various standards. People feel pride at getting an A in calculus, guilt over having sexual intercourse with a neighbor's spouse, anger over a perceived inequity in sports officiating, and sadness over a drop in stock prices, none of which is an innate pattern of response.

It is hardly controversial to suggest that people internalize many of these standards and go through life with many goals, values, and expectations. Inevitably, however, some events and performances will fall short of these standards. Life simply does not offer an uninterrupted series of successes and fulfillments.

Happiness depends very heavily on comparing one's perceived circumstances against standards (e.g., Argyle, 1987). Because events often fall short of standards, it is not easy to remain happy; this is consistent with Freud's (1930) observation that human beings do not seem to be designed to be happy. But, of course, people *desire* to be happy. Therefore, a pervasive problem in applying meaning to life is constructing some interpretation that will resolve or conceal these shortfalls. Some distortions occur—to be happy and well-adjusted, people tend to have to misperceive events to some degree (Taylor & Brown, 1988; also Taylor, 1983)—but it is clearly no simple matter to convince oneself that events have passed standards when they manifestly fell short. People may exaggerate their SAT scores or romantic successes *somewhat* in memory, but it is hard for beginners to convince themselves that they are experts, or for obscure, unknown individuals to convince themselves that they are internationally famous stars. Indeed, there is some evidence that gross distortions in social perception can cause unrealistic aspirations, self-defeating behaviors, and other problems (e.g., Baumeister & Scher, 1988). One resolution is to suggest that there is an "optimal margin of illusion" that involves seeing self and events as *slightly* better than they are (Baumeister, 1988c, 1989b).

The most common strategy, then, appears to be to come reasonably close to one's goals and standards, and then rely on a dose of illusion to make up the difference. Brutal, realistic, honest assessment of one's life circumstances is fairly rare among nondepressed individuals, and substantial distortions and fabrications are vulnerable to disconfirmation.

Four Needs for Meaning

The basis for my approach to understanding the problem of life's meaning is the assumption that people need their lives to make sense in certain basic ways. These ways can be conceptualized as a set of *needs for meaning*.

My approach uses a list of four needs for meaning, that is, there are four main ways in which people need their lives to make sense. There is nothing magical or sacred (in this connection) about the number four. These four needs overlap to some extent, and they could probably be expressed as three basic needs or subdivided further into six or seven. This is not important; what is important is the total conceptual space they cover. If a person manages to satisfy these needs, he or she is likely to find life adequately meaningful. If a person is unable to satisfy one or more of these needs, that person is likely to experience some distress that could be resolved by finding new sources of meaning or further elaborating other sources of meaning.

The first need is for purpose; people need purposes in life. This was the focus of Klinger's (1977) work on how people find meaning in life, in his discussion of incentives. Human behavior is goal-directed, and people interpret their own and others' behavior in relation to goals.

Purposes can be subdivided into extrinsic and intrinsic ones. Extrinsic purposes are goals. Intrinsic purposes are fulfillment states. Life can derive meaning from either the pursuit of external goals or the pursuit (or enjoyment) of various forms of fulfillment—in either case, the purpose gives meaning and direction to present activities.

Modern life offers a wide assortment of extrinsic goals for structuring individual life. On the other hand, its ideals of fulfillment are relatively few and problematic. Christianity dominated Western society for many centuries and accustomed people to having a powerful and compelling model of fulfillment—salvation in heaven, which meant everlasting bliss beginning immediately after death. As many individuals began to live their lives by more secular patterns and meanings, Christianity retreated from its central place in the life of the society, and this led to a general perception of a need for new ideas of fulfillment. The search for new, secular, this-worldly concepts and methods of fulfillment has continued down to the present, with uneven success (Baumeister, 1986).

The second need is for efficacy. This is a need to feel that one is making a difference in or having some impact on the world. Motivations to seek, increase, and maintain control have been widely noted in psychology (e.g., Brehm, 1966; Rothbaum, Weisz & Snyder, 1982; White, 1959). By emphasizing efficacy rather than control, I want to call attention to the importance of the subjective appearance of control. That is, people need to interpret their lives in some way that gives them the belief that they have control. Often this control may be illusory (e.g., Langer, 1975; Taylor, 1983), but it is nonetheless satisfactory, at least as long as the illusion is sustained. The important thing is not the actual control but the belief in one's control.

The third need is for value or justification. People need to be able to justify their actions as right and good. Moral values are a common and important source of legitimation, but moral rules are predominantly negative, whereas people also need positive source(s) of value in their lives.

Value is typically derivative: One justifies one's acts on the basis of some general principles about what is right and good, and these principles are in turn based on more general and fundamental notions of value and goodness. The process of justifying something on the basis of something else can continue until it reaches something that is accepted as good in its own right, without appeal to any other source of goodness. A Christian, for example, may justify a particular action on the basis of his intentions, which are justified on the basis of his general moral principles, which are justified in relation to the Ten Commandments, which are justified on the basis of God's will. The reasoning stops there: God's will does not require further justification.

These factors that can justify other things without themselves needing justification can be called *value bases*. In the above example, God's will is a value base. Value bases are important, and they are precious because they are difficult to create. Some thinkers have noted that the accelerated progress of social change in recent centuries has undermined several major value bases (such as traditions) without offering viable replacements. As a result, modern life suffers from a potentially critical shortage of sources of value (e.g., Habermas, 1973). In addition, the transition from a heavily religious society to a more secular society has clearly reduced the reliance on religious legitimation, and this too has contributed to the shortage of viable value bases.

The last need is for self-worth. This is the need to understand the self as having positive value, as deserving esteem and approval. In practice, the need for self-worth generally seems to take the form of a need to feel superior to others. Self-worth can be based either collectively (i.e., belonging to a superior or valued group) or individually (i.e., being valued or superior as an individual). Most traditional societies appear to have relied heavily on collective sources of self-worth. Membership in a valued social class or religious group enabled people to feel superior to others. Indeed, the stratified social structure was a very important basis for self-worth; aristocrats felt superior to the middle classes, who felt superior to the peasants, who felt superior to the slaves. An important function of slavery was thus the enhancement of the self-worth of the owner (Patterson, 1982). Slaves themselves struggled relentlessly to find some basis for self-worth, either by forming their own social groups (e.g., house slaves might feel superior to field slaves; Patterson, 1982), or by joining esteemed religious groups (Raboteau, 1978).

Our own society has placed self-worth on a much more individual basis. By sustaining the ideal and the appearance (if not the reality) of a classless society, one major collective basis for self-worth was eliminated. The individualistic ideology, economics, and political structure of the U.S.A. has fostered an emphasis on individual comparison as the main basis for evaluating self-worth.

Self and the Value Gap

The preceding overview of the needs for meaning provides a basis for evaluating the current problems of life's meaning in modern Western society. It is readily apparent that our society offers abundant sources of self-worth and efficacy, and that the society is heavily oriented toward a well-defined system of extrinsic goals. On the other hand, the widespread decline of religious faith has created deficiencies in firm sources of value or conceptions of fulfillment.

In the early stages of my work on meanings and life, I assumed that when people lost a major source of meaning in life they would immediately seek to find a new source of meaning to replace it. This was repeatedly contradicted by the empirical evidence, however. The first response to a loss of meaning appears to be the attempt *to elaborate one's remaining sources of meaning* to make up the deficiency. For example, if someone lost a major basis for self-worth, he or she might try to elaborate his or her source of value or purpose to furnish a basis for self-worth—instead of immediately searching for some new activity which might, if added to one's life, furnish a new basis for self-worth.

The individual self has gained importance over the past few centuries as a source of meaning in life. As already stated, self-worth has been put on an increasingly individualistic basis, as has efficacy. Furthermore, the concept of personal identity has been extended and elaborated (Baumeister, 1986, 1987).

The modern individual thus has a very meaningful self but confronts shortages in other areas of meaning. It is consistent with the general pattern, therefore, for self to be further elaborated to take over the function of supplying the deficits in meaning, notably value and fulfillment. In other words, when deficits cropped up with respect to value and fulfillment, people turned to their main available sources of meaning—notably the self—and sought to make the self furnish value and fulfillment in addition to its other functions.

To serve as a source of value, the self has been redefined as a value base. Today, self is regarded as a high value and a source of quasi-moral duties and obligations. Knowing oneself and fulfilling one's potentials (e.g., cultivating one's talents) are considered good things in their own right. Asserting oneself, seeking esteem, being unique, and pursuing one's own self-interests are similarly regarded as good things, or at least as moral rights.

Transforming the self into a value base has revolutionized the relationship between self and morality. Throughout most of history, morality was seen as essentially opposed to self (e.g., Rosenthal, 1984). Pursuit of self-interest was considered the root of much evil, and the social function of morality was to place checks and limits on the self. Moral virtue meant overcoming the self. Now, in contrast, self has become allied with morality to the point where self is an important basis for deciding what is right, good, and desirable.

There are several possible ways in which the self can be elaborated into a source of fulfillment. The cultivation of one's inner potential, such as in some conceptions of artistic creation, was a central fascination for the Romantics (Baumeister, 1986, 1987). More recently, however, emphasis has fallen on egotistical pride as the main form of self-based fulfillment. The search for a meaning of fulfillment in life thus elaborates the pursuit of self-worth (one of the other needs for meaning); thinking that one is terrific becomes a much-sought form of fulfillment. The pursuit of fame and celebrity (e.g., Braudy, 1986; Lasch, 1978) and the quest for esteem take on added urgency and meaning as they come to be perceived as necessary ingredients of a fulfilled life.

The elaboration of self into a source of legitimation and fulfillment returns this discussion to the issues addressed in the opening paragraphs. It is no accident that the modern problems of meaning in life are often experienced and discussed in terms of problems of the self. In addition to all the other demands that our culture has placed on the construction of personal identity, identity is now also supposed to serve as an important source of meaning in life by satisfying two of the most problematic needs for meaning.

Author's Note. This material was presented at the Michigan Personality Miniconference in March 1988 and at the American Psychological Convention in August 1988 (Atlanta), under the title "Conceptual Scheme for Meanings of Life." It is based on a forthcoming book, *Meanings of Life,* scheduled for completion in 1989.

References

Argyle, M. (1987). *The psychology of happiness.* London, England: Methuen.
Baumeister, R.F. (1986) *Identity: Cultural change and the struggle for self.* New York: Oxford University Press.

Baumeister, R.F. (1987) How the self became a problem: A psychological review of historical research. *Journal of Personality and Social Psychology, 52,* 163–176.

Baumeister, R.F. (1988a). Masochism as escape from self. *Journal of Sex Research, 25* (1), 28–59.

Baumeister, R.F. (1988b). Gender differences in masochistic scripts. *Journal of Sex Research, 25* (4), 478–499.

Baumeister, R.F. (1988c). The optimal margin of illusion. Paper presented at the convention of the American Psychological Association, August, Atlanta, GA.

Baumeister, R.F. (1989a). *Masochism and the Self.* Hillsdale, NJ: Erlbaum.

Baumeister, R.F. (1989b). The optimal margin of illusion. *Journal of Social and Clinical Psychology,* **8,**176–189.

Baumeister, R.F. (in press). Anxiety and deconstruction: On escaping the self. In J. Olson & M. Zanna (Eds.), *Self-inference processes: The Ontario Symposium, Vol. 6.* Hillsdale, NJ: Erlbaum.

Baumeister, R.F., & Scher, S.J. (1988). Self-defeating behavior patterns among normal individuals: Review and analysis of common self-destructive tendencies. *Psychological Bulletin, 104,* 3–22.

Bowlby, J. (1969). *Attachment and loss: Vol 1. Attachment.* New York: Basic Books.

Bowlby, J. (1973). *Attachment and loss: Vol 2. Separation anxiety and anger.* New York: Basic Books.

Braudy, L. (1986). *The frenzy of renown: Fame and its history.* New York: Oxford University Press.

Brehm, J. (1966). *A theory of psychological reactance.* New York: Academic Press.

Cantor, N., & Kihlstrom, J. (in press). Social intelligence. In R.S. Wyer & T.K. Srull (Eds.), *Advances in social cognition: Vol. III. Social intelligence and cognitive assessments of personality.* Hillsdale, NJ: Erlbaum.

Freud, S. (1930). *Civilization and its discontents.* (J. Strachey, Trans.) New York: Norton.

Habermas, J. (1973). *Legitimation crisis.* Boston, MA: Beacon Press.

Jones, E.E., & Nisbett, R.E. (1971). *The actor and the observer: Divergent perceptions of the causes of behavior.* Morristown, NJ: General Learning Press.

Klinger, E. (1977). *Meaning and void: Inner experience and the incentives in people's lives.* Minneapolis, MN: University of Minnesota Press.

Langer, E. (1975). The illusion of control. *Journal of Personality and Social Psychology, 32,* 311–328.

Lasch, C. (1978). *The culture of narcissism.* New York: Norton.

Patterson, O. (1982). *Slavery and social death.* Cambridge, MA: Harvard University Press.

Raboteau, A. (1978). *Slave religion.* New York: Oxford University Press.

Rosenthal, P. (1984). *Words and values: Some leading words and where they lead us.* New York: Oxford University Press.

Ross, L. (1977). The intuitive psychologist and his shortcomings: Distortions in the attribution process. In L. Berkowitz (Ed.), *Advances in experimental social psychology: Vol 10.* New York: Academic Press.

Rothbaum, F., Weisz, J.R., & Snyder, S. (1982). Changing the world and changing the self: A two process model of perceived control. *Journal of Personality and Social Psychology, 42*, 5-37.

Taylor, S.E. (1983). Adjustment to threatening events: A theory of cognitive adaptation. *American Psychologist, 38*, 1161-1173.

Taylor, S.E., & Brown, J.D. (1988). Illusion and well-being: Some social psychological contributions to a theory of mental health. *Psychological Bulletin, 103*, 193-210.

White, R.W. (1959). Motivation reconsidered: The concept of competence. *Psychological Review, 66*, 297-333.

CHAPTER 10

Conditional Patterns, Transference, and the Coherence of Personality Across Time

Avril Thorne

The study of personality coherence across time has been limited mostly to nonconditional attributes. By nonconditional attributes, I mean traits such as dominance and extraversion, moods such as happiness, and behaviors such as talking and smiling. These kinds of concepts can be contrasted with explicitly conditional categories such as: My dominance shows when my competence is threatened; I fall apart when people try to comfort me; I talk the most when I am nervous.

The difference between nonconditional and conditional attributes is that the latter are explicitly contextualized. For example, dominance has been defined as a summary of behavioral acts (Buss & Craik, 1983), but the conditions under which such acts are displayed are not part of the definition of dominance. Dispositions such as dominance or extraversion can, of course, be studied under specified conditions in order to discover the circumstances that accentuate dispositional expression. For example, friends have been found to elicit more consistent patterns of dominance than do strangers (Moscowitz, 1988), and extraverts have been found to elicit sociability (Thorne, 1987). In these cases, however, as in other experimental research, the eliciting conditions were imposed independently of the subjects.

Although the independent specification of conditions underlying the expression of personality is important, such specification is independent in a limited sense. The conditions are technically independent in that the conditions are selected by the experimenter. However, whether subjects are ignorant of the links between their dispositional displays and the imposed conditions——whether the conditions are 'phenomenologically' independent——is another matter.

My interest in working from subjects' own specifications of the conditions surrounding their characteristic expressions of personality derives, in part, from my feeling that an adequate understanding of personality coherence needs more grounding in personal experience. In many cases, we still do not know much about the conditions that are tied to particular expressions of personality. I made this case in regard to theory and research on extraversion-introversion (Thorne, 1983), and I think that similar cases can be made for other commonly studied dispositions. Studies of interpersonal complementarity, for example, have eluded the theoretical prediction that dominance begets submission (Orford, 1986). By citing these limitations, I do not mean to imply that formal theory should be discarded, or that we should no longer conduct experiments, but only that we do not know enough about the contingencies that people perceive as surrounding their personological expression, and that such understandings might be a good place to start (Jones & Thorne, 1986; Thorne, 1985).

There are two basic, and presumably interrelated, viewpoints from which people perceive the conditions that are linked to particular dispositions——an observer-view, and a self-view. Wright and Mischel (1987, 1988) have pursued an observer-view by examining the conditions that observers consider relevant to their dispositional attributions. Working with counsellors and boys at a summer camp, they found that observers are able to specify accurately some of the contexts in which children display aggression and withdrawal. Content analysis of the counsellors' contingency statements revealed that two kinds of aversive events were associated with aggression and withdrawal——interpersonal events (e.g., criticism), and internal states (e.g., feeling angry).

In this chapter, I explore some possibilities of self-views. A self-view of conditional patterns would seem to enjoy a large, and relatively unique, data base, since only one's self has been with oneself as long as oneself has lived. The conceptual advantage of studying self-views of conditional attributes is that such patterns may parallel, phenomenologically, the process by which personality coheres across time. Beginning with Freud, many personality theorists have posited the internalization of interpersonal conditions as a fundamental feature of personality development. Consistent with some of these approaches (e.g., Sullivan, 1940), I view personality as a working representation of the self in relation to specific, repeated, interpersonal conditions. This definition, of course, is only one of several generally accepted definitions of personality, and centers on psycho-social and emotional aspects of personality development.

Having been encouraged at this conference to speculate, I have chosen to address the question of whether people perceive that their dispositional displays are tied to certain contingencies and, if so, how we might approach, identify, and put these perceptions to use. Before considering the kinds of conditional statements that people spontaneously produce, however, I should justify using the term "condition" instead of the more customary term "situation." "Condition," in dictionary usage, means anything called for as a requirement for the performance, completion, or effectiveness of something else. "Situation," on the other hand, is a more general term referring to the place of something in relation to its surroundings. There is no necessary link between a situation and its contents; the contents may just happen to be located in the situation. By contrast, there is a compelling link of some sort between a condition and an attribute. Thus, "condition," as opposed to "situation," more readily implies explicitly represented relations of attributes and ecological requirements.

A Pursuit of Conditional Patterns

The first problem to consider is whether the notion of conditional patterns of personality makes intuitive sense. The notion of conditionality, at least for some adults in our culture, seems to make sense. This is apparent when subjects are asked to account for their responses to true-false personality inventory items. At such times, it is not unusual for subjects to balk at questions by saying, "Well, it depends." When asked on what it depends, I have found that subjects are not often very forthcoming. Of course, this does not mean that people do not perceive themselves to have any conditional patterns, but only that, in this instance, a specific pattern does not come to mind.

Where else might one find spontaneous conditional self-statements? Stories that people tell about themselves sometimes have them, and complaints often seem to have them. Stories and complaints can be found in conversations, letters, diaries, and other kinds of personal narratives. Because the data were readily available, I will focus on interactants' accounts of conversations with strangers that I collected in a previous study (Thorne, 1983). I collected the accounts to examine the reciprocal impact of introverts and extroverts on conversational style, and, at the time, did not intend to use the accounts to study conditional self-statements. Compared to the method of asking subjects to explain the conditions that led them to answer true, false, or "it depends" to personality inventory items, having people listen to their own conversations and provide play-by-play accounts of what they were doing seemed to have more potential for activating conditional self-statements.

In examining the transcribed accounts, I looked for self-statements that could be reduced to an if-then, or when-then, rule linking characteristic behaviors to conditions (Alston, 1975). It quickly became clear that conditional statements vary in elaboration. Compare the following four utterances. What I hope is a reasonable if-then or when-then reduction follows each of the statements.

(A) I am shy when I meet strangers.

   [If I meet strangers, then I am shy.]

(B) I was hoping you would put us in a group so that I could just sit back and take it easy.

   [If I am in a group of strangers, then I can take it easy, and I wish you had put me in a group.]

(C) I'm not usually attracted to independent people like her because then I'd be competing with them. I like people to feel awed and inferior to me.

[When I am with independent people like her, then I have to compete with them; I prefer people to feel awed and inferior to me.]

(D) I guess I get jealous of outgoing people, not jealous, but my mom's always telling me "you should be more outgoing like your sister and not so shy and quiet," and it makes me feel bad when I can't be the way she wants me to be.

[When I am with outgoing people, then I get jealous or feel bad because I wish I could be outgoing like my mom wants me to be.]

Whereas pattern (A) can be reduced to a fairly simple if-then statement without loss of information, the other patterns cannot. Patterns (B), (C), and (D) each contain additional information about the wishes or desires of the person, and in each case the wishes are frustrated. In patterns (B) and (C), the frustration seems temporary, whereas in (D), the frustration seems more enduring. Pattern (D) is also interesting because the condition is a function of two conditions——mom, and the outgoing conversational partner. Conditional self-statements of any form, and especially the more complex ones, were not frequent in the accounts, emerging on the average no more than once or twice per one-hour session. Despite their infrequency, however, the more complex patterns are more personologically informative because they specify the person's feelings about the contingencies.

Another kind of conditional pattern was so perfunctorily declared that the person might have been describing moves in a chess game. The perfunctory patterns did not include the element of frustrated wishes, and primarily referred to behavioral routines. An example of such a self-statement is Sally's description of how she maneuvered through the situation of getting acquainted with a stranger:

When I meet strangers, I assume we have a lot in common so I just try to explore its extent. Like, if she'd said she was in a sorority, I would say, "Which one," and if I knew someone in it, I would ask her about her, and. . . .

Although the low base rate of any kind of conditional self-statement precluded statistical comparisons, extraverts (versus introverts) seemed more likely to declare this perfunctory kind of pattern. These subjects were also more comfortable in the situation and, perhaps partly for that reason, were less likely to talk about frustrations.

So far, we have seen that conditional self-statements can vary in complexity and in affect. The more complex statements explicitly include the element of a wish or desire. The affect accompanying the statement may be negative (explicit dissatisfaction with the pattern), neutral (e.g., perfunctory), or, presumably, positive (explicit satisfaction with the pattern). For reasons that I will increasingly elaborate, the remainder of this chapter focuses on patterns of the complex, dissatisfied sort.

Extending Conditional Patterns Backwards in Time

My study of interactants' accounts provided a very limited view of personality because the interaction was stuck in time. I had to rely on the inclinations of the subjects to generalize their patterns to other contexts, and the rare cases of such extensions were not very elaborated.

To begin to explore the question of how people extend conditional patterns across time, I decided to try a direct approach. I asked my students, all of whom are women, to select naturally occurring events from memory. Because of the apparent salience of frustrating events, I asked for a particular kind of pattern. The task was to describe a recent encounter in which the outcome wasn't what the subject wanted, and then to describe any other past encounters that seemed to show a similar pattern. In order to avoid activating painful memories, I also offered students several other, less personal, options. The women were given a week to complete the narratives. Here is an example from Alice, which I have shortened and, as usual, altered slightly to protect the subject's identity.

I was talking on the phone to my boyfriend last night. Even though he was unfairly critical of me, I responded in a placating manner. . . . I knew that he had misunderstood me, but rather than continue the discussion with him, I allowed him to change the subject and did not stand up for myself. . . . The next day, I realized how upset I was about the phonecall. I realized this is a pattern of mine. When I do not like what is being said, I do not stand up for myself. Instead I appear to agree with it and only later do I allow myself to feel angry, and then I keep my anger to myself. What I wished to happen in this conversation was for me to be honest and tell my boyfriend that he was being unfair, and tell him that I did not enjoy his teasing.

This pattern of my denying my true feelings in order to placate another person started when I was very young. The first example that I can recall occurred when I was in the third grade, when my mother kept telling me I was fat and made me lose weight even though the doctor said I was okay; though I knew it to be untrue, I did nothing to protest her assertion that I was fat.

When I come to think of it, I remember an even earlier incident around this pattern when I learned my mother would approve of me if I agreed with her. When I was about seven, she was showing me a puzzle and I told her she wasn't doing it right; she threw a fit and ran out of the room; my dad came in and punished me for contradicting her.

Karen, another student, attributed her failure to initiate a reconciliation with her boyfriend, as well as her failure to fully express her enthusiasm for a competition to a high school teacher (and her subsequent failure, in each case, to get what she wanted), to her parents' edict that "a good child is polite and patient." Karen, one of seven children, said that as a child when she and her siblings screamed and fought over who would get to sit in the front seat of the car, the quiet and obedient child was always chosen. She thus learned to dampen her expression of enthusiasm.

Unfortunately, Karen has found, since leaving home, that good things do not necessarily come to those who sit and wait.

A final example comes from Joanne, who said she was surprised to find a tantrum reaction connecting several early memories; in each case the tantrum occurred when she felt unfairly treated. What distinguishes Joanne's pattern from that of Alice is that Joanne's response to the condition of being unjustly treated is immediate and vocal; she does not retreat quietly.

I would like to highlight two "findings" from this exploratory enterprise. One is that a good deal of reflection may be necessary for the self-perception of personality coherence. In the case of Alice, the episode with her boyfriend did not seem like a pattern to her while the episode was happening; only afterward did it seem like a pattern (and perhaps more so because she had been asked to find one!). Substantial self-reflection on the part of subjects, although relatively infrequent in personality research, may be necessary methodologically to reveal the phenomenology of personality coherence. Secondly, these few examples suggest that people perceive coherence across several features of their conditional episodes; in each case, the nature of the frustrated wish, and the reactions of self and of other, are constant. In the case of Alice, for example, each episode contains a wish to be treated fairly, an unfair criticism from another person (boyfriend, mother, father), and Alice's failure to express what she calls her true feelings. In essence, the occurrence of such episodes requires the repeated cooperation of self and other in frustrating one's own wishes.

The Importance of Conditional Patterns that are Frustrating

The study of conditional patterns that are frustrating is important because such patterns seem to be particularly stable across time, difficult to change, and yet desirable to change. Several studies suggest that these kinds of patterns, or at least aspects of them, tend to be especially stable. Markus and Nurius (1986) found that the aspects of themselves that people expected to endure into the future were more likely to be negative or conflictual past selves than positive past selves. Only the negative past selves showed a substantial correlation with the selves imagined as possible ($r = .55$). Further evidence of the staying power of negative patterns comes from Emmons and King (1988), who reported that the content of conflictual strivings tended to be stable over a one-year follow up. Although Emmons and King studied nonconditional attributes, their subjects' concerns seem to be similar to those cited here in descriptions of frustrating episodes: examples of conflictual strivings included keeping jealousy under contol and dealing with anger constructively.

What accounts for the apparent stability of these patterns? Negative patterns may be especially enduring because such patterns function to maintain the emotional life of an individual on an even, if less than satisfactory, keel. The stability may be a function of early learning about the consequences of emotional expression. Duhl and Duhl (1981, p. 493) note that children need "the validation of knowing that feeling mad, sad, and bad" is "okay, not unique to themselves, felt by mom and dad too, not a cause for punishment, and not the cause of others' illness or leaving." Unfortunately, few of us gain such complete validation, and protection against vulnerabilities begins early. Duhl and Duhl (1981, p. 501) describe such patterns as "core images." Core images, they speculate, are "held in the repository of the mind like movie archives. . . . enactments of actual past experiences or rebuttals of them, plotted and rehearsed" again and again.

In thinking about such patterns, several old-fashioned concepts come readily to mind: inner conflict (Horney, 1945), unity theme (Murray, 1938), parataxic distortion (Sullivan, 1940), and the oldest formal concept of them all, transference (Freud, 1912/1976). As Freud's revisionists have shown, one need not accept certain orthodox assumptions, such as unconscious instinctual motivation and the universality of the Oedipal drama, to appreciate the worth of Freud's clinical insights. The psychosocial dynamics of transference are consistent with the kind of conditional patterns that I have been discussing, in that the transference pattern is said to be well developed, to be triggered by the frustration of a desired gratification from someone else, and repeated over and over again with different people. Freud (1912/1976, p. 105) referred to transference as "a special individuality in the exercise of [one's] capacity to love, in the conditions one sets up for loving." This individuality is said to occur as a result of conditions imposed by parents in interaction with the special requirements of the child. The requirements are never fully met, according to Freud, and frustration is a necessary aspect of becoming socialized. Thus, the pattern endures because certain needs are never fully satisfied, and one comes to perceive, tolerate, and negotiate the frustration in particular ways.

Although the notion of transference has been central to clinical psychology since Freud, only recently have transference-like concepts been systematically studied. Several personologists in the last decade have shown an empirical interest in the kinds of conditional patterns I am describing. The label "conditional pattern" is my own, because I wish to emphasize the utility of thinking about personality in mutually contingent and episodic rather than singular units. Compatible if somewhat differently aimed approaches can, however, be found in studies of core conflictual relationship themes (Luborsky, 1978), nuclear scripts (Carlson, 1981; Tomkins, 1979), life stories (McAdams, 1985), personal projects (Little, 1983), and personal strivings (Emmons, 1986). These approaches share an interest in analyzing subjects' narrative accounts to formulate a conception of what individuals are trying to do psychologically, emotionally, and, to a lesser extent, interpersonally.

As an example of the empirical promise of recent work, Luborsky and his colleagues (1985) have corroborated several of Freud's original observations about transference, including that each person has a distinct transference pattern, that the pattern relates to the content of one's emotional life, and that the pattern is repeated in other important relationships beyond the therapy room. In a more recent study, Luborsky, Crits-Christoph, Mintz, and Auerbach (1988) found that particular changes in the transference pattern coincided with successful outcomes in psychotherapy, suggesting that core conditional patterns are implicated in personality change as well as personality consistency.

Summary and Implications

The problem of personality coherence—how to identify and account for individual differences in the organization of behavior and experience—has puzzled personality psychologists for decades (e.g., Block, 1977; Mischel, 1968; Murray, 1938). In the field of personology, one solution has been especially persistent. This is the notion of a core conditional pattern that motivates individuals to perceive and construct experience in such a way as to fashion contingencies that are familiar and relatively comfortable. Conditional patterns are an important and neglected way in which individuals repeatedly construct their personalities. The construals can be pursued historically and idiographically (as with the concept of transference), locally and nomothetically (as with the work of Wright and Mischel (1988)), or, as I have tried to illustrate, through a combination of local and historical approaches.

The present approach focuses on personal accounts of frustrating encounters as the ground on which to uncover secrets of personality coherence and change. In studying interactants' accounts and the conversations on which they are based, it appears that the character of at least some individual differences is manifest in what we characteristically want from others and characteristically fail to get. The frustrating patterns that we develop, such as not standing up for ourselves as a way of weathering conditions of unfair treatment, define not only who we are in relation to our inner selves, but also who we are in relation to those around us. One's sense of personological coherence may partly derive from the kinds of wishes that others repeatedly fail to gratify, and for which one's own efforts never seem to be enough.

At this early stage of research, there is a lot left to know about the structure, function, and expression of conditional patterns. It is probably the case, for example, that the idea of one core conditional pattern is oversimplified and that, despite some evidence to the contrary (Luborsky, et al., 1985), people have more than one enduring pattern, and that the patterns serve different functions. The rules of reciprocity, for example, seem to require patterns that mesh with the special requirements of the other person (e.g., Thorne, 1987). Another problem is that conditional patterns may be difficult to detect. Some people may be more likely to disclose conditional patterns than are others; the most revealing group may be clinical or troubled populations, the samples that seem to have been preferred as subjects so far (Carlson, 1986; Luborsky, et al., 1985; Wright & Mischel, 1988).

Certain kinds of problems also attend the use of personal narratives. The use of narratives as basic data is relatively time-consuming, more so than structured personality inventories, but then the data are also more flexible and can be used for more purposes. A second problem is that the use of narratives invites an abundance of coding schemes that may have little apparent relation to one another; however, at this exploratory phase, new schemes should be welcome, and their relative informativeness should be a matter of empirical inquiry facilitated by a common data base. A third problem is that explicit statements about conditional patterns may be relatively rare, certainly more rare than are many behaviors, such as talking and smiling. Conditional patterns seem to be highly condensed and would profit from elaboration from other sources, such as the views of the other person involved in the episode and the views of outside observers.

A final problem with relying on self-views about conditional patterns is that self-perceptions may be less articulated than are outsiders' views. Also, due to self-deception, selective inattention, repression, or whatever one wishes to call lack of enlightenment, self-views may be less accurate than are outsider's views. Assumptions about the greater articulateness, accuracy, and insight of the expert outside observer are the grounds on which many insight-oriented psychotherapies proceed, although the basic data for such enterprises necessarily consist of self-views. Claims about the inaccuracy and inarticulateness of self-views, although interesting, are beyond the reach of the present endeavor. In this chapter, I have been content to address the question of whether people perceive that their dispositional displays are tied to certain contingencies, and, if so, how we might approach, identify, and put these perceptions to use in understanding personality coherence and change.

References

Alston, W.P. (1975). Traits, consistency, and conceptual alternatives for personality theory. *Journal for the Theory of Social Behavior, 5,* 17–48.

Block, J. (1977). Advancing the science of personality: Paradigmatic shift or improving the quality of research? In D. Magnusson and N.S. Endler (Eds.), *Psychology at the crossroads: Current issues in interactional psychology* (pp. 37–63). Hillsdale, N.J.: Erlbaum.

Buss, D.M., & Craik, K.H. (1983). The act frequency approach to personality. *Psychological Review, 90,* 105–126.

Carlson, R. (1981). Studies in script theory: Adult analogs of a childhood nuclear scene. *Journal of Personality and Social Psychology, 40,* 501–510.

Carlson, R. (1986). After analysis: A study of transference dreams following treatment. *Journal of Consulting and Clinical Psychology, 54,* 246–252.

Duhl, B.S., & Duhl, F.J. (1981). Integrative family therapy. In A.S. Gurman & D.P. Kniskern (Eds.), *Handbook of family therapy* (pp. 483–513). New York: Brunner/Mazel.

Emmons, R.A. (1986). Personal strivings: An approach to personality and subjective well-being. *Journal of Personality and Social Psychology, 51,* 1058–1068.

Emmons, R.A., & King, L.A. (1988). Conflict among personal strivings: Immediate and long-term implications for psychological and physical well-being. *Journal of Personality and Social Psychology, 54,* 1040–1048.

Freud, S. (1976). *Therapy and technique.* New York: MacMillan. (Original work published 1912)

Horney, K. (1945). *Our inner conflicts: A constructive theory of neurosis.* New York: Norton.

Jones, E.E., & Thorne, A. (1987). Rediscovery of the subject: Intercultural approaches to clinical assessment. *Journal of Consulting and Clinical Psychology, 55,* 488–495.

Little, B.R. (1983). Personal projects: A rationale and method for investigation. *Environment and Behavior, 15,* 273–309.

Luborsky, L. (1978). *The Core Conflictual Relationship Theme (CCRT) method: Guide to scoring and rationale.* Unpublished manuscript, Hospital of the University of Pennsylvania, Philadelphia.

Luborsky, L., Mellon, J., van Ravenswaay, P., Childress, A.R., Cohen, K.D., Hole, A.V., Ming. S., Crits-Christoph, P., Levine, F.J., & Alexander, K. (1985). A verification of Freud's grandest clinical hypothesis: The transference. *Clinical Psychology Review, 5,* 231–246.

Luborsky, L. Crits-Christoph, P., Mintz, J., & Auerbach, A. (1988). *Who will benefit from psychotherapy?* New York: Basic Books.

McAdams, D.P. (1985). *Power, intimacy, and the life story: Personological inquiries into identity.* Homewood, IL: Dorsey Press.

Markus, H., & Nurius, P. (1986). Possible selves. *American Psychologist, 41,* 954–69.

Mischel, W. (1968). *Personality and assessment.* New York: Wiley.

Moskowitz, D.S. (1988). Cross-situational generality in the laboratory: Dominance and friendliness. *Journal of Personality and Social Psychology, 54,* 829–839.

Murray, H. (1938). *Explorations in personality.* New York: Oxford University Press.

Orford, J. (1986). The rules of interpersonal complementarity: Does hostility beget hostility and dominance, submission? *Psychological Review, 93,* 365–377.

Sullivan, H.S. (1940). *Conceptions of modern psychiatry.* New York: Norton.

Thorne, A. (1983). *Disposition as interpersonal constraint.* Unpublished doctoral dissertation, University of California, Berkeley.

Thorne, A. (1985, August). Using interactants' accounts to interpersonalize personality theory. In P.F. Secord (Chair), *Uses of interactants' accounts in interpersonal research*. Symposium conducted at the meeting of the American Psychological Association, Los Angeles.

Thorne, A. (1986, August). Toward an interpersonology. In J.M. Cheek (Chair), *Evolutionary biology and future directions in personality psychology*. Symposium conducted at the meeting of the American Psychological Association, Washington, D.C.

Thorne, A. (1987). The press of personality: A study of conversations between introverts and extraverts. *Journal of Personality and Social Psychology, 53*, 718–726.

Tomkins, S.S. (1979). Script theory: Differential magnification of affects. In H.E. Howe, Jr., & R.A. Dienstbier (Eds.), *Nebraska Symposium on Motivation* (Vol. 26, pp. 741–746). Lincoln: University of Nebraska Press.

Wright, J.C., & Mischel, W. (1987). A conditional approach to dispositional constructs: The local predictability of social behavior. *Journal of Personality and Social Psychology, 53*, 1159–1177.

Wright, J.C., & Mischel, W. (1988). Conditional hedges and the intuitive psychology of traits. *Journal of Personality and Social Psychology, 55*, 454–469.

CHAPTER 11

The Development of a Narrative Identity

Dan P. McAdams

My own research and theorizing over the past ten years may be situated within that maverick tradition in the social sciences called "the study of lives" or "the personological tradition"—historically associated with the approaches advanced by Murray (1938), White (1966, 1981), and Tomkins (1987), among others. As Murray envisioned it over fifty years ago, the personologist should endeavor to study the whole person and to comprehend the structure and the content of his or her life in its full socio-historical context. Following Murray's (1938) lead in *Explorations in Personality,* personologists have traditionally placed prime emphasis on *motivation* and *biography* in their own empirical explorations of the whole person.

Motivation and Biography

Murray understood human motivation in terms of a collection of psychogenic needs, each of which was viewed as an enduring underlying disposition which energizes, directs, and selects behavior, though always within an environmental context, or what Murray termed a "press." I have focused on two needs, or "motives," ultimately derived from Murray's list. Both motives are measured through objective content analysis of the Thematic Apperception Test (TAT), an assessment device invented by Murray and Morgan (Morgan & Murray, 1935). The first of these is the *intimacy motive,* defined as a recurrent preference or readiness for warm, close, and sharing interaction with other people (McAdams, 1980). The intimacy motive is an underlying desire to share oneself with another—to engage in the kind of intimate and intensive quality of interpersonal experience described by Buber (1970) as the I-Thou encounter. Research has suggested that people who are high in intimacy motivation, as assessed on the TAT, spend more time thinking about other people and their relationships with them, engage in more mutual conversations with people, smile and show more eye contact in friendly encounters, disclose more about themselves when they are with their friends, and even show slightly higher levels on certain dimensions of psychological well-being, compared to people low in intimacy motivation (McAdams & Bryant, 1987; McAdams & Constantian, 1983; McAdams, Healy, & Krause, 1984; McAdams, Jackson, & Kirshnit, 1984; McAdams & Vaillant, 1982; Zeldow, Daugherty, & McAdams, 1988).

The second is the *power motive,* defined as a recurrent preference for having an impact on other people and on one's environment (Winter, 1973). A large body of research investigating individual differences in power motivation supports the construct validity of the TAT-system developed by Winter (1973). People high in power motivation seek to make strong impacts on their worlds in many ways—rising to positions of leadership in organizations, influencing others in authoritative ways in decision-making groups, collecting prestige possessions, speaking out and taking big risks, and so forth (Fodor & Smith, 1982; McClelland, 1975; McClelland & Boyatzis, 1982; Veroff, 1982; Winter, 1973; Winter & Stewart, 1978).

With respect to the personological emphasis on biography, Murray wrote, "the history of the organism *is* the organism"—"this proposition calls for biographical studies" (p. 39). For Murray, however, biographical studies meant more than merely collecting life histories. The personologist was to construct biographies, too. White (1981) describes Murray's commitment to biography:

Murray envisioned a time when scientific psychology would be able to write abstract biographies, expressed in a generalized notation derived from a common conceptual scheme. Such biographies would be the scientific contribution to understanding personality, in contrast to, though much indebted to, the literary contribution. (p. 12).

My own approach to the study of lives is in fact doubly biographical. First, I record autobiographies, as people relate them to me in lengthy interviews. Second, I listen to these accounts with the ear of a biographer, as described by Edel (1978): "When the biographer can discover a myth, he has found his story. He knows the meaning of his material and can choose, select, sift, without deceiving himself about the subject of his work" (p. 2). To "find the story" is to discover what Erikson (1959) calls *identity*. This is the main thesis of my work: *Identity is a life story*—an internalized narrative integration of past, present, and anticipated future which provides lives with a sense of unity and purpose (McAdams, 1985, 1987, in press). Let us interpret Murray quite literally: "The history of the organism *is* the organism." A person is, among other things, a history. A person's internalized and idiosyncratic historical rendering of his or her own life defines the person.

As a person constructs his or her own identity over the life span, he or she consciously and unconsciously composes a narrative of the self, a mythological integration of setting, scene, character, plot, and theme. MacIntyre (1981) writes, "The unity of a human life is the unity of a narrative quest" (p. 219). Similarly, Sartre suggests, "This is what fools people: a man is always a teller of tales, he lives surrounded by his stories and the stories of others, he sees everything that happens to him through them; and he tries to live his life as if he were telling a story" (in Charme, 1984, p. 9). Erikson, too, implies that the identity configuration that is consolidated in adulthood may take the form of an historical narrative when he writes, "the adult is able to selectively reconstruct his past in such a way that, step for step, it seems to have planned him, or better, he seems to have planned it" (1958, p. 112). A major task for the personologist, therefore, is discerning the story, interpreting the autobiographical text, ultimately cataloguing and classifying stories, to determine how a particular life story is, in certain aspects, like all other stories, like some other stories, and, finally, like no other story (Kluckhohn & Murray, 1953).

How is it that, over the human life span, the person comes to compose a self-defining story which confers upon life a sense of unity and purpose? After Erikson, I submit that the story-making becomes an explicit and self-conscious affair in late adolescence and young adulthood—during that period Erikson deems to be critical for identity formation. For the first time in the life cycle, the young person adopts an historical perspective on the self. But the origins of story-making reside in childhood, I believe, and the process of composing the narrative may extend into old age. Let me sketch briefly, then, my current provisional view of this process of creating and recreating a narrative identity over the life span. (A substantially more detailed presentation appears in McAdams, in press). Figure 11.1 provides a schematic outline of the main concepts to be discussed.

Infancy and Childhood: Tone, Image, Theme

Erikson (1963) and others (Bowlby, 1969; Sroufe, 1979) have argued that the psychosocial centerpiece of the first years of life is the developing bond of love between the caregiver and the infant. The development of caregiver-infant attachment organizes experiences of trust and mistrust, security and anxiety in the first year of life. The lifelong legacy of attachment is a pervasive and unconscious attitude about people, the world, and the self (Shaver & Rubenstein, 1980). Erikson calls this attitude "hope." He writes, "Hope is the enduring belief in the attainability of fervent wishes, in spite of the dark urges and rages which mark the beginning of existence" (1964, p. 118). The infant emerges from the first year of life in the family with an unconscious and "enduring belief"

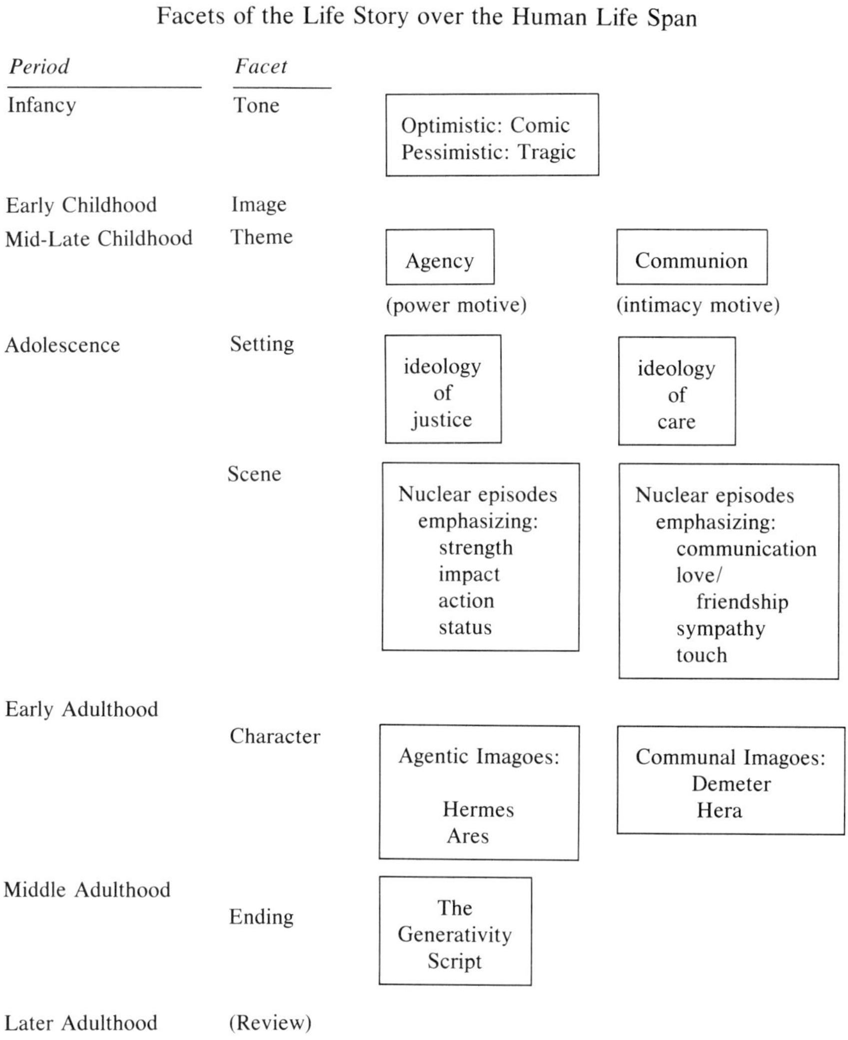

Facets of the Life Story over the Human Life Span

Period	Facet		
Infancy	Tone	Optimistic: Comic Pessimistic: Tragic	
Early Childhood	Image		
Mid-Late Childhood	Theme	Agency (power motive)	Communion (intimacy motive)
Adolescence	Setting	ideology of justice	ideology of care
	Scene	Nuclear episodes emphasizing: strength impact action status	Nuclear episodes emphasizing: communication love/ friendship sympathy touch
Early Adulthood	Character	Agentic Imagoes: Hermes Ares	Communal Imagoes: Demeter Hera
Middle Adulthood	Ending	The Generativity Script	
Later Adulthood	(Review)		

FIGURE 11.1

concerning the extent to which wishes, or intentions, are "attainable." According to Bruner (1986), the essence of a story is that it "deals with the vicissitudes of *intention*" (p. 17). To the extent, therefore, that the bond of love between infant and caregiver provides an enduring belief in the attainability of human intentions, Erikson's hope is fundamentally a perspective *on narrative* as well. A hopeful, optimistic narrative *tone* or attitude suggests that human beings are capable of attaining their "fervent wishes," that human intentions may be realized over time. It suggests that the world is relatively predictable, that things work out in the long run, that stories have happy endings, as they often do in *comedy* and *romance* (Frye, 1957). A relatively hopeless, pessimistic narrative tone or attitude suggests that human beings do not get what they wish for, that human intentions are repeatedly foiled over time. From a more pessimistic perspective, the world is capricious and unpredictable, narratives take unforeseen turns, things rarely work out over time, and stories have unhappy endings, as they often do in *tragedy* and *irony* (Frye, 1957).

Secure attachment in the first year of life may plant the seeds of hopeful and trusting stories to come. Even though the infant does not yet know what a story is, secure attachment may predispose him or her in later years to imbue narrative—stories of all kinds, including those constructed about the self—with a generally hopeful quality or tone. The infant whose attachment bond is relatively insecure, by contrast, may be predisposed to imbue narrative with a negative, pessimistic quality. This does not mean that secure attachment guarantees a happy life or an especially coherent identity. Indeed, stories with negative tone may be just as integrative—just as unifying and purposeful—as stories that are more positive. A well-formed identity in adulthood does not have to be a story suggesting that "they all lived happily ever after." But the quality of the attachment bonds in infancy may, in concert with other as-yet-undetermined early influences, play a subtle role in the development of a characteristic intonation in narrative identity. Attachment may exert a long-term and perhaps indirect influence on identity through a legacy of trust vs. mistrust—a general and preverbal feeling/belief about the "storied" nature of human life (Sarbin, 1986).

For nursery-school children in Piaget's cognitive stage of "preoperational thought," stories provide a rich stock of *images* that may become the raw stuff, later transformed and refined, of narratives of the self. Preoperational thinking is fluid and magical, unrestrained by the dictates of logical operations. The child represents the world in symbols and images, but he or she does not insist that these semiotic representations remain true to logic or context. For the four-year-old, Cinderella can be dead one minute and alive the next. She can perform actions that are completely at odds with her original narrative context. Although Cinderella is forever dutiful and sweet, preferring dancing to fighting in the fairy tale itself, the child may decide in her fantasy play that Cinderella should do battle one afternoon with the Wicked Witch of the West—with swords yet—and that the two of them should sit down afterwards to have tea with Jesus. What appeals most to four-year-olds about stories is their egocentric appropriation of image, not the coherent narrative itself. This kind of fantasy-based egocentrism is a hallmark of preoperational thought.

The child's world of make-believe is populated with figures, symbols, pictures, and other idiosyncratic mental representations that are heavily laden with affect. The major sources of these images are the family, peers, schools and churches, books, and especially the media. Fowler (1981) writes that religious traditions provide some of the most enduring images for stories. For example, children raised in Christian families develop rich imagery associated with angel, serpent, devil, star, lamb, cross, etc. In Fowler's view, religious meaning is conveyed through image in the preoperational stage. God is an old man with a white beard. Jesus is a soft baby.

Later in the elementary-school years, as the child enters concrete operations, images are situated in narrative context. The eight-year-old may know that Jesus was a baby born in a manger because there was no room in the inn. He grew up and did a lot of things. God created the heaven and earth in six days and then rested on the seventh. After that, he did a lot of things, too. In elementary school, children come to understand implicitly that narratives organize human intentions in time, as Bruner (1986) maintains. In short, the older child's approach to story moves beyond image to *theme*.

Themes are recurrent patterns of motivational content in stories, as when characters repeatedly strive to attain a particular goal over time. Indeed, a story is more than a collection of images: a story gives form to *human motivation*. Stories tell us what characters are trying to do, what they want, and how they go about getting or not getting what they want over time.

Elementary-school children, therefore, are able to organize the "vicissitudes of human intention" (Bruner, 1987) into coherent narratives with beginnings, middles, and endings (Applebee, 1978). The story is the most natural vehicle for transporting the meaning and the course of human intentions. Until children understand what a story is, they may be unable to comprehend the world and themselves in terms of human intentions organized in time. This does not mean, however, that even infants do not "intend" to do things. Indeed, Piaget (1952) has traced the origins of intentionality back to the primary circular reactions of ages one to four months. But infants and very young children do not conceptualize intentions as springing from internal wants and desires that they "have" and upon which they may act over time in order to achieve a desired end state (Kegan, 1982). They are not able to sustain the kind of distance of consciousness which suggests that I (a subject, a character) have (possess, own) an intention (an object), or that the intention exists "inside of me," as something upon which I may, or may not, act. Narrative action is guided by intentions, as characters choose to pursue certain goal states over time. Goal-directed activity ends when the goal is achieved or when the achievement is blocked, or when the character's intentions change.

Two superordinate end states in stories of many sorts—goals recurrently desired by many different kinds of characters—are what Bakan (1966) has termed *agency* and *communion*. Agency denotes themes of power, separation, mastery, control, and isolation. Communion denotes themes of intimacy, love, cooperation, and merger. In most general terms, many of the greatest stories in Western cultures concern agency and communion, tales in which characters strive for *glory* and *love, separation and closeness, mastery and merger*. These two general thematic lines are partially captured in the TAT scoring systems for power and intimacy motivation respectively. People high in power motivation should fashion relatively agentic life stories; people high in intimacy should emphasize communal themes in identity. The origins of power and intimacy motivation—as enduring underlying dispositions of personality—may reside in the school-child's relation to narrative. Largely through the stories they hear and create, children in elementary school may be gathering together their motivational resources, eventually consolidating their various wants, desires, and intentions within broad motivational dispositions, such as the power and intimacy motives.

Adolescence and Young Adulthood: Setting and Scene

The boy or girl on the brink of adolescence has already formed conscious and unconscious preferences and inclinations regarding the narrative aspects of tone, image, and theme. Now the child is ready to begin the work of formulating a setting for his or her own life story. The setting is ideological. The emergence of formal operational thinking in adolescence catalyzes the development of ideology. The formal thinker is blessed now with the power of abstract thought and the ability to reason about what is hypothetical and what is real from many different perspectives (Inhelder & Piaget, 1958). As a result, the adolescent is inclined to ponder such abstract questions as "What is good and evil?" and "What is true?" The young person may initially latch on to conventional religious creeds and ethical dogmas that systematize abstract answers to questions of ultimate concern. And he or she may eventually question such systems, developing alternative and more personalized ideologies as he or she matures into young adulthood (McAdams, Booth, & Selvik, 1981). Erikson considers the formation of a coherent ideology to be a prerequisite for identity formation. The adolescent mind "is an ideological mind, indeed, it is the ideological outlook of society that speaks most clearly to the adolescent who is eager to be affirmed by his peers, and is ready to be confirmed by rituals, creeds, and programs which at the same time define what is evil, uncanny, and inimical" (Erikson, 1963, p. 263).

One's more or less systematic solution to ideological concerrns—generally crystallized in late adolescence—functions as an *ideological setting* or backdrop for the emerging life story—a story that is a partial integration of story elements from the past. The ideological setting situates the action of the story within a particular locus of belief and value—a locus shaped by society's conventions regarding the good and the true and the individual's struggles to find meaning within or outside of convention. There are many different ways to map the ideological terrain in a given life story. A very simple and useful approach, however, is suggested by Gilligan (1982) and Forsyth (1985). Gilligan distinguishes between an ideology of justice and individual rights on the one hand and an ideology of care and social responsibilities on the other. The two approaches mirror Bakan's distinction between agency and communion. An ethic of justice suggests an agentic ideological setting in which individuals are viewed as autonomous agents who, in their ultimate individuality, are likely now and again to clash. Justice sorts out what is fair when independent agents, each granted basic individual rights, come into conflict with each other. Gilligan's ethic of care suggests a communal ideological setting in which individuals are interdependent parts of larger networks. One's duties to specific others within the network must be evaluated according to standards of care and compassion. These two approaches to ideology may be understood as making up orthogonal dimensions of ideology, yielding four different types of ideological settings, as shown in Figure 11.2.

If ideology forms a setting for one's emerging narrative identity in late adolescence, then some of the critical action of the narrative is captured in key life story *scenes,* or what I call *nuclear episodes.* For reasons that are cognitive, physiological, and societal, it is in adolescence that the person is likely to view his or her life in historical terms for the first time (Elkind, 1981; Hankiss, 1981; McAdams, 1985a). As an adolescent, I know that I am no longer a child. I am now something different—indeed, I even look very different. But I am not exactly sure what I am. I now have a history: I was something, and now I am something else. What was I? What am I now? What will I be in the future? What is the relation between past, present, and future? Hankiss (1981) writes that the adolescent "mythologically re-arranges" his or her own past in order to develop a story of the self that explains who he or she is, was, and will be. Certain scenes from the past are imbued with strong symbolic meaning; others are neglected, even forgotten. The key scenes may be viewed as origin myths, telling how I first came to be a certain way, or as transformation scenes, telling how I quit being one way and started being another. Nuclear episodes, therefore, stand out in bold print in the life story, as narrative high points, low points, and turning points explaining how the person has remained the same and how he or she has changed over time.

In adolescence, one's initial narrative renditions of self may assume fantastical forms. Elkind (1981) writes of the *personal fable* of adolescence. A personal fable is a fantastical story of greatness and uniqueness that some teenagers make up about themselves. Elkind views these unrealistic narratives as cognitive mistakes or egocentrisms of adolescence, inevitable results of not quite knowing how to reign in the power of formal operational thought. The personal fable fades with experience and maturity. In my view, the personal fable may be seen as a first and very

Four Types of Ideological Settings

Hi Agency

Ethic of justice; individual rights	Ethic of justice and care; "situationist" (Forsyth)
Ethic of pragmatics; "exceptionist" (Forsyth)	Ethic of care; communal responsibilities

Lo ——————————————————— Hi Communion

Lo

FIGURE 11.2

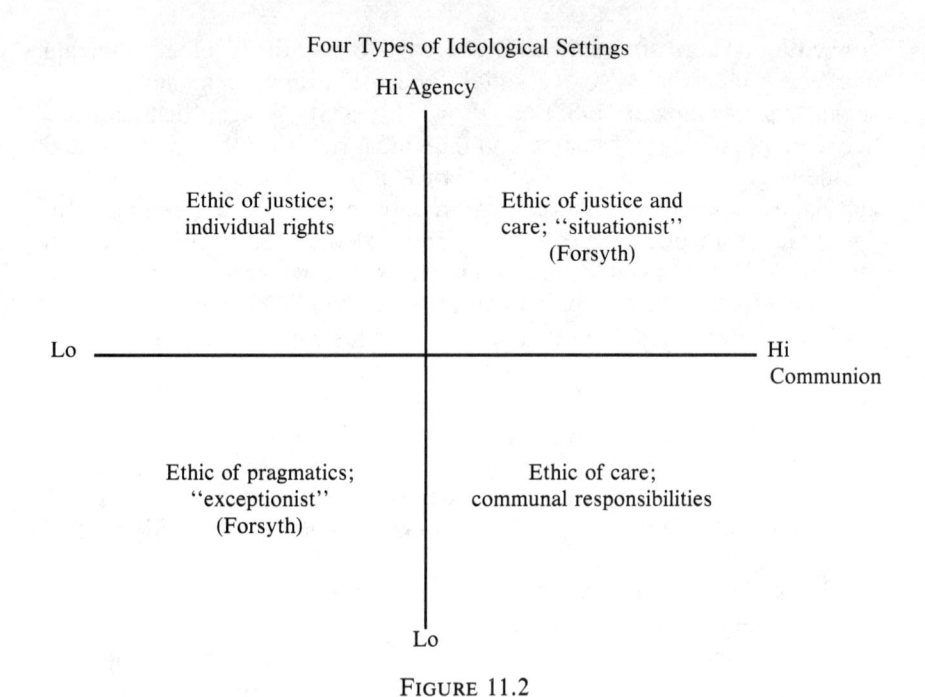

rough draft of identity, incorporating the tone, images, and themes most prevalent in childhood. It is eventually edited, rewritten, reworked, and made more realistic as the young person becomes more and more knowledgable about the opportunities and limitations of defining the self in his or her particular society. As we formulate more mature life stories, we come to realize that other people have their own stories—both similar to and different from ours—and that we all live within a historical and social matrix embodying its own narrative parameters. Fashioning a life story is always a psycho-*social* endeavor. In a sense, society and the individual work on the story together. Bruner (1960) writes that the "mythologically instructed community provides its members with a library of scripts" against which the individual may judge his or her own "internal drama" (p. 281). "Life, then, produces myth, and finally imitates it" (p. 283).

The scenes that stand out in bold print in a person's historical rendering of self reflect the dual thematic lines of agency and communion. For instance, persons high in power motivation tend to recall and describe nuclear episodes from their life stories emphasizing themes of strength, impact, action, and status. Individuals high in intimacy motivation, by contrast, highlight themes of love and liking, communication, sympathy for others, and tender interpersonal touch (McAdams, 1982, 1985a; McAdams, Booth, & Selvik, 1981).

Adulthood: Character, Ending

In the years of early and middle adulthood, the emphasis in identity work shifts from setting and scene to the refinement of narrative *character* (McAdams, 1985b, in press). The identity task during this time involves identifying, articulating, and refining the main character(s) in one's own life story. The main characters are *idealized and personified images of self,* or what I have termed *imagoes* (McAdams, 1984, 1985b). The concept of the imago shares meaning with such concepts as "personification" (Sullivan, 1953), "subself" (Martindale, 1980), and "possible selves" (Markus & Nurius, 1986). Each life story may contain one or more imagoes, functioning as semi-autonomous protagonists whose actions and conflicts determine the major movements of the plot. In his analysis of the identity structure of George Bernard Shaw, Erikson (1959) identified three such protagonists in Shaw's story: Shaw "the snob," Shaw "the noisemaker," and Shaw "the diabolical one." As Shaw matured and his identity took on a more integrated form, these three imagoes coalesced into one: Shaw "the actor."

As idealized and personified images of the self, imagoes cut across many different life and life-story domains. They are larger than situationally specific roles, and rather integrate numerous roles to suggest unity and purpose in life. For example, an individual may see him- or herself as the sophisticated and intellectual professor, the rough-around-the-edges working boy or girl from the wrong side of town, the consummate caregiver always available to those in need, the corporate executive playing out the American dream, the worldly traveller in search of the new and exotic, the athlete, the sage, the soldier, the teacher, the clown, or the peacemaker. Each of these is larger and more encompassing than a socially defined role, integrating a wide variety of information about the self. Each might qualify as an imago. Imagoes exist as highly personalized and intricately crafted parts of the self, and they may be highlighted as protagonists in certain chapters of the adult's life story, expressed through a particular subset of the adult's values and interests, and often embodied in external role models and other significant people in the adult's life.

I have delineated a provisional taxonomy of imago types, organized along the content dimensions of Bakan's (1966) agency and communion. Names for the imago types are derived from the mythology of ancient Greece (McAdams, 1985b). For instance, two prominent agentic imagoes are Ares the warrior/soldier and Hermes the adventurer/explorer. Two prominent communal imagoes are Demeter the caregiver/martyr and Hera the loyal friend/confidante. Analyzing the life-story interviews of fifty men and women in their 30s and 40s, I found that adults displaying prominent agentic imagoes in their life stories tend to score very high on the power motive, assessed via TAT, whereas adults displaying communal imagoes are high in intimacy motivation (McAdams, 1984, 1985a).

Having established an ideological setting and developed an historical perspective for identity in late adolescence and young adulthood, the adult then faces the narrative challenge of characterization. What are the main characters in my life story? How were they born? How will they develop? How will they flourish and fail? How do they relate to each other? What kind of story are they trying to tell? Watkins (1986) conceives of the adult self as a grand chorus of internalized characters who engage in "imaginal dialogues" with each other. She argues that the adult who seeks psychological maturity must engender and promote the "animation," "articulation," and "specification" of each of the many characters within the self (pp. 114–116). These characters may conflict with each other, revealing major rifts and contradictions within the self. Two hallmarks of mature identity in the adult years are (1) the full articulation and expression of different imageos in a life story and (2) the integration or reconciliation of conflicting imageos. An example of the latter is Erikson's characterization of Shaw, whose life story integrated three subordinate images into a larger personified and idealized image of self as "the actor."

As many scholars of narrative point out, the ending of a story shapes all that comes before it (Charme, 1984). A good story leaves the reader with the impression that the scenes, the characters, and the plot were all developed by the author to lead up to a particular and appropriate ending. If identity is an integrative life narrative establishing unity and purpose in the self, then the adult who seeks to define who he or she is and how he or she fits into the adult world must be concerned with how all of this is going to end. The concern may be something of a preoccupation at mid-life when one comes to realize that one's life is probably at least half over, and that time can now be understood in terms of how much is left rather than how much has passed (Jacques, 1965; Marshall, 1975). As one grows older, experiences of loss become more salient, as in loss of others through the death of one's parents and friends and through separations from children who have moved away, loss of vitality through changes in athletic and reproductive abilities, and loss of hopes and aspirations through the inevitable instrumental and interpersonal disappointments accompanying adult life (Levinson, 1978).

Many of the salient and troubling issues of mid-life, therefore, may revolve around one's inescapable mortality. Many psychologists have outlined developmental trends in mid life—some adaptive (Gutman, 1982; Jung, 1961) and some less so (Lownethal, Thurnher, & Chiriboga, 1975)—that appear, on one level or another, to be psychological responses to the increasing awareness of one's mortality. Many normative and individual changes at this time may make their way into the life story, transforming the past, present, and expectations for the future, and rewriting the narrative to accomodate the growing realization that the *end* is nearer than one would like.

The aspect of the life story that is directly implicated in the construction of narrative endings is what I call the *generativity script*. The generativity script is the adult's plan or outline specifying what he or she hopes to *do* in order to leave legacy of the self for the next generation. According to Kotre (1984), generativity involves "the desire to invest one's substance in forms of life and work that will *outlive the self*" (p. 10). Becker (1973) describes a similar concept, which he calls *heroism*. Through heroism, human beings affirm "that the things [and the ideas and the people] that man creates in society are of lasting worth and meaning, that they outlive or outshine death and decay, that man and his products count" (p. 5). Cognizant that one's life is at least half over, the adult at mid-life and after may seek to fashion a legacy of the self that lives on—that outshines death and decay. To be generative is to fashion some life product (a career, a child, a family business, an idea, a legacy of hard work, a piece of advice), to care for and nurture the product, and ultimately to give the product up, to grant it its own autonomy—indeed, its own identity—in order to promote some aspect of the human enterprise. One's generativity script may be as humble as a foreman's plan to improve working conditions in a factory in order to benefit those under him, or a woman's regular service as a girl-scout leader. Or it can be as grand as Mahatma Gandhi's mission to care for an entire nation, as described by Erikson (1969):

From the moment in January of 1915 when Gandhi set foot on a pier reserved for important arrivals in Bombay, he behaved like a man who knew the nature and the extent of India's calamity and that of his own fundamental mission. A mature man of middle age has not only made up his mind as to what, in the various compartments of his life, he does and does not *care for,* he is also firm in his vision of what he *will* and *can* take *care of*. He takes as his baseline what he irreducibly is and reaches out for what only he can, and therefore, must do. (p. 255).

Although Erikson views generativity as a stage separate from identity, I view the generativity script as a key life story component that is likely to occupy one's story-telling efforts in middle adulthood and after. Thus, generativity is part and parcel of identity, especially in mid-life and after. The generativity script functions to extend the life story line into an envisioned future beyond the limits of one's own lifetime. It provides a satisfying story ending, if you will, while suggesting at the same time that the story does not *really* end. In light of the major concerns of the middle years, the generativity script may serve as a narrative answer to the problem of the mortality of the self. Thus, the envisioned ending of a person's life story generates new stories which outlive the person, assuring the continuity of the original story, the original identity, into the next generation and, maybe, beyond.

References

Applebee, A.N. (1978). *The child's concept of story*. Chicago: The University of Chicago Press.
Bakan, D. (1966). *The duality of human existence: Isolation and communion in Western man*. Boston: Beacon Press.
Becker, E. (1973). *The denial of death*. New York: The Free Press.
Bowlby, J. (1969). *Attachment and loss: Vol. 1. Attachment*. New York: Basic Books.
Bruner, J.S. (1960). Myth and identity. In H.A. Murray (Ed.), *Myth and mythmaking*. New York: George Braziller.
Bruner, J.S. (1986). *Actual minds, possible worlds*. Cambridge, MA: Harvard University Press.
Buber, M. (1970). *I and Thou*. New York: Charles Scribner's Sons.
Charme, S.L. (1984). *Meaning and myth in the study of lives: A Sartrean perspective*. Philadelphia: University of Pennsylvania Press.
Edel, L. (1978). Biography: A manifesto. *Biography: An Interdisciplinary Quarterly, 1,* 1–3.
Elkind, D. (1981). *Children and adolescents: Interpretive essays on Jean Piaget* (3rd ed.). New York: Oxford University Press.
Erikson, E.H. (1958). *Young man Luther: A study in psychoanalysis and history*. New York: Norton.
Erikson, E.H. (1959). Identity and the life cycle: Selected papers. *Psychological Issues, 1* (1), 5–165.
Erikson, E.H. (1963). *Childhood and society* (2nd ed.). New York: Norton.
Erikson, E.H. (1964). *Insight and responsibility*. New York: Norton.
Erikson, E.H. (1969). *Gandhi's truth: On the origins of military nonviolence*. New York: Norton.
Fodor, E.M., & Smith, T. (1982). The power motive as an influence on group decision making. *Journal of Personality and Social Psychology, 42,* 178–185.
Forsyth, D.R. (1985). Individual differences in information processing during moral judgment. *Journal of Personality and Social Psychology, 49,* 264–272.
Fowler, J.W. (1981). *Stages of faith: The psychology of human development and the quest for meaning*. New York: Harper & Row.
Frye, N. (1957). *The anatomy of criticism*. Princeton, NJ: Princeton University Press.
Gilligan, C. (1982). *In a different voice*. Cambridge, MA: Harvard University Press.
Gutmann, D.L. (1980). The postparental years: Clinical problems and developmental possibilities. In W.H. Norman and T.J. Scaramella (Eds.), *Mid-life: Developmental and clinical issues* (pp. 38–52). New York: Bruner/Mazel.
Hankiss, A. (1981). Ontologies of the self: On the mythological rearranging of one's life history. In D. Bertaux (Ed.), *Biography and society: The life history history approach in the social sciences* (pp. 203–209). Beverly Hills, CA: Sage.
Inhelder, B., & Piaget, J. (1958). *The growth of logical thinking from childhood to adolescence*. New York: Basic Books.
Jacques, E. (1965). Death and the midlife crisis. *International Journal of Psychoanalysis, 46,* 502–514.
Jung, C.G. (1961). *Memories, dreams, reflections*. New York: Random House.

Kegan, R. (1982). *The evolving self: Problems and process in human development.* Cambridge, MA: Harvard University Press.

Kluckhohn, C., & Murray, H.A. (1953). Personality formation: The determinants. In C. Kluckhohn, H.A. Murray, and D.M. Schneider (Eds.), *Personality in nature, society, and culture* (pp. 53–67). New York: Alfred A. Knopf.

Kotre, J. (1984). *Outliving the self: Generativity and the interpretation of lives.* Baltimore, MD: Johns Hopkins University Press.

Levinson, D.J. (1978). *The seasons of a man's life.* New York: Alfred A. Knopf.

Lowenthal, M.F., Thurnher, M., Chiriboga, D., & Associates. (1975). *Four stages of life: A comparative study of men and women facing transitions.* San Francisco: Jossey-Bass.

MacIntyre, A. (1981). *After virtue.* Notre Dame, IN: University of Notre Dame Press.

Markus, H., & Nurius, P. (1986). Possible selves. *American Psychologist, 41,* 954–969.

Marshall, V. (1975). Age and awareness of finitude in developmental gerontology. *Omega, 6,* 113–129.

Martindale, C. (1980). Subselves: The internal representation of situational and personal dispositions. In L. Wheeler (Ed.), *Review of personality and social psychology* (Vol. 1, pp. 193–218). Beverly Hills, CA: Sage.

McAdams, D.P. (1980). A thematic coding system for the intimacy motive. *Journal of Research in Personality, 14,* 413–432.

McAdams, D.P. (1982). Experiences of intimacy and power: Relationships between social motives and autobiographical memory. *Journal of Personality and Social Psychology, 42,* 292–302.

McAdams, D.P. (1984). Love, power, and images of the self. In C.Z. Malatesta and C.E. Izard (Eds.), *Emotion in adult development* (pp. 159–174). Beverly Hills, CA: Sage.

McAdams, D.P. (1985a). *Power, intimacy, and the life story: Personological inquiries into identity.* New York: Guilford.

McAdams, D.P. (1985b). The "imago": A key narrative component of identity. In P. Shaver (Ed.), *Review of personality and social psychology: Vol. 6. Self, situations, and social behavior* (pp. 115–141). Beverly Hills, CA: Sage.

McAdams, D.P. (1987). A life-story model of identity. In R. Hogan and W.H. Jones (Eds.), *Perspectives in personality* (Vol. 2, pp. 15–50). Greenwich, CT: JAI Press.

McAdams, D.P. (in press). Unity and purpose in human lives: The emergence of identity as a life story. In A.I. Rabin (Ed.), *Studying persons and lives.* New York: Springer.

McAdams, D.P., Booth, L., & Selvik, R. (1981). Religious identity among students at a private college: Social motives, ego stage, and development. *Merrill-Palmer Quarterly, 27,* 219–239.

McAdams, D.P., & Bryant, F.B. (1987). Intimacy motivation and subjective mental health in a nationwide sample. *Journal of Personality, 55,* 395–413.

McAdams, D.P., & Constantian, C.A. (1983). Intimacy and affiliation motives in daily living: An experience sampling analysis. *Journal of Personality and Social Psychology, 45,* 851–861.

McAdams, D.P., Healy, S., & Krause, S. (1984). Social motives and patterns of friendship. *Journal of Personality and Social Psychology, 47,* 828–838.

McAdams, D.P., Jackson, R.J., & Kirshnit, C. (1984). Looking, laughing, and smiling in dyads as a function of intimacy motivation and reciprocity. *Journal of Personality, 52,* 261–273.

McAdams, D.P., & Vaillant, G.E. (1982). Intimacy motivation and psychosocial adjustment: A longitudinal study. *Journal of Personality Assessment, 46,* 586–593.

McClelland, D.C. (1975). *Power: The inner experience.* New York: Irvington.

McClelland, D.C., & Boyatzis, R.E. (1982). The leadership motive pattern and long-term success in management. *Journal of Applied Psychology, 67,* 737–743.

Morgan, C.D., & Murray, H.A. (1935). A method of investigating fantasies: The Thematic Apperception Test. *Archives of Neurology and Psychiatry, 34,* 289–306.

Murray, H.A. (1938). *Explorations in personality.* New York: Oxford University Press.

Piaget, J. (1952). *The origins of intelligence in children.* New York: International Universities Press.

Sarbin, T.R. (1986). (Ed.). *The storied nature of human conduct.* New York: Praeger.

Shaver, P., & Rubenstein, C. (1980). Childhood attachment experience and adult loneliness. In L. Wheeler (Ed.), *Review of personality and social psychology* (Vol. 1, pp. 43–73). Beverly Hills, CA: Sage.

Sroufe, L.A. (1979). The coherence of individual development: Early care, attachment, and subsequent developmental issues. *American Psychologist, 34,* 834–841.

Sullivan, H.S. (1953). *The interpersonal theory of psychiatry.* New York: Norton.

Tomkins, S.S. (1987). Script theory. In J. Aronoff, A.I. Rabin, and R.A. Zucker (Eds.), *The emergence of personality* (pp. 147–216). New York: Springer.

Veroff, J. (1982). Assertive motivations: Achievement versus power. In A.J. Stewart (Ed.), *Motivation and society* (pp. 99–132). San Francisco: Jossey-Bass.

Watkins, M. (1986). *Invisible guests: The development of imaginal dialogues.* Hillsdale, NJ: The Analytic Press.

White, R.W. (1966). *Lives in progress* (2nd ed.). New York: Holt, Rinehart & Winston.

White, R.W. (1981). Exploring personality the long way: The study of lives. In A.I. Rabin, J. Aronoff, A.M. Barclay, and R.A. Zucker (Eds.), *Further explorations in personality* (pp. 3–19). New York: Wiley.

Winter, D.G. (1973). *The power motive.* New York: The Free Press.

Winter, D.G., & Stewart, A.J. (1978). The power motive. In H. London and J.E. Exner, Jr. (Eds.), *Dimensions of personality* (pp. 391–447). New York: Wiley.

Zeldow, P.B., Daugherty, S.R., & McAdams, D.P. (1988). Intimacy, power, and psychological well-being in medical students. *Journal of Nervous and Mental Disease, 176,* 182–187.

Part III
Advances in Assessment

CHAPTER 12

A Process Approach to Personality Psychology: Utilizing Time as a Facet of Data

Randy J. Larsen

An emerging issue in the psychology of personality is an increased use of research that involves extensive observation of subjects over time (see Hormuth, 1986 for review). Semi-longitudinal designs, where measurements are made on many occasions for each subject, have generated a great deal of interest and enthusiasm within our field. Perhaps this is due to an implicit acknowledgment that the subjects of our investigations are embedded within time, that time is fundamentally important to life as it is lived, and that personality processes take place over time. Research on such personality processes must, therefore, include the temporal dimension. Researchers are beginning to ask if personality functioning is patterned over time or irregular, temporally lawful or unpredictable.

This chapter suggests an approach to personality research based on the study of behavior and experience in the ongoing stream of time— —an approach that represents not only a research strategy for combined person- and time-sampling, but also presents a way of thinking about questions important to personality psychology. For example, how do we reconcile the traditional concern for consistency as a defining aspect of personality with a research approach that emphasizes change and fluctuation? How do we reconcile the traditional concern over individual difference comparisons with a research approach that emphasizes the extensive study of single cases over time? How do we reconcile the need for precise assessment with a research approach that seeks to capture the temporal ebb and flow of human behavior, affect, and cognition?

I believe that such reconciliations can occur, but they will demand a new way of conceptualizing aspects of personality. This conceptualization will focus on personality processes as stable but nonstatic phenomena— —as consistent *patterns* of change. These consistent patterns of change represent what I will call second-order consistencies that may, in turn, be useful for describing differences among individuals, but we are getting ahead of ourselves. Let us build up to this process approach by considering some of the more traditional conceptions of personality.

Conceptualizing Personality

Personality theories differ in terms of which aspects of human nature are deemed appropriate foci of concern for our discipline and may be distinguished in a variety of ways, as demonstrated in most personality textbooks. Such distinctions may be evaluated with reference as to how we go about studying personality, and, in terms of conducting scientific inquiry, one important distinction is between those approaches that emphasize consistency (personality as fixed) and those approaches that emphasize change (personality as fluid).

Personality as Fixed

Traditional trait conceptions are good examples of the fixed approach to personality. Trait approaches hold that the focus of concern for our discipline lies in discovering various fundamental trait entities. Such entities can be discovered and documented in the more or less stable and enduring aspects of behavior, affect, and cognition. Based upon at least some evidence of consistency and stability, trait researchers ascribe theoretical existence to entities 'within' the person. Personality is thus conceived as a collection of fundamentally fixed entities that determine (Hirschberg, 1978), or at least describe or summarize (Buss & Craik, 1980), classes of behavioral, affective, and cognitive consistencies that are useful for making distinctions among persons, as well as for making predictions about their futures.

The fixed approach to personality has clear implications for determining the agenda of scientific personality research. Certain key questions naturally follow from the fixed approach to personality. One important question concerns the nature and number of the fundamental personality entities. For example, different researchers have argued that consistencies can be represented as sixteen (Cattell, 1973), three (Eysenck, 1966), or five (McCrae & Costa, 1987; Norman, 1963) fundamental, fixed trait entities. Another important line of inquiry consists of elaborating the nomological network that surrounds each personality entity. Thus, much of modern personality research is "construct-driven," in that the goal is to elaborate and expand the scientific meaning and utility of various trait entities by linking them to other aspects of behavior, affect, or cognition. Another agenda from the fixed approach is to document the origin or locus of the entities themselves. That is, from where do these consistencies emerge, and what causes these consistencies to be maintained? Examples of this line of inquiry can be found in the biological approach to personality traits, as well as in some aspects of the social learning approach.

Although the view that personality entities are *completely* consistent is out of date (Diener & Larsen, 1984; Ozer, 1986), the modern conception of traits still conforms to the notion that some degree or type of consistency is a necessary condition for defining aspects of personality (see discussion of different types of consistency in Cantor & Kihlstrom, 1987, p. 237). Personality entities are currently viewed as averaged tendencies (e.g., Epstein, 1979) or summary descriptions of behaviors that people exhibit with some degree of consistency and, hence, predictability. This approach has generated a great deal of reliable information about human functioning and represents an enduring contribution by personality theory to psychological knowledge. The emphasis on consistency, however, limits this approach by ignoring those aspects of human functioning that are more changing and fluid in nature. There is another view that takes change as the starting point for the study of personality.

Personality as Fluid

A fluid approach to personality holds that the focus of concern for our discipline lies in understanding adaptation, adjustment, growth, and dynamic change. The emphasis here is on the evolution or unfolding of behavioral, affective, or cognitive patterns over time. The search is for patterning in lives, and the goal is to specify the psychological processes or mechanisms that generate such patterns. Examples of fluid-oriented theorists would include Allport (1942), Denzin (1978), Murray (1938), Runyon (1982), and White (1972). Rather than being concerned with consistent entities that are fixed in time, the hallmark of the fluid approach to personality is a concern with understanding changes and adjustment over time. Apter (1982, p. 9), for example, discusses several different types of change that are appropriate topics of research by personality psychologists.

The fluid approach to personality also generates its own agenda for scientific personality research. Questions generated by this orientation are well-summarized by Runyon (1982, p. 82): What kinds of order or regularity can be found in the sequence of events in lives?; What is the probabilistic structure of the course of lives?; What are the meanings of events through the life span?; What processes are responsible for the flow of subjective experience over time?

From the above concerns, we see that this fluid approach to personality is the result of a direct acknowledgment of the importance of time in understanding human nature. Time is the medium through which change and adjustment is realized and made manifest. Thus, we see that phrases common to this approach—the life course, temporal story, biographical sequence, life history, the course of experience—all contain explicit reference to time. In the fluid approach, scientific meaning is given to key psychological terms (e.g., adjustment) by comparing individuals to themselves at different points in time. In contrast, the fixed approach gives scientific meaning to key psychological terms (e.g., traits) by comparing individuals to each other at the same point in time.

The fluid approach to studying personality through time is often practiced at the individual level of analysis. More often than not, researchers interested in the fluid aspects of human nature study these processes in the course of individual human lives: the methods of case study, idiography, and psychobiography are often employed to study lives through time; the search for temporal order, patterning, trends, and associations that evolve through time is often done with single subjects.

The fluid approach to personality is well-suited for describing, explaining, predicting, and generalizing at the level of the individual. Runyon (1982) makes a strong case for the value of knowledge generated through intensive study of lives over time. The tradition of studying individuals has always been a part of personality psychology, and the knowledge and methods so generated also represent enduring contributions to psychological theory. The drawback of this approach, as most researchers see it, is that it fails to obtain the level of generality afforded by making comparisons across persons. It would seem advantageous to construct an approach to personality that employs some form of process analysis at the individual level, in order to examine temporal patterning, and that then returns to the group level of analysis to search for meaningful individual differences in the temporal patterns identified.

Integrating the Fixed and Fluid Approaches to Personality: The Notion of Second-Order Consistency

The fluid approach emphasizes change, whereas the fixed approach emphasizes consistency. Might we not think of some third, hybrid category of phenomena that can be conceptualized as fluid in fixed form, or as nonstatic consistencies? Is there a category of phenomena that can be viewed as *consistencies* in *patterns* of change? For example, would we say that a rapidly cycling manic-depressive is exhibiting consistency? Or would we say that such a person is exhibiting constant change? Both views are correct. At one level, such a person is exhibiting change and flux, but at another level these fluctuations reveal a pattern. It is this *pattern of change that is consistent,* and such consistency in the patterning of mood change describes a useful and clinically important individual difference. It is, however, a nonstatic consistency that is described with the concept of manic depression, so that I would refer to the phenomenon of manic depression as a *stable but nonstatic* phenomenon. Such stable but nonstatic patterns of change make up the hybrid category of consistencies that I am talking about.

Let me give another example of consistencies in patterns of change.

Assume that people try to regulate their moods in such a way that they maintain positive affective states and remediate negative affective states. The process might be much like a homeostatic process, where the goal is to maintain one's emotional life at a desired affective setpoint. Assume further that life intrudes randomly and disrupts the person by causing negative affect. Since negative affect has a way of getting one's attention, it acts much like feedback that calls for corrective or regulative action. In order to observe such a process, we would need to study at least one person fairly intensively over time, paying careful attention to mood changes, to the events from the environment, and to what the person does to regulate his or her moods. By observing *one person* for a period of time, we might be able to model his or her mood regulation system, perhaps using concepts and even the mathematics from cybernetic control theory (Apter, 1982; Carver & Scheier, 1981; Hyland, 1987) or chaos theory (Pool, 1989). On a day-by-day basis, we would observe what might seem to be chaotic changes in mood, but using a model that incorporates a longer time frame, we might see a consistent *pattern* of mood regulation that appears somewhat purposeful, intelligent, and predictable. That is, there may be some nonstatic stability at the level of the individual's efforts to maintain emotional equilibrium.

Now, if we observe many people in this same manner over time, we might begin to notice important individual differences in regulatory patterns of mood change. That is, some people might consistently exhibit one pattern of mood regulation, while others exhibit another consistent pattern of mood regulation. Perhaps some individuals begin to take corrective action when their moods are only slightly different from their desired setpoint. Others might tolerate larger deviations from their desired state before attempting to regulate their moods. Thus, what defines the individual difference of interest is the *temporal pattern of change* that is occurring in the ongoing and fluctuating moods among the sample of individuals. This example highlights how we may, on a case-by-case basis, search for order or patterning in what might otherwise look chaotic, and the order or patterns that we find—consistent patterns of change—may indeed turn out to reveal important differences among the individuals we are studying.

I will refer to such consistent patterns of change as second-order consistencies. That is, a second-order consistency is defined as a temporal regularity or pattern identified at the individual level of analysis that is useful for describing reliable differences among persons. I suggest that such second-order consistencies form a class of phenomena that can be profitably studied by personality psychologists. To study such hybrid phenomena, we will need a hybrid approach—one that blends aspects of the fluid and fixed approaches to personality research. The remainder of this chapter describes just such an approach, which I will refer to as the process approach. It focuses on the assessment of patterns of temporal change observed at the level of the individual (characteristic of the fluid approach) and then looks for consistencies in these patterns that might in turn be useful for making comparisons among individuals (characteristic of the fixed approach). The blending of these two approaches will allow us, I believe, to ask questions about personality that neither approach used alone is capable of asking.

What can be concluded at this point is that there exists a category of individual-difference phenomena that refer to particular *patterns* of change, or what I call second-order consistencies. The fixed approach fails to conceptualize such individual differences because it is concerned with primary consistencies or averaged tendencies. The purely fluid approach would also miss such individual differences because it typically stops at the individual level of analysis. The process approach is well-suited for such phenomena because it begins with the individual level of analysis in a search for temporal patterns and then goes to the group level to search for meaningful differences among individuals in those temporal patterns.

The Process Approach to Personality Psychology

A defining characteristic of the process approach is that it consists of two steps: first, each case is analyzed separately over the temporal dimension to assess some form of temporal pattern; secondly, an estimate of the degree to which each subject exhibits the temporal pattern is used as an individual-difference variable for comparison across subjects. This approach represents a concern for within-individual temporal organization balanced with a concern for similarities/differences among individuals and has much in common with the idiographic-nomothetic pardigm proposed by Epstein (1983) and employed by Zevon and Tellegen (1982). I prefer the term process to idiographic-nomothetic, however, because there are several ways to conduct an idiographic analysis that *do not* take into account the temporal dimension (e.g., Bem & Allen, 1972; Lamiell, Foss, Larsen, & Hemple, 1983; Runyon, 1983). The process approach, on the other hand, demands that the first step at the individual level of analysis be performed *across time* to identify temporal patterns for each subject. Also, in my discussion of the process approach, I will provide an extensive framework of analytic tools for quantifying temporal patterns at the individual level of analysis. This framework should serve as a heuristic for researchers who may be considering the temporal aspects of some substantive topic. Any phenomenon that fluctuates over time (e.g., mood, self-esteem) or exhibits development, adaptation, adjustment, regulation, rhythm, learning, reversal, or any form of temporal covariation with one or more other variables would be appropriate topics for research using the process approach. The crucial point is that the

Time as a Facet of Data

Because the process approach is concerned with patterns of change, measurement over time is crucial. The inclusion of time in data collection demands that we think differently about the nature of psychological data. A typical study generates a two-dimensional data set, with persons as rows and variables as columns. With the process approach, assessment over time is extensive enough that a temporal or occasions dimension must be added to the data set. This results in a three-dimentional data set as the starting point for the process approach. Quite simply, if we measure many subjects on many variables over many occasions, the resulting data set will have three dimensions: persons by variables by occasions. Such a data set is schematized in Figure 12.1, which represents the covariation chart or "data box" first proposed by Cattell in 1946 (and which he revised several times during his career, (e.g., Cattell, 1966). Cattell used the data box to demonstrate heuristically the combination of different dimensions over which one may perform correlational analyses. Cattell's most recent version (1966) of the data box contains ten dimensions. Although conceptually thorough, the ten-dimensional data box has been called "inordinately impractical" (Ozer, 1986). However, Cattell's contribution of the data box is valuable in that it highlights and conceptually organizes the many sources of variation that contribute to a single score, although few researchers ever go beyond the practical consideration of three sources of variance. In fact, besides persons and variables, the most commonly sampled third source of variance is the temporal dimension. The inclusion of time is used to capture the temporal or

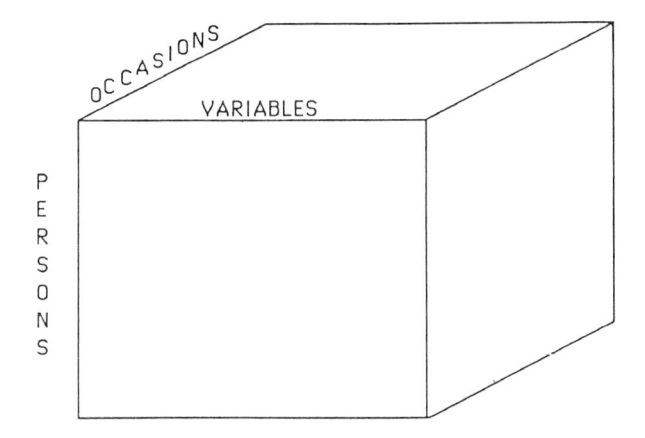

FIGURE 12.1. The Three-Dimensional Data Box.

sequential nature of behavior and experience and allows for concepts such as process, lability, growth, and change to emerge from *each* subject's data. Thus, the practical implication of Cattell's very thorough treatment of the dimensions of data relations is a return to the heuristic simplicity of the three-dimensional data box.

In the present chapter, the data box provides a conceptual starting point for clarifying and organizing the individual-subject phase of the process approach by providing a scheme for classifying the various within-subject temporally-derived parameters that, potentially, represent second-order consistencies. By starting with the data box, we can generate process-descriptive variables at the individual level of analysis, which can then be examined for meaningful differences across individuals.

Generating Process-Descriptive Variables at the Individual Level of Analysis

Now that we have both time and persons in the same data set, we can turn to the question of how to go about capturing process-descriptive variables at the level of the individual. That is, what are the ways by which we can capture process-descriptive variables for each subject? What are the methods by which we can assess second-order consistencies?

We must proceed by analyzing each case separately; in terms of the data box, we peel off one subject at a time. Treating each subject as an individual time series (Gottman, 1981), we can examine patterns of change in a number of ways. Figure 12.2 retains the data box analogy to illustrate three potential forms of process analysis. For each subject, we may examine temporal patterns for single variables, temporal covariation between two variables, or patterns of relationships among many variables over time for each subject. The important point is that, during this phase of the process approach, each subject's data are analyzed separately to look for patterns of variation over time.

Table 12.1 presents a collection of quantitative strategies for generating process-descriptive variables by analyzing single subjects over time—— these strategies represent ways of capturing second-order consistencies. The various analytic stragteies are capable of representing specific patterns of change at the level of the individual, and the way to think about these analytic strategies is that they generate 'scores' for each subject. These scores, however, refer to specific patterns of change for each subject over time.

It is worth repeating that the statistical concepts presented in Table 12.1 are applied *within subjects* (Battig, 1979) over the temporal dimension of their data. Each strategy in Table 12.1 captures a psychologically different aspect of change over time at the level of the individual case. For

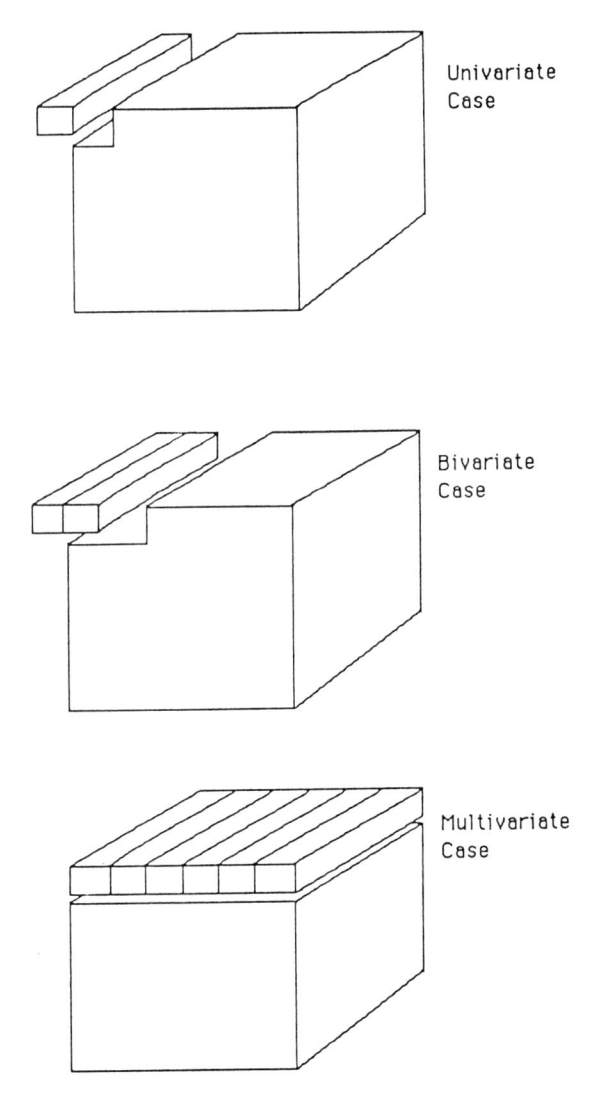

FIGURE 12.2. Three Approaches to Generating Process-Descriptive Variables at the Individual Level of analysis.

example, the within-subject standard deviation quantifies the degree to which each subject exhibits temporal fluctuation on the measured variable. The within-subject correlation quantifies the degree to which two variables are linked over time for each subject. Within-subject factor analysis (p-technique) quantifies the degree to which several variables show temporal coherence for each subject.

TABLE 12.1 Within-subject methods for generating process-descriptive variables at the level of the individual over time.

I. Univariate Process-Descriptive Variables
   A. Within-Subject Standard Deviation
   B. Within-Subject Skew
   C. Within-Subject Kurtosis
   D. Within-Subject Time-Series Models
      1. Frequency Models, e.g., Spectral Analysis
      2. Time Models, e.g., ARIMA Analysis
II. Bivariate Process-Descriptive Variables
   A. Within-Subject Correlation
   B. Within-Subject Auto-Regressive Models
   C. Within-Subject Cross-Spectral Analysis
III. Multivariate Process-Descriptive Variables
   A. Within-Subject Multiple Regression (lagged or unlagged)
   B. Within-Subject Fit Statistic
   C. Within-Subject Factor Analysis
      1. P-Technique
      2. Three-Mode

The choice of which analytic strategy from Table 12.1 to utilize in any given research project is entirely dependent on the researcher's questions. The process approach——like any general approach to psychological research——does not exist in a substantive vacuum. It must be applied to substantive questions, and its use must be guided and informed by those questions. Of itself, the process approach is only a collection of possibilities and ways of thinking about data. It is up to the researcher to translate his or her substantive questions into process-approach terms. For example, if a researcher wonders if there are temporal cycles in peoples' moods, and if such cycles relate to other characteristics of those individuals, then spectral analysis might be the appropriate analytic strategy to employ. As another example, perhaps a researcher is interested in whether one variable (e.g., physical symptoms) lags behind another variable (e.g., stress), and whether or not there are meaningful individual differences in the length of this lag relationship (i.e., the 'incubation' period for the effect of stress on health). In this case, within-subject ARIMA models might be useful for quantifying the lagged relationship for each subject with enough precision to make comparisons across subjects.

These analytic strategies might also be employed in research on critical transitions or shift points in people's lives. The notions of critical life transitions, shift points, or life stages incorporate time as an essential feature. For example, the birth of a child in the study of ongoing marital life (Stewart, Sokol, Healy, & Chester, 1986), or entry into college in the study of young adult life (Cantor, Norem, Niedenthal, Langston, &

Brower, 1987) represent studies of critical shift points in the ongoing stream of time within individual lives. The researcher might center the temporal perspective around such critical shift points. In such cases, the discovery strategies of Table 12.1 could be time-linked to include observation of the shift point, plus observations on both temporal sides of the shift point, for all subjects. In such a manner, the researcher can examine if the critical event influences the form of the temporal process giving rise to patterning in the observations. Theoretical rationale and researcher interest will dictate which shift points are important to study. Shift points that may be theoretically important to certain researchers might include: when life contexts change; when new goals emerge; when physiological states surpass some level of stress; the onset of illness; when significant persons enter one's life space.

What I am suggesting is that theoretical questions of interest must always come first in the researcher's thinking. Once the question is focused, the analytic strategies in Table 12.1 can be considered for which one might be most useful in addressing the question. A perusal of the possibilities represented in Table 12.1 might, however, lead the researcher to consider different possibilities and questions about psychological processes over time. That is, Table 12.1 can, perhaps, represent a heuristic collection of 'ways of thinking' about the temporal implications of various psychological phenomena. The different within-subject techniques presented in Table 12.1 are useful for characterizing different psychological processes at the level of the individual. They can be used to test different theoretical predictions about what sorts of people are likely to exhibit different temporal patterning in the variables of interest. For example, what sorts of people are likely to show a short lag relationship between stress and illness in the ongoing stream of time that defines their life course?

In Table 12.1 the univariate strategies are useful for assessing the distributional properties of some variable over time for each subject. The pattern of change may concern the temporal distribution of the variable, its variability over time, its pattern of occurrence (skew or kurtosis), or its rhythmic nature (spectral analysis). The bivariate strategies are useful for assessing covariation between two variables of interest over time for each subject. The focus may be on the concurrent occurrence of those variables (first-order, within-subject correlation), the lead-lag relations between those variables (bivariate auto-regression), or the rhythmic coherence between variables that are themselves rhythmic but differ with respect to their phase relationship (cross-spectral analysis). The multivariate strategies are useful for assessing the pattern of temporal covariation among a collection of variables of interest over time for each subject. The focus of concern may be on the temporal relation between one variable and a collection of others (multiple regression), the multivariate fit of each subject's temporal pattern of covariation to some target, or the temporal structure of each subject's pattern of covariation among a number of variables (within-subject or three-mode factor analysis).

Elsewhere (Larsen, 1988), I give examples of each of the analytic strategies outlined in Table 12.1. Due to space limitations here, I will give only one example each of univariate, bivariate, and multivariate applications of the process approach. As a univariate example, consider the possibility of cycles in peoples' moods. Using spectral analysis, Larsen and Kasimatis (in press) examined each of seventy-six subjects for cyclicity in mood over a three-month period of daily mood reporting. It was found that most college student subjects exhibited at least some degree of weekly cyclicity in mood, generally peaking during the weekend and lowest around mid-week. By analyzing the rhythmic distribution of mood for each subject over time with spectral analysis, we were able to assess the degree to which *each subject* exhibited this weekly cycle. We took this within-subject 'score', derived from spectral analyzing each subject's data, to represent how "entrained" each subject was to a weekly calendar. Without going into the details, we predicted that this specific pattern of change should relate to the individual difference variable of extraversion. More specifically, we predicted that extraverts should show less weekly cyclicity in mood due to their tendency to avoid routine by seeking arousal throughout the week (i.e, extraverts don't wait for the weekend to enliven their lives). This prediction was supported by the finding that extraversion scores correlated negatively (across subjects) with the degree of weekly mood cyclicity (computed within-subject). In this example, the process variable generated at the individual level of analysis is the spectral estimate of seven-day periodic variation in mood. Cycles or rhythmic changes are good examples of second-order consistencies since they describe nonstatic consistencies (Larsen, 1985).

As a bivariate example of the process approach, consider the temporal relationship between life events and mood. We might imagine that, for each subject, when good things happen they will be happy and when bad things happen they will be sad. Larsen and Cowan (1988) examined the temporal covariation between mood and life events for each of sixty-two subjects over two months of consecutive daily reporting of mood and life events. For all subjects, this pattern of covariation was positive. At the individual level of analysis, there was at least some degree of temporal match between changes in life events and concurrent changes in mood. Across subjects, however, there were wide individual differences in the strength of this within-subject linkage between mood and life events. As it turns out, we found that individual differences in depression (assessed by standard questionnaire measures) correlated negatively with the process variable, i.e., the temporal linkage between mood and life events. That is, the more depressed individuals showed a pattern of mood change that was less linked to their life events than nondepressed individuals. Depressed individuals appear to have day-to-day moods that are less tightly linked to the objective events of their daily lives than nondepressed individuals. In this example, the process variable is a within-subject correlation, and the psychological meaning of this variable is that it assesses the *temporal linkage* between the subject's daily moods and what is happening in his or her daily life.

As a multivariate example of the process approach, consider the following study we have underway currently. In this study, we assessed moods for each of forty-five subjects over 180 consecutive occasions during a two-month period. Mood assessments were made by having subjects rate the degree to which they were feeling each of twenty-four mood adjectives on each occasion. We then factor analyzed *each subject's data* separately over the 180 occasions (i.e., *p*-technique factor analysis). Such an analysis tells us, for each subject, how his or her moods covary over time. That is, to what extent does each subject's mood-states form coherent patterns over time? How many factors are needed to describe each subject's temporal pattern of mood covariation, and are there meaningful individual differences in the factor structures of peoples' day-to-day moods?

Preliminary analyses reveal individual differences in the number and nature of the factors that emerged from each subject's data. Some subjects have fairly simple factor structures to their moods, with only a few factors accounting for much of the variance. Such subjects tend to have an 'all-or-nothing' emotional life. Other subjects have a more complex factor structure to their moods, requiring more factors to account for an equal amount of variance. That is, the emotionally complex subjects have more independent units of affective covariation over time than the less emotionally complex subjects. Our goal will be to learn more about such individual differences in affective complexity by examining the relation between the number of emotion factors that emerged for each subject and their scores on several standard measures of personality. In this example, the process variable of interest is the within-subject factor structure of the emotion ratings obtained over time for each subject.

Conclusions

A major journal in our field, the *Journal of Personality and Social Psychology,* has one of its sections entitled "Personality Processes and Individual Differences." Scanning the articles published in this section, one quickly comes to the conclusion that the majority of articles concern individual differences and very few are related to personality processes. This may be due to the fact that our field has developed a consensual approach for the study of individual differences, but we have yet to agree upon an approach for the study of personality processes. The concept of process, as defined in the *American Heritage Dictionary,* refers to (1) a series of actions, changes, or functions that bring about an end or result, (2) the course or passage of time, (3) ongoing movement. The aspects of this definition suggest that whatever approach we develop to study personality processes, it will necessarily concern the temporal dimension of our subjects' lives.

The process approach suggested in this chapter represents not only a research strategy for combined time- and person-sampling, but also a new way of thinking about psychological questions. The psychological meanings of the various temporally generated, process-descriptive variables discussed in this chapter become apparent to those researchers who consider how such an approach might apply to his or her own research questions. There is a sense that this process approach gives us a new strategy for asking and answering questions within personality psychology. The emphasis in this approach is on how time may be used theoretically to think about patterns and processes in the lives of our subjects. Time is then utilized methodologically to generate process-descriptive variables for research. Such temporally generated variables, indexed at the level of the individual, have the appeal of 'the dynamic' while retaining the precision afforded by quantification. The flexibility of this approach to represent second-order consistencies allows us to grapple with a wide variety of old, and new, questions.

Renewed interest in the intensive study of individual personalities brings with it a renewed debate about the purpose of science and the credibility of an individual level of analysis (Sechrest, 1986). Certainly, most scientists would agree that the purpose of science is to identify general principles rather than to collect observations of specific individuals or events. We want to know, for example, what people are like in general. Sampling theory tells us that intensive knowledge of one individual is not a sufficient basis from which to generalize about a given population of persons, and so we demand multisubject research because of our desire for generalizability from the sample to the population.

When we think of the concept of a population, we typically think of a population of persons. There are, however, many facets to the concept of a population, and we might alternatively ask whether the population of occasions was adequately sampled in a given study. This generalizability question——temporal generalizability——becomes increasingly important to the extent that the phenomenon under investigation changes over time (Nesselroad & Ford, 1985).

The subjects we study are changing and fluctuating as we study them. Time is an important aspect of the lived experience of our subjects. Time is ubiquitous in the lives of our subjects and is at least implicitly operative in our methodology (Kelly & McGrath, 1988). Even our language is structured by temporal factors. *Roget's Thesaurus* lists Time as a major subclass of Abstract Relations, along with other such scientifically important concepts as Quantity, Cause, and Order, yet the practice of scientific personality research is relatively "timeless."

The process approach represents one way to put time back into personality research. The various temporally generated variables discussed in this chapter allow researchers to test predictions about how some personality process manifests itself over time. This is not just a generalizability issue; the inclusion of the temporal dimension potentially provides a greater likelihood of understanding time-relevant personality processes than does the typical cross-sectional research design. Our understanding of inherently temporal personality processes will be hampered to the extent that they are studied cross-sectionally (Runyon, 1978). To gain an understanding of such personality processes, it may be necessary to study persons the long way (i.e., over time) and to think differently about the possibilities inherent in data generated from such research.

Acknowledgments. Preparation of this chapter was supported, in part, by Research Scientist Development Award #K01-MH00704 and grant #R01-MH42057 from the National Institute of Mental Health.

I would like to acknowledge helpful comments on an earlier draft of this paper received from Michael Apter, Nancy Cantor, Ed Diener, Seymour Epstein, David Funder, Janice Kelly, Mac Runyon, and Bob Thayer.

References

Allport, G.W. (1942). *The use of personal documents in psychological science.* New York: Social Science Research Council.

Apter, M.J. (1982). *The experience of motivation: The theory of psychological reversals.* New York: Academic Press.

Battig, W.F. (1979). Are the important "individual differences" between or within individuals? *Journal of Research in Personality, 13,* 546–558.

Bem, D. & Allen, A. (1972). On predicting some of the people some of the time: The search for cross-situational consistencies in behavior. *Psychological Review, 81,* 506–520.

Buss, D.M., & Craik, K.H. (1980). The frequency concept of disposition: Dominance and prototypically dominant acts. *Journal of Personality, 48,* 379–392.

Cantor, N., & Khilstrom, J. (1987). *Personality and social intelligence.* Englewood Cliffs, NJ: Prentice-Hall.

Cantor, N., Norem, J.K., Niedenthal, P.M., Langston, C.A., & Brower, A.M. (1987). Life tasks, self-concept ideals, and cognitive strategies in a life transition. *Journal of Personality and Social Psychology, 53,* 1178–1191.

Carver, C.S., & Scheier, M.F., (1981). *Attention and self-regulation: A control-theory approach to human behavior.* New York: Springer.

Cattell, R.B. (1966). Patterns of change: Measurement in relation to state dimension, trait change, lability, and process concepts. In R.B. Cattell (Ed.), *Handbook of multivariate experimental psychology*. Chicago: Rand McNally.

Cattell, R.B., (1973). *Personality and mood by questionnaire*. San Francisco: Jossey-Bass.

Denzin, N.K. (1972). *The research act*. New York: McGraw-Hill.

Diener, E., & Larsen, R.J. (1984). Temporal stability and cross-situational consistency of affective, behavioral, and cognitive responses. *Journal of Personality and Social Psychology, 47*, 580–592.

Epstein, S. (1979). The stability of behavior: I. On predicting most of the people much of the time. *Journal of Personality and Social Psychology, 37*, 1097–1126.

Epstein, S. (1983). A research paradigm for the study of personality and emotions. *Nebraska Symposium on Motivation, 1982*, 91–154.

Eysenck, H.J. (1966). *The biological basis of personality*. Springfield, IL: Thomas.

Gottman, J.M. (1981). *Time series analysis: A comprehensive introduction for social scientists*. Cambridge, England: Cambridge University Press.

Hirschberg, N. (1978). A correct treatment of traits. In H. London (Ed.), *Personality: A new look at meta-theories* (pp. 45–68). New York: Wiley.

Hormuth, S.E. (1986). The sampling of experience *in situ*. *Journal of Personality, 54*, 262–293.

Hyland, M.E., (1987). Control theory interpretation of psychological mechanisms of depression: Comparison and integration of several theories. *Psychological Bulletin, 102*, 109–121.

Kelly, J. & McGrath, J. (1988). *On time and method*. Newbury Park, CA: Sage.

Lamiell, J.T., Foss, M.A., Larsen, R.J., & Hempel, A.M. (1983). Studies in intuitive personology from an idiothetic point of view: Implications for personality theory. *Journal of Personality, 51*, 438–467.

Larsen, R.J. (1985). Individual differences in circadian activity rhythm and personality. *Personality and Individual Differences, 6*, 305–311.

Larsen, R.J. (1987). The stability of mood variability: A spectral analytic approach to daily mood assessments. *Journal of Personality and Social Psychology, 52*, 1195–1204.

Larsen, R.J. (1988). *Analytic strategies in the idiographic/nomothetic paradigm*. Unpublished manuscript, Purdue University.

Larsen, R.J., & Cowan, G.S. (1988). Internal focus of attention and depression: A study of daily experience. *Motivation and Emotion, 12*, 237–149.

Larsen, R.J., & Kasimatis, M. (in press). Individual differences in entrainment of mood to the weekly calendar. *Journal of Personality and Social Psychology*.

McCrae, R. R., & Costa, P.T. (1987). Validation of the five-factor model of personality across instruments and observers. *Journal of Personality and Social Psychology, 52*, 81–90.

Murray, H.A. et al. (1938). *Assessment of men*. New York: Rinehart.

Nesselroade, J.R., & Ford, D.H. (1985). P-technique comes of age: Multivariate, replicated, single-subject designs for research on older adults. *Research on Aging, 7*, 46–80.

Norman, W.T. (1963). Toward an adequate taxonomy of personality attributes: Replicated factor structure in peer nomination personality ratings. *Journal of Abnormal and Social Psychology, 66*, 574–583.

Ozer, D.J. (1986). *Consistency in personality: A methodological framework.* Berlin: Springer.

Pool, R. (1989). Is it chaos, or is it just noise? *Science, 243,* 25-28.

Runyon, W.M. (1978). The life course as a theoretical orientation: Sequences of person-situation interaction. *Journal of Personality, 46,* 569-593.

Runyon, W.M. (1983). Idiographic goals and methods in the study of lives. *Journal of Personality, 51,* 413-437.

Runyon, W.M. (1982). *Life histories and psychobiography.* New York: Oxford University Press.

Sechrest, L. (1986). Modes and methods of personality research. *Journal of Personality, 54,* 318-331.

Stewart, A.J., Sokol, M., Healy, J.M., & Chester, N.L. (1986). Longitudinal studies of psychological consequences of life changes in children and adults. *Journal of Personality and Social Psychology, 50,* 143-151.

White, R.W. (1972). *The enterprise of living.* New York: Holt, Rinehart & Winston.

Zevon, M.A., & Tellegen, A. (1982). The structure of mood change: An idiographic/nomothetic analysis. *Journal of Personality and Social Psychology, 43,* 111-122.

CHAPTER 13

Metatraits: Interitem Variance as Personality Assessment

Dianne M. Tice

Many researchers studying individual differences conduct studies in which they ask a large number of individuals to complete a questionnaire designed to measure a specific trait. The researchers then examine whether the individuals receiving a high score on the trait measure will perform differently on a behavioral measure, or other questionnaire, than individuals receiving a low score on the trait. An implicit assumption of this methodology is that the trait dimension being measured applies equally well to all individuals. In other words, a particular individual participating in the study may receive a high score on the trait (or may receive a medium score or a low score), but every individual's score is equally meaningful as a representation of that individual's personality.

In contrast, other researchers such as Allport (1937) and Bem and Allen (1974) have suggested that not all trait dimensions apply equally well to all individuals. Individuals may differ not only in their levels of a given trait, but also according to which trait dimensions are most predictive of behavior. Allport suggests that the personality dimension of introversion-extroversion, for example, is applicable for some individuals (who can be described as introverts and extraverts, varying in their levels of the trait), but for other individuals the dimension of introversion-extroversion is simply irrelevant. Bem and Allen (1974) built upon Allport's earlier work by proposing methods to operationalize the concept that personalities differ in the trait dimensions they contain. Their findings proved difficult to replicate, however (see Chaplin and Goldberg, 1984, for failure to replicate Bem and Allen's original study). Thus, the purpose of this paper is to discuss an alternative methodolgy for quantifying and operationalizing the concept that different trait dimensions apply to different people. This proposed method has been called metatrait analysis (Baumeister & Tice, 1988).

What is Meant by the Term Metatraits?

A metatrait is the trait of having versus not having a particular trait. In other words, it refers to the presence versus the absence of a trait dimension in an individual's personality. To continue with Allport's example, a researcher may be interested in the metatrait of introversion-extroversion—that is, whether the introversion-extroversion dimension is applicable for a given individual or whether it is irrelevant for the individual. If the individual's personality does contain the (particular) trait, the individual is referred to as *traited* on that trait dimension. If the individual's personality does not contain the (particular) trait, the individual is referred to as *untraited* on that trait dimension. Thus, an individual whose personality contains the dimension of introversion would be labeled as traited on the dimension. A person who is neither an introvert nor an extrovert (nor consistently intermediate between the two), whose personality may seem introverted at some times and in some respects and extraverted at others, is referred to as untraited on the introversion-extroversion dimension.

A metatrait is always associated with a particular trait. Thus, we may look for the presence versus the absence of the introversion-estroversion dimension in the personalities of our subjects; we may also look for the presence versus the absence of self-consciousness, religiosity, self-monitoring, the dominance-submissive dimension, or other personality traits or trait dimensions that have been identified by researchers.

The metatrait approach argues that one can be strongly traited at an intermediate or moderate level of a trait. In other words, a person may score in the middle range on a personality scale (as opposed to scoring very high or very low on the scale) and still be rated as traited on that dimension if that dimension is highly relevant to the person's personality structure. In the same way that a person having a "middle-of-the-road" political belief may feel that his or her moderate belief is very central, important, and relevant to his or her overall political philosophy, intermediate or moderate trait scores do not necessarily imply that the trait is not relevant to the individual's personality.

In an earlier paper (Baumeister & Tice, 1988), we argued that attitudes are a better analogue than physical traits to personality traits. Not everyone has an attitude about every issue. Although it may be possible, using a forced-choice format, to get an individual to respond to an attitude scale, the number circled by the respondent may not give an accurate indication of how well thought-out and central the attitude is to the respondent. For example, although two respondents may both circle 4 on a ten-point scale for the question "Do you believe that abortion is immoral?," the first repondent may have put a lot of thought into the question to develop a well-reasoned, coherent view on the sanctity of life, while the second responded to the question perfunctorily due to ignorance of and indifference to the issues. In a similar manner, one individual may receive a moderately high score on a personality scale, and the trait it measured may be highly relevant to that individual's personality. Another individual may receive exactly the same score on the measure, but for that individual the trait is not a good predictor of behavior.

Recent work on attitudes has developed a concept similar to metatraits. Fazio, Sanbonmatsu, Powell, and Kardes (1986) revived the attitude/ nonattitude distinction discussed in earlier work by Hovland (1959) and Converse (1970). They suggest a continuum, with nonattitude at one end and a strong salient attitude at the other. In past work (Baumeister & Tice, 1988), we have suggested that the attitude analogy for metatraits makes the most sense for high-level, abstract attitudes or ideological positions, such as being liberal or conservative. These high-level attitudes may be assessed by asking someone's opinions on a large set of issues. Some people may respond with traditional political consistency, but others might hold some very conservative and some very liberal opinions simultaneously. The former group of people corresponds to traited individuals and the latter group corresponds to untraited individuals in the domain of political conservatism.

Metatraits may frequently act as a moderator variables. Traited individuals may show a relationship between trait score and behavior, thus indicating that the trait caused the behavior. In our initial paper on metatraits (Baumeister & Tice, 1988), we found an overall correlation between Locus of Control scores and behavior of $r = +.096$, ns. When we separated traited individuals from untraited individuals, we found that the traited individuals showed a significant positive correlation between trait scores and behavior, $r = +.502$, whereas the untraited individuals showed a nonsignificant negative correlation between trait scores and behavior, $r = -.297$. In this study, therefore, the metatrait acted as a moderator variable. The relationship between trait scores and behavior was found to be substantially and significantly different in the traited and untraited groups.

Untraited individuals may show fluctuations dependent on state manipulations and situational influences. By definition the trait-relevant behavior of untraited individuals is considerably less stable and consistent in untraited than traited individuals, so that untraited individuals may be more prone to situational pressures. Untraited individuals do not, however, show less test-retest reliability than traited individuals over a two week period of time (Baumeister, 1988).

Although metatraits frequently function as moderators, we have also cited an example (Baumeister & Tice, 1988) in which the metatrait predicts behavior directly—independent of the trait. We found that public situations increased the behavioral differences between subjects who were traited versus untraited on the dimension of self-esteem. Specifically, in the public condition, self-esteem traited subjects (regardless of their *level* of self-esteem) requested significantly less advice on problem solving than untraited subjects. There was no difference between the groups in the private condition. In this example, the metatrait directly predicted the advice-seeking behavior of the subjects. Thus, metatraits usually function as, but are not necessarily, moderators; they may also have predictive utility independent of trait level.

How are Metatraits Measured?

Bem and Allen (1974) attempted to quantify and operationalize Allport's (1937) insight that different trait dimensions apply to different people. One of their operationalizations consisted of developing a new and detailed measure of behavioral consistency (the Cross-Situation Behavior Survey; Bem & Allen, 1974). The principal drawback of this method is inconvenience. It means that a new instrument must be developed and validated for every trait scale. A second measure of behavioral consistency developed by Bem and Allen (1974) was the "ipsatized variance index." This measure requires the simultaneous assessment of several traits. For each subject, one computes the ratio of interitem variance on the target dimension (Trait A) to the interitem variance on all dimensions measured by the researcher (Traits A, B, & C). A principal objection to the ipsatized index is that an individual's classification of consistency on Trait A is dependent on his responses to the others traits that happened to be measured by the researchers (Traits B & C; cf. Tellegen, Kamp, & Watson, 1982). Although Bem and Allen's (1974) methodology was a real advance in opening up the possibilities for empirical research, their findings proved difficult to replicate (Chaplin & Goldberg, 1984).

In our first paper on metatraits (Baumeister & Tice, 1988), we proposed the use of interitem variance of scale responses on the personality scale of interest. Low interitem variance suggests that the individual is traited, in that the person responded consistently to all the items. High interitem variance suggests that the individual is untraited on the personality dimension measured by the scale, because the person responded variably to items meant to tap a single personality construct.

Other researchers have proposed refinements of the variability measurement, such as computing variance of standardized rather than raw scores, or computing each item score as a deviation from the sample mean for that item (e.g., Tellegen, 1988). I would not argue that interitem variance is a perfect technique for measuring trait relevance; it is not. It is, however, a simple methodology that can be used with a wide variety of existing scales (thereby reducing the necessity of constructing new scales to measure trait relevance) to help determine for which subjects in a sample the trait being measured is most relevant or predictive of behavior. The refinements proposed by Tellegen (1988) and others may increase the accuracy of assignment to traited and untraited conditions.

The metatrait approach is similar to the approach of a variety of other researchers). Markus (1977) and Swann (e.g., Swann & Hill, 1982; Swann & Predmore, 1985) have both used extremity of self-rating on the dimension to classify individuals. Extremity may be the most appropriate method for classification of self-schemas (which consist of the organization of self-knowledge) but may not be as appropriate outside the self-schema area. Use of interitem variance as a classification method rather than extremity in the areas of personality and behavior will help to reduce the confound between extremity and traitedness, so that intermediate scores will not imply the absence of the trait. We found correlations of $r = -.17$ and $r = +.01$ between extremity and interitem variance, which is similar to other researchers who have either found no correlation (Underwood & Moore, 1981) or have suggested that the correlation may hover around $-.20$ (Paunonen and Jackson (1985).

Use of interitem variance rather than extremity or certainty ratings will also enable personality researchers to assess traitedness on dimensions that might be unfamiliar to laypersons. Because most common personality scales can lend themselves to metatrait analysis, personality researchers are not dependent only on traits of which laypersons have common knowledge to determine trait relevance. In addition, event though most laypersons have a definition of the trait self-consciousness, for example, they may not be referring to the same dimension as researchers using the self-consciousness scale developed by Fenigstein, Scheier, and Buss (1975). Thus, the use of interitem variance rather than extremity for the study of trait relevance (outside the area of self-knowledge) may reduce the confound between extremity and relevance and allow researchers to assess traits not familiar to laypersons.

When is the Metatrait Approach Not Advisable?

Interitem variance may prove unreliable if the scale is very short. In traditional personality research, the researcher is often interested in the subject's level of a given trait. The more items that the trait scale has, the more confident the researcher is that the trait score for each individual subject is reliable. This issue of scale length becomes even more important when the researcher is computing interitem variance as well as level of the trait. If the scale contains too few items, interitem variance will be quite unreliable. It is important, therefore, to use only scales with enough items to result in reasonable reliability of the interitem variance. Recent work by Johnson (1988), for example, found no effect for metatraits using a group of very short scales, each of which was only seven items in length. Baumeister (1988) found that metatrait scores were more stable and reliable over time with longer scales than with shorter subscales, even though the subscales were supposedly more homogeneous.

Another scale feature of which to be aware when computing metatraits is the response format. Although it is technically possible to compute metatraits when the response format is dichotomous, the interitem variance is much more valid and reliable using an expanded response format (e.g., on a scale of 1 to 11 rather than a yes-no response).

One of the benefits of the use of interitem variance over extremity as a measure of trait relevance is that interitem variance reduces the confound of the correlation between extremity and variance, so that moderate scores are not necessarily classified as untraited. The researcher should examine the correlation between extremity and variance to assure himself or herself that the correlation is low (usual correlations range from close to zero to around $-.20$; e.g., Baumeister & Tice, 1988; Paunonen & Jackson, 1985).

It is important when conducting computer simulations of metatrait experiments to model the subject data after data collected from real subjects so that an accurate correlation of extremity and variance is computed. If computer simulations include responses at the very highest and lowest extremes of the scale (responses which may rarely or never been given by real subjects), then the correlation between extremity and variance will be artificially increased.

Summary

Interitem variance (with possible refinements such as standardization of scores or correction for item means) is a suggested operationalization of Allport's concept of trait relevance. Variance is preferable to extremity scores because it is possible for an individual with an intermediate or moderate score on a trait scale to be traited on that dimension. Interitem variance can be used with many existing trait scales to determine whether respondents are traited or untraited on the given trait dimension.

References

Allport, G.W. (1937). *Personality: A psychological interpretation*. New York: Holt.

Baumeister, R.F., & Tice, D.M. (1988). Metatraits. *Journal of Personality, 56*, 571–598.

Baumeister, R.F. (1988). On the stability of variability: Retest reliability of metatraits. Unpublished manuscript, Case Western Reserve University.

Bem, D.J., & Allen, A. (1974). On predicting some of the people some of the time: The search for cross-situational consistencies in behavior. *Psychological Review, 81*, 506–520.

Chaplin, W.F., & Goldberg, L.R. (1984). A failure to replicate the Bem and Allen study of individual differences in cross-situational consistency. *Journal of Personality and Social Psychology, 47*, 1074–1090.

Converse, P.E. (1970). Attitudes and non-attitudes: Continuation of a dialogue. In E.R. Tufte (Ed.), *The quantitative analysis of social problems* (pp. 168–189). Reading, MA: Addison-Wesley.

Fazio, R.H., Sanbonmatsu, D.M., Powell, M.C., & Kardes, F.R. (1986). On the automatic activation of attitudes. *Journal of Personality and Social Psychology, 50*, 229–238.

Fenigstein, A., Scheier, M.F., & Buss, A.H. (1975). Public and private self-consciousness: Assessment and theory. *Journal of Consulting and Clinical Psychology, 43*, 522–527.

Hovland, C.I. (1959). Reconciling conflicting results derived from experimental and survey studies of attitude change. *American Psychologist, 14*, 8–17.

Markus, H. (1977). Self-schemata and processing information about the self. *Journal of Personality and Social Psychology, 35*, 63–78.

Paunonen, S.V., & Jackson, D.N. (1985). Idiographic measurement strategies for personality and prediction: Some unredeemed promissory notes. *Psychological Review, 92*, 486–511.

Swann, W.A., & Hill, C.A. (1982). When our identities are mistaken: Reaffirming self-conceptions through social interaction. *Journal of Personality and Social Psychology, 43*, 59–66.

Swann, W.A., & Predmore, S.C. (1985). Intimates as agents of social support: Sources of consolation or despair? *Journal of Personality and Social Psychology, 49*, 1609–1617.

Tellegen, A. (1988). The analysis of consistency in personality assessment. *Journal of Personality, 56*, 621–663.

Tellegen, A., Kamp, J., & Watson, D. (1982). Recognizing individual differences in predictive structure. *Psychological Review, 89*, 95–105.

Underwood, B., & Moore, B.S. (1981). Sources of behavioral consistency. *Journal of Personality and Social Psychology, 40*, 780–795.

CHAPTER 14

Socially Desirable Responding: Some New Solutions to Old Problems

Delroy L. Paulhus

Perhaps the most irritating critics of one's theory or data are those who say "it's just self-presentation" or "it's just impression management." Such critics are like gadflies——they nip away at you while you are trying to do serious psychologizing. We often think they are taking cheap shots and try to ignore them.

In personality assessment, the version we hear is "it's just social desirability." Your critic is alleging that the measure you have developed to assess some content variable, such as anxiety or self-esteem, is, in fact, measuring individual differences in socially desirable responding (SDR). That is, those respondents who are simply trying to look good are getting systematically different scores on your test; for example, they will disclaim any symptom of anxiety because such an admission would make them look bad. Thus, respondents engaging in SDR will tend to score systematically lower than other respondents on your new anxiety scale.

Your critic will often have evidence——typically that your scale correlates with some standard measure of socially desirable responding, such as the Edwards SD scale (Edwards, 1957) or the Marlowe-Crowne scale (Crowne & Marlowe, 1964). Unfortunately, this evidence has to be taken seriously. Because anxiety is confounded with SDR, there will always be two explanations for any correlation found between your measure and a criterion——even a behavioral criterion. As confounds go, SDR is among the worst because it takes only a modicum of imagination to devise an SDR explanation for any correlation found with your new instrument.

Some History

The measurement of SDR began with the comprehensive effort of Hartshorne and May (1928) to assess the rate of dishonest behavior and its generality. Among the measures they developed was a self-report measure of SDR very similar to the Marlowe-Crowne scale. It was not until the development of the MMPI, however, that SDR scales came into prominence. (The Lie-scale and K-scale continue to play an important role in the MMPI, even in the 1989 revision.)

The disputes over SDR scales became full-blown during the sixties. Eventually, most of the major figures in personality assessment were dragged into the controversy. One side was led by Doug Jackson, Sam Messick, and Allen Edwards, who decried the confounding of SDR with major dimensions of personality and psychopathology (e.g., Edwards, 1957; Jackson & Messick, 1962). More specifically, they showed that the Edwards SD scale and similar SDR measures correlated highly with major dimensions of personality such as anxiety, dominance, self-esteem, and many of the MMPI clinical scales. Thus, these substantive measures were alleged to be an artifact of stylistic tendencies.

On the other side, Jack Block and other MMPI experts responded either that the claims for confounding were exaggerated (e.g., Crowne & Marlowe, 1964), or that the putatively confounded scales were demonstrably valid (e.g., Block, 1965). That is, measures of anxiety, for example, could be demonstrated to measure anxiety. Indeed, some turned the attack around to argue that SDR scales were also measuring anxiety. Other major figures such as Lew Goldberg, Jerry Wiggins and Warren Norman participated vigorously in the debates, but took more qualified positions.

Ironically, the two sides eventually settled on similar positions: both agreed that SDR scales must be measuring some consistent aspect of personality on their own—in other words, there must be some substance in the style. Nonetheless, the animosity seemed to induce a pact of obstinate silence on both sides. The non expert was left to wonder—is it a problem if my scale is correlated with SDR? Perhaps worse, the divisiveness in personality assessment led some to abandon the field in disgust and tainted the credibility of those who remained.

Current Status

Partly because of the pact of silence, déjà vu is a frequent experience as neophyte test constructors are doomed to relive the past. After laboring to develop a new personality test, they discover high correlations with SDR and cry out, "the horror, the horror!"

The reactions of veteran personality assessors seem to fall into one of three general categories. Hardcore cynics are adamant that personality is mostly SDR. (Selective cynics apply this criticism only to scales they dislike). Escapists know about the controversy but repress the fact: seeing the problem as unsolvable, they advise one to ignore it. The Pragmatists emphasize validity: if one's measure can be demonstrated to perform as claimed in predicting behavior then the problem of SDR is effectively bypassed.

Two Factor Theories of SDR

Some of my own work has been directed at reconciling the polarized positions on SDR. A number of disputes may be resolved by noting the long-standing evidence that there are two distinct clusters of SDR scales: I have labeled these *self-deception* and *impression management* (Paulhus, 1984, 1986). Scales falling into the self-deception cluster include the Edwards SD scale (Edwards, 1957), the Self-Deception Scale (Paulhus, 1984, in press; Sackeim & Gur, 1978) and the MMPI K-scale (Meehl & Hathaway, 1946). These measures tap an honest, positivistic bias that contributes to good psychological adjustment. A typical item is, "My first impressions of people usually turn out to be right." Scales falling into the impression-management cluster include the Sd scale (Wiggins, 1959) and the Impression Management Scale (Paulhus, 1984, in press; Sackeim & Gur, 1978). These scales appear to tap a naive form of conscious self-presentation. A typical item is, "I have never pretended to be sick to avoid work or school." Interestingly, the most commonly-used SDR measure, the Marlowe-Crowne scale, appears to lie in between the two major clusters of SDR scales.

The separation of SDR into self-deception and impression management helps resolve two critical problems. First, are those who score high on SDR scales really healthy or not? According to my analysis, those who score high on self-deceptive positivity are generally well-adjusted individuals who are biased in the sense that they are overly optimistic and play down the negative aspects of their personality. Those who score high on impression management measures are trying to appear conventionally nice out of a fear of social disapproval (but see Johnson & Hogan, 1981).

The second resolvable issue is whether SDR should be controlled in assessing personality (e.g., Paulhus, 1981). My work has suggested that controlling SDR using self-deception type measures is seldom appropriate. It tends to remove valid variance because self-deceptive positivity is a central component of many personality dimensions (e.g., anxiety, self-esteem, dominance).[1] On the other hand, impression management can contaminate the assessment of these dimensions and should usually be controlled. More details on the various methods of control and their application are provided in a recent review paper (Paulhus, in press).

The Self- and Other-Deception Questionnaires, developed by Sackeim and Gur (1978), originally came to my attention as a graduate student. I subsequently showed that they paralleled the Alpha and Gamma factors found in early factor analyses of SDR measures, thus providing a simple interpretation of the latter (Paulhus, 1984). Since then I have spent some

---

[1] Norman (1988) argues that removal of a general factor of SDR clarifies the Big Five factor structure and, therefore, should increase validity. My own position is that there are several factors of perceived desirability (Messick, 1960) with two being particularly important. They must be dealt with separately.

time validating the measures and refining them into what I now call the Self-Deception and Impression Management Scales to distinguish them from the originals (see Paulhus, in press).

The association found between measures of self-deception and measures of psychological adjustment warrants further comment. Consistent with Taylor and Brown's review (1988), I hold that self-deceptive positivity helps the individual to cope with negative events, and, therefore, promotes adjustment. It may be that some individuals are so self-deceptive that they are maladjusted, but there is not yet any evidence that current measures can discriminate such cases. As it stands, self-deception and adjustment are conceptually distinct but cannot be measured independently.

In the most recent development, we have found that the tendency to claim certain *positive* attributes is more closely linked to adjustment than is the tendency to disclaim *negative* attributes (Paulhus & Reid, 1988). To further explore the construct of self-deception, I have reviewed the many conceptions in the literature and collected reviews of the major positions in a recent book (Lockard & Paulhus, 1988).

Experimental Work

With a view to clarifying these concepts, my recent empirical work has moved in the direction of experimentally manipulating socially desirable responding. In one paradigm, subjects are asked to respond "me" or "not me" to traits presented on a microcomputer screen. When threatening words were presented off to the side, an increased level of SDR was observed (Paulhus & Levitt, 1987); that is, subjects claimed more of the positive and fewer of the negative traits. In a subsequent study (Paulhus & Murphy, 1987), subjects who were instructed to "fake bad" showed an even more dramatic increase in SDR under threat. In the condition where subjects were instructed to "fake good," however, threatening distractors caused a *decrease* in SDR. Also reported in Paulhus and Murphy (1987) were studies showing that both threat and speed instructions eliminate the impression-management factor, leaving the self-deception factor predominant.

Reconciliation of all these findings necessitated the development of a new theory: Automatic and Controlled Self-Presentation (Paulhus, 1988). Following the terminology used in cognitive psychology (Schneider & Shiffrin, 1977; Posner & Snyder, 1975), controlled processes are those that require attentional resources to continue. Controlled selfpresentation, then, is equivalent to the familiar strategic variety known as impression management. In contrast, automatic processes are those that are stimulus-driven and proceed even without attention. Automatic self-presentation is a highly practiced, generally positivistic self-description. It is the default evaluation available even without attentional resources.

Controlled self-presentation is very flexible and is tailored to the audience; one may fake-good, fake-bad, fake-mad, and so on. There is, however, but one automatic self, which appears under stress in the form of impulsive bursts of SDR known as defensiveness.[2] Given its impulsive rather than strategic character, this automatic self-presentation may often be inappropriate and maladaptive.

One problem in studying the automatic self is understanding its origin. Our latest series of studies have been jokingly labeled the Frankenstein studies because they involve creating new selves in the laboratory. They were inspired by studies reporting that automatic responses (e.g., attitudes, stereotypes) can be conditioned in the laboratory (e.g., Smith & Lerner, 1986). Our subjects practice arbitrary self-presentations (e.g., fake-good) until they reach asymptotic levels of speed and consistency. These subjects are later tested under the distractor paradigm to see if the automatized self re-appears under stress.

As a whole, the studies reviewed above have provided a link between (a) the two-factor theories of SDR found in questionnaire responses and (b) laboratory studies of reaction to threat. In summary, self-deceptive positivity occurs when the default self-belief, which is biased toward a favorable self-description, is emitted. Individuals with a negative automatic self are likely to be maladjusted (anxious, depressed, etc.).[3] Impression management is a controlled process that is tailored to the audience. The interplay between the two modes is governed by the individual's changing emotional state (for a detailed description, see Paulhus, 1988).

Individual Differences in Motivated Bias

The above conception of self-deception as a default self-presentation does not embrace the full flavor of the concept. In most conceptions, self-deception is not so passive. Indeed, it has to be much more flexible to protect self-esteem.

This second paradigm entails a more direct approach: Make subjects distort answers and measure that distortion. The concept was derived from a manipulation used by Quattrone and Tversky (1983). They had subjects take a cold-pressor test and rate its painfulness. Half the subjects

---

[2] The automatic self may appear to be unitary and stable because it is goverened by a global self-evaluation. Alternatively, the automatic self may comprise a number of important self-schemas, which will all tend to be positive.

[3] The inculcation of a negative automatic self is particularly debilitating because of its appearance under arousal, which would be experienced as anxiety. Under nonemotional circumstances, this individual would simply be depressed. Thus the inactivity of depression would be functional in avoiding anxiety.

were advised that a person who experiences the cold-pressor as painful has a sensitive nervous system susceptible to heart disease and, therefore, can expect a lowered life-span. These subjects reported much less pain and kept their arm in the cold water longer than subjects not given this warning.

We have used a milder version of this manipulation in a questionnaire format (Paulhus & Van Selst, 1988). The questionnaire asks subjects to rate themselves on thirty traits selected to be as diverse as possible. The first page of traits is preceded by the following message:

The 15 traits listed below have been found to predict happiness in middle age. That is, people who have these traits, for some reason, end up being happy in later life.

A second page also contains 15 traits with the following message:

The 15 traits listed below have been found to predict poor success in marriage. That is, people who have these traits, for some reason, end up in unhappy marriages.

Unknown to the subject, the traits on the two pages are actually pairs of synonyms. The positive bias tends to increase ratings above those obtained under standard conditions, and the negative bias tends to lower them. Thus, the fact that the two pages contain synonyms makes the scoring procedure easy. Any increase in score from the negative to positive instructions must be a motivated bias. We have found that the order of the pages has no effect on the overall effect size or external correlates.

The sum of the differences across fifteen pairs of items is labeled the Index of Motivational Bias (IMB). Because the questionnaire is completed anonymously, any observed distortion is presumably for intrapsychic goals. The IMB may be used as a standard instrument for comparing the motivational impact of various outcomes (e.g., fear of death, aspirations for success or wealth). Alternatively, the IMB may be administered together with various measures of personality to determine their contamination with a tendency for self-deception.

In one study, the IMB was administered along with measures of the Big Five personality dimensions. Results showed that the IMB correlates positively with intellectance and negatively with anxiety and conscientiousness. The negative correlation with anxiety is consistent with theories suggesting that individuals low in anxiety employ more intrapsychic defensive processes.

The IMB also correlates positively with the Principalization defense ($r = .40$) from the Defense Mechanisms Inventory (Ihilevich & Gleser, 1986), and the Self-Deception Scale ($r = .43$), but minimally with the Impression Management Scale ($r = .09$). It is noteworthy that motivated distortion is linked to self-deception, now operationalized as excessive cognitive confidence (Paulhus, in press).

A Positive Note

The central issues in SDR have not been resolved to everyone's satisfaction. In part, the reason is a lingering animosity between polarized camps. In part, the reason is an intractable problem. Whatever its cause, the deadlock in clarifying the nature of response styles may well be broken by the joint experimental/correlational methods described here. This eclectic approach has been encouraged by a growing interest in the *process* of self-reporting (e.g., Cantor & Kihlstrom, 1987; Cliff, 1977; Jackson, 1986; Rogers, 1971). Much of the research exploits the techniques of modern cognitive psychology, for example, computer-controlled manipulation of stimuli and measurement of reaction times (e.g., Holden, Fekken, & Jackson, 1985; Knowles, 1988; Paulhus & Levitt, 1987).

My own research is part of this movement to apply social cognition techniques to issues in personality assessment. The two experimental analyses of self-deceptive positivity have converged with the traditional factor-analytic research. My hope is that these techniques contribute to the construction of a general cognitive model of the process of self-description. These, I believe, are the new solutions required to solve the old problems.

References

Block, J. (1965). *The challenge of response sets*. New York: Appleton-Century-Crofts.

Cantor, N., & Kihlstrom, J.F. (1987). *Personality and social intelligence*. Englewood Cliffs, NJ: Prentice-Hall.

Cliff, N. (1977). Further study of cognitive processing models for inventory response. *Applied Psychological Measurement, 1*, 41–49.

Crowne, D.P., & Marlowe, D.A. (1964). *The approval motive*. New York: Wiley.

Edwards, A.L. (1957). *The social desirability variable in personality assessment and research*. New York: Dryden Press.

Hartshorne, H., & May, M. (1928). *Studies in deceit*. New York: Macmillan.

Holden, R.R., Fekken, G.C., & Jackson, D.N. (1985). Structured personality test item characteristics and validity. *Journal of Research in Personality, 19*, 386–394.

Ihilevich, D., & Gleser, G.C. (1986). *Defense Mechanisms: Their classification, correlates, and measurement with the Defense Mechanisms Inventory*. Owosso, IL: DMI Associates.

Jackson, D.N. (1986). The process of responding in personality assessment. In A. Angleitner & J.S. Wiggins (Eds.), *Personality assessment via questionnaire* (pp. 123–142). New York: Springer.

Jackson, D.N., & Messick, S. (1962). Response styles and the assessment of psychopathology. In S. Messick, & J. Ross (Eds.), *Measurement in personality and cognition*. New York: Wiley.

Johnson, J.A., & Hogan, R. (1981). Moral judgments as self-presentations. *Journal of Research in Personality, 15*, 57–63.

Knowles, E.S. (1988). Item context effects on personality scales: Measuring changes the measure. *Journal of Personality and Social Psychology, 55,* 312–320.

Lockard, J.S., & Paulhus, D.L. (Eds.). (1988). *Self-deception: An adaptive mechanism?* Englewood, Cliffs, NJ: Prentice-Hall.

Meehl, P.E., & Hathaway, S.R. (1946). The K-factor as a suppressor variable in the MMPI. *Journal of Applied Psychology, 30,* 525–546.

Messick, S. (1960). Dimensions of social desirability. *Journal of Consulting Psychology, 14,* 287–297.

Norman, W.T. (1988). On separating substantive, stylistic, and evaluative components in personality measurements: A cross-national comparison. Unpublished manuscript.

Paulhus, D.L. (1981). Control of social desirability in personality inventories: Principal-factor deletion. *Journal of Research in Personality, 15,* 383–388.

Paulhus, D.L. (1984). Two-component models of socially desirable responding. *Journal of Personality and Social Psychology, 46,* 598–609.

Paulhus, D.L. (1986). Self-deception and impression management in test responses. In A. Angleitner, & J.S. Wiggins (Eds.), *Personality assessment via questionnaire* (pp. 142–165). New York: Springer.

Paulhus, D.L. (1988, August). *Automatic and controlled self-presentation.* Paper presented at meeting of the American Psychological Association, Atlanta, Georgia.

Paulhus, D.L. (in press). Measurement and control of response bias. In J.P. Robinson, P. Shaver, & L. Wrightsman (Eds.), *Measures of social attitudes and personality.* New York: Academic Press.

Paulhus, D.L., & Levitt, K. (1987). Desirable responding triggered by affect: Automatic egotism? *Journal of Personality and Social Psychology, 52,* 245–259.

Paulhus, D.L., & Murphy, G. (1987). *Disruption of impression management.* Unpublished study, University of British Columbia.

Paulhus, D.L., & Reid, D.B. (1988). *Attribution and denial in socially desirable responding.* Manuscript submitted for publication.

Paulhus, D.L., & Van Selst, M. (1988). *The Index of Motivated Bias.* Unpublished study, University of British Columbia.

Posner, M.I., & Snyder, C.R.R. (1975). Attention and cognitive control. In R.L. Solso (Ed.), *Information processing and cognition: The Loyola symposium.* Hillsdale, NJ: Erlbaum.

Quattrone, G.A., & Tversky, A. (1984). Causal versus diagnostic contingencies: On self-deception and the voter's illusion. *Journal of Personality and Social Psychology, 46,* 236–248.

Rogers, T.B. (1971). The process of responding to personality items: Some issues, a theory and some research. *Multivariate Behavioral Research Monographs,* 6(Whole No. 2).

Sackeim, H.A., & Gur, R.C. (1978). Self-deception, self-confrontation and consciousness. In G.E. Schwartz & D. Shapiro (Eds.), *Consciousness and self-regulation: Advances in research* (Vol. 2, pp. 139–197). New York: Plenum.

Schneider, W. & Shiffrin, R.M. (1977). Controlled and automatic human information processing: I. Detection, search, and attention. *Psychological Review, 84,* 1–66.

Smith, E.R., & Lerner, M. (1986). Development of automatism of social judgments. *Journal of Personality and Social Psychology, 50,* 246–259.

Taylor, S.E., & Brown, J.D. (1988). Illusion and well-being: A social-psychological perspective on mental health. *Psychological Bulletin, 103,* 193–210.

Wiggins, J.S. (1959). Interrelationships among MMPI measures of dissimulation under standard and social desirability instructions. *Journal of Consulting Psychology, 23,* 419–427.

CHAPTER 15

Accuracy in Personality Judgment and the Dancing Bear

David C. Funder

This is a symposium devoted to the future of personality research, and one development that seems likely to emerge in that future is an increasing integration of personality with social psychology. What a relief. Over the past two decades these supposedly neighboring subfields have practically been at each other's throats. In part, this antagonism was an unpleasant side effect of the "person-situation debate," and, in part, it arose out of sheer ignorance, by members of each subfield, about the aims and methodological tools of the other. As a result, as Kenrick and Funder (1988) wrote, "the two subdisciplines [have] sometimes seemed intent on defining each other out of existence" (p. 31).

More recently, however, we have begun to see something of a *rapproachement*. Once recent symbol of an improving situation was the issue of *JPSP* devoted to "integrating personality and social psychology" (Kihlstrom, 1987). Another manifestation can be seen at this conference: a surprising number of social psychologists have jumped the fence and begun conducting personality research. This latter trend has aroused a certain amount of resentment among personality's old guard, some of whom have welcomed their new colleagues with scornful remarks about "social psychologists [who] have abandoned their own fields to become . . . amateur personalogists" (Carlson, 1984, p. 1304).

Such grouchiness aside, it seems hard to doubt that the integration of personality and social psychology is a good thing (Kenrick, 1986), one reason being that each subfield has important methodological lessons to learn from the other. Social psychologists are showing an increased appreciation of matters of measurement reliability and construct validity, to which they used to think their research was immune (when the issues occurred to them at all). For their part, personality psychologists are finally breaking free of their fascination, indeed obsession, with questionnaires and the mathematical tricks you can play with them. I am greatly encouraged by the number of presentations at this symposium that examine relations between personality variables and real life outcomes in academic, work, and marital settings, and even a few that point cameras at subjects to see, from moment to moment, what they actually do. I am equally encouraged by the *scarcity* of studies that do no more than correlate questionnaire responses with other questionnaire responses. I think the influence of social upon personality psychology can take some of the credit for this methodological broadening.

Another reason that the integration of personality and social psychology is a good thing is that a number of important topics lies right at their intersection. One of these topics is the accuracy of interpersonal judgment, which I study. I am sometimes asked whether I am a personality "or" a social psychologist. (I must warn graduate students that questions like that are frequently asked at job interviews.) All I can reply is, when you study accuracy you cross that border, if there is a border, several times a day.

If one prefers, my research can be viewed as being concerned with a traditional old topic of personality psychology—assessment. My research tries to learn about the best ways to correctly characterize what a person is like, but the assessment technique that is examined by accuracy research is one each of us uses every day—intuitive judgment based on informal observation of behavior in real life settings. Researchers such as Jackson and Goldberg used to investigate (and argue about) which techniques for constructing and administering questionnaires led to the most valid assessments (e.g., Hase & Goldberg, 1967; Jackson, Neill & Bevan, 1973). My own research can be viewed as having the same basic purpose, with the twist being that, where these earlier investigators focused on questionnaires, I focus upon peer judgments.

I think that, in general, these peer judgments offer a valuable source of information about personality. I am certainly aware of the vast amount of research documenting the various "errors" people make (e.g., Nisbett & Ross, 1980), and the fact that many psychologists regard the accuracy of ordinary human judgment as rather pitiful (e.g., Dawes, 1988). But research on error, in fact, tells us very little about judgmental accuracy,[1] and defining good judgment in terms of its match to normative, quantitative models is likely not only to be oversimplifying, but fundamentally misleading. I have written about these issues elsewhere (Funder, 1987). In this chapter I would like to accentuate the positive and illustrate a few reasons why I am so impressed by the abilities displayed every day by the ordinary, intuitive judge of personality.

---

[1] Specifically, laboratory demonstrations of error establish that judgment is not perfect under all possible circumstances. Such demonstrations are informative about accuracy in daily life only to the extent that the research settings in which they are conducted can be shown to be representative of real-life settings. To date, researchers on error have put more effort into the design of clever experimental situations that elicit error than into providing evidence that these experimental situations are realistic.

Not that the intuitive judge of personality is perfect—far from it. Somebody once said that what makes a dancing bear so impressive is not that it dances well, but that it dances at all. I am impressed by human judgments of personality for roughly the same reason—not because the judgments are perfect, but because in the face of enormous difficulties it seems remarkable they manage to have any accuracy at all.

Let me be concrete about these difficulties in the context of my own research. A procedure I have used many times requires undergraduates to come into the lab and provide a Q-sort of their own personalities. After about two minutes of instruction in Q-technique, they sort one hundred cards into a forced distribution across nine categories ranging from "not all characteristic" to "highly characteristic." Each card bears a general, descriptive phrase such as "is critical and skeptical" or "is a genuinely dependable and responsible person" (Bem & Funder, 1978; Block, 1978). Each subject then provides the names of two people who know him or her well, and we bring those individuals into the lab and ask them to construct Q-sorts of the subject (we call these individuals "informants").

Many times during the course of such studies, I have walked past an experimental room in which sits a typical undergraduate, one of my informants, silently placing Q-sort cards on a table. The sight always causes me to worry: what is he (or she) doing in there?; How well is he or she doing it? After all, the whole success of my research program hinges on these informants providing accurate information.

There are many reasons to doubt such accuracy will be forthcoming. First of all, the large literature on judgmental error, while it does not tell us anything about the ratio of correct to incorrect judgments in real life, does establish that the basic processes of human reason are less than perfect. People forget things, and the way they interpret the facts they do remember is heavily influenced by biases, expectations, and tendencies to oversimplify complex phenomena. My undergraduate Q-sorters are certainly afflicted by every heuristic and bias that has ever been documented (e.g., Nisbett & Ross, 1980).

Moreover, each of these Q-sorters has had limited and idiosyncratic experience with the person he or she is trying to describe. The informant might know the subject in a couple of classes, but not in the dorm, or vice versa; he or she may be a team-mate, or a dating partner, or a drinking buddy. Each of these relationships leads the informant to see the subject in a different kind of social environment, in which the behavior that can be observed is not necessarily representative of the subject's behavior in other settings or in general. No two informants will see the subject in exactly the same settings; and no informant at all may be able to tell us about aspects of the subject's personality that he or she chooses to keep secret.

My undergraduate Q-sorters also have no particularly strong motivation to be accurate. There are no penalties or other consequences for bad performance, and the informants are sometimes in a hurry or, not surprisingly, feel they have better things to do. Some informants may also be less than totally honest. Perhaps they hate, or love, the subject they are describing, perhaps the Q-technique is asking them for information they feel is none of the researcher's business. If the informants distort or withhold information for any of these reasons, there is not a thing we can do about it.

Then there are the difficulties inherent in the technique itself. Q-sorting is no easy task, and it is not always a sure bet that informants completely understand the basis by which they should assign items to categories 1, 5, or 9. Even more importantly, the Q-items themselves are neither unambiguous nor self-explanatory. What behaviors, exactly, are referred to by "is critical and skeptical" or "is a genuinely dependable and responsible person?" Informants surely differ from each other in how they interpret items such as these, and these differences add yet another source of distortion and noise to the data.

In fact, the more one thinks about an informant doing a Q-sort of a close acquaintance, the more the procedure looks like a disaster waiting to happen. What kind of valid information about personality could possibly emerge from circumstances like these? I am not just being rhetorical. I have worried about this question more than a few times.

I am not so worried any more, however. My experience with Q-sort data has, to some degree, restored my faith in human nature, or at least in human judgment. The bear does dance. He's not ready for the Bolshoi, but he doesn't do badly, for a bear.

The evidence that the human judge of personality can do a pretty good job, despite all the obvious obstacles, comes in two forms. The first is interjudge agreement. The second consists of the specific behaviors that peer judgments of personality are able to predict. For now, let me present just one example of each kind of evidence.

Interjudge Agreement

The best way I can illustrate the findings on interjudge agreement is with Table 15.1, which was taken from Funder and Dobroth (1987). This table lists the fifteen Q-sort items with the best and worst agreement between self-judgments and peer judgments (self-other agreement), and among peer judgments (other-other agreement). The data come from several different samples, so you can see the relative stability of these correlations from one sample to the next.

First, it should be noted that, overall, eighty-seven of the one hundred Q-sort items manifest a significant degree of average interjudge agreement. In other words, two of the fifteen *worst* items still manage to attain significant agreement. The fifteen *best* items span a wide portion of the

TABLE 15.1. Traits with highest and lowest interjudge agreement

No. Trait	Average total agreement	Self-other Sample 1 (n = 41)	Self-other Sample 2 (n = 64)	Interpeer Sample 1 (n = 37)	Interpeer Sample 2 (n = 69)	Interpeer Sample 3 (n = 50)
		Most agreement				
90. Is concerned with philosophical problems	.50***	.68***	.31*	.52***	.53***	.54***
84. Is cheerful	.43***	.42**	.36**	.35*	.45***	.58***
31. Regards self as physically attractive	.43***	.35*	.40**	.55***	.35**	.57***
28. Tends to arouse liking and acceptance	.41***	.50***	.41***	.45**	.31**	.40**
52. Behaves in an assertive fashion	.40***	.38*	.30*	.36*	.55***	.44**
4. Is a talkative individual	.40***	.40**	.33**	.38*	.37**	.59***
80. Interested in opposite sex	.40***	.39*	.21	.58***	.43***	.52***
62. Rebellious and nonconforming	.40***	.50***	.33**	.57***	.30*	.36**
33. Is calm, relaxed	.39***	.44*	.32**	.15	.50***	.48***
29. Turned to for advice and reassurance	.38***	.59***	.33**	.36*	.27*	.32*
91. Is power oriented	.37***	.40**	.22	.52***	.34**	.50***
81. Physically attractive	.36***	.36*	.28*	.51**	.39***	.36**
51. Values intellectual matters	.36***	.34*	.48***	.52***	.04	.42**
66. Enjoys aesthetic impressions	.36***	.46**	.20	.33*	.23	.64***
18. Initiates humor	.36***	.46**	.31*	.12	.40***	.41**
		Least agreement				
46. Engages in personal fantasy and daydreams	.05	.08	.00	.00	.16	.02
87. Interprets clear-cut situations in particularizing ways	.07	.18	.00	.00	.16	.02
89. Compares self to others	.07	.05	.00	.00	.25	.01
12. Tends to be self-defensive	.08	.02	.05	.19	.16	.02
34. Overreactive to minor frustrations	.08	.05	.00	.22	.15	.07
23. Extrapunitive: transfers and projects blame	.09	.10	.00	.22	.00	.25

TABLE 15.1. *Continued*

	No. Trait	Average total agreement	Self-other Sample 1 (n = 41)	Self-other Sample 2 (n = 64)	Interpeer Sample 1 (n = 37)	Interpeer Sample 2 (n = 69)	Interpeer Sample 3 (n = 50)
10.	Anxiety and tension produce bodily symptoms	.10	.01	.02	.28	.10	.19
69.	Sensitive to demands	.10	−.22	.00	.15	.02	.43**
76.	Projects own motives onto others	.10	−.10	.00	.36	.13	.15
13.	Thin-skinned; sensitive to criticism	.11	.17	.00	.31	.09	.11
36.	Subtly negativistic	.11	.16	.00	.15	.06	.30
77.	Appears straightforward and candid	.11	−.05	.07	.19	.19	.16
50.	Unpredictable and changeable	.11	−.06	.12	.22	.00	.31
30.	Withdraws from adversity	.13*	.32*	.00	.26	.08	.10
70.	Is ethically consistent	.13*	.10	.10	.14	.21	.11

*p<.05. two-tailed.
**p<.01. two-tailed.
***p<.001. two-tailed.
From Funder, D. C. & Dobroth, K. M. "Differences Between Traits: Properties Associated with Interjudge Agreement." *Journal of Personality and Social Psychology, 52.* Copyright ©1987. Reprinted with permission.

personality domain. They include "concerned with philosophical problems," "cheerful" and "rebellious and nonconforming." So good interjudge agreement is not restricted to just one kind of trait; nor is good agreement "flukey." The high correlations hold up well across different samples of judges and targets.

Still, one can notice a difference between the best and worst items. The best items include traits such as "talkative," whereas the worst items seem more likely to include such traits as "engages in personality fantasy and daydreams" and "is sensitive to demands." In the study by Funder and Dobroth (1987), we operationalized the dimension of difference as a composite variable we named "subjective visibility." The essence of this dimension is captured by a question we asked a group of undergraduate raters about each of the Q-items: "How easy (or hard) do you think it would be to judge this trait?" It turns out that such ratings correlate well with the actual agreement with which these traits are applied to real individuals, as is illustrated in Table 15.1 (across all one hundred items, the r between visibility and average agreement was .42, $p < .001$). For related findings, see Cheek (1982), Kenrick and Stringfield (1980), and Norman and Goldberg (1966).

We recently extended this finding to judges who do not know their targets nearly so well. It turns out that even when judges have viewed their target for just a few minutes, the visibility dimension discriminates well between the traits that will be judged with better and worse self-other and other-other agreement (Funder & Colvin, 1988). This is the case even though, as might be expected, these "strangers" ratings agree with self-ratings much less than do ratings by well-acquainted informants.

Unfortunately, the woefully incomplete literature review by Shrauger and Schoeneman (1979) continues to be cited as having established that agreement between self- and peer judgments of personality is low or nonexistent. The data just summarized, and findings by many other investigators, establish instead that good agreement can be routinely found (e.g., Andersen, 1984; Cheek, 1982; Edwards & Klockars, 1981; Funder, 1980b; Goldberg, Norman & Schwartz, 1980; Hase & Goldberg, 1967; McCrae, 1982; Monson, Tanke & Lund, 1980; Paunonen & Jackson, 1985; Woodruffe, 1985), and that this agreement occurs despite all the obstacles I listed earlier that stand in the way of two judges of the same personality managing to agree with each other. The agreement is not perfect, but I stand amazed that the judges do so well.

Correlations with Behavior

Another example of what peer judgments of personality can do is provided by their correlations with direct behavioral measurements. Many investigators, including myself, have obtained peer personality judgments of our subjects and then viewed the subjects' behavior in some kind of laboratory situation. There are good reasons to doubt that any correlations between personality judgments and behavior could arise in such circumstances. All the problems with peer judgments cited earlier still apply. Moreover, the behavior measured is often of a sort the peer judges have never seen, and is measured at one time, at one place, and under one idiosyncratic set of circumstances. No matter how strong one's faith is in the essential coherence of personality, one can find reasons to wonder whether meaningful correlations between general peer judgments of personality and single laboratory behaviors could ever emerge.

I am always amazed, therefore, when they do emerge. Examples in my own research have included strong and meaningful correlations between informants' Q-sort judgments and behaviors so diverse as attributional style (Funder, 1980a), attitude change (Funder, 1982), delay of gratification (Bem & Funder, 1978; Funder, Block & Block, 1983; Funder & Block, in press), and even the tendency to make the so-called "fundamental attribution error" (Block & Funder, 1986), so I don't think the point needs belaboring here. I cannot, however, resist illustrating the point with one set of correlations that has emerged from the computer only recently.

In our research, an experimenter stays in the room with the subject while he or she completes the self Q-sort, just in case questions or problems arise. Because the experimenter has to sit there anyway, in one study we decided to have him write down how long the subject took to complete the self Q-sort. No time limit was imposed, and the subject did not know that he or she was being timed. The range was anywhere from twenty minutes to two-and-a-half hours. We correlated this variable, which we dubbed "Q-time," with the Q-sort descriptions of the subjects that were provided by their friends and acquaintances.

Again, there seems no good reason to expect these correlations to be significant or numerous. The "behavior," if you can call it that, was nothing that peers had ever seen the subject do. At least, it seems unlikely that a subject's roomates ordinarily had a chance to observe how much time he or she required to complete a formalized self-description task. Their Q-sort judgments had to be based, instead, on whatever idiosyncratic, *other* behaviors they happened to observe, and the relationship between their judgments and "Q-time" were then limited by (1) the extent to which these behaviors were indeed informative about relevant personality characteristics and (2) the extent to which these personality characteristics were indeed predictive of the "Q-time" behavior. Of course, these limitations are just added to the other problems associated with the individual ways the informants interpreted each item, had difficulties with the technique, and so on.

Nonetheless, an interesting set of correlates did emerge and is shown in Table 15.2. I must hasten to acknowledge that these correlates are not particularly large. Much larger correlations between personality judgments and behavior abound in the literature, including those references cited above. Nevertheless, the present results clearly go beyond chance, are consistent across the sexes, and tell an interesting story; according to may "dancing bear" philosophy, I find it impressive that they managed to appear at all.

The subjects who took the longest to complete a self Q-sort were described by their acquaintances as tending to "particularize situations . . . interpret basically simple situations in complex ways." That tendency would slow one down when doing a self Q-sort, wouldn't it? The slow Q-sorters also were described as having a "readiness to feel guilt," and as being considerate, sympathetic, and warm. We get a picture of a subject considerably trying to help the experimenter, to the point of overdoing it somewhat.

The negative correlates of the "Q-time" variable are even more interesting. The subjects who took the *least* time to complete their self Q-sorts were described by their acquaintances as over-reactive, irritable,

TABLE 15.2 Informants' Q-sort correlates of Q-time (time taken to complete self Q-sort.)

Q-item	All S (n=121)	Females (n=61)	Males (n=60)
Positive correlates			
Particularizes situations (interprets simple situations in complex ways)	.26★★	.12	.40★★
Has a readiness to feel guilt	.21★	.24	.19
Considerate and sympathetic	.20★	.25	.17
Evaluates motives of others	.20★	.25	.17
Warm	.19★	.29	.08
Negative correlates			
Projects own feelings/motives onto others	−.24★★	−.36★★	−.11
Gives up in face of adversity	−.22★★	−.23★★	−.21
Over-reactive; irritable	−.22★★	−.20	−.24
Tends to be self-defensive	−.21★	−.11	−.32★★
Guileful and deceitful	−.19★	−.29	−.10
Fluctuating moods	−.19★	−.14	−.28★
Feels lack of personal meaning in life	−.18★	−.23	−.14

Two tailed probabilities
★★ $p < .01$
★ $p < .05$

self-defensive, deceitful, moody, and feeling a lack of meaning in life. And they give up in the face of adversity! It would appear that the self-descriptive task confronted these subjects with a lot of negative information about themselves that they had difficulty facing, so they simply got out of the situation, as quickly as they could.

Remember where these peer judgments came from. They resulted from whatever behaviors the subjects' acquaintances happened fortuitously to view in the dorm, in class or wherever, and from the way these observations were combined by the acquaintances' intuitive judgment processes. The behaviors could have been "similar" to the Q-time variable only in the most general sense; judging from Table 15.2 they involved expressions of guilt and sympathy, irritability, moodiness, and defensiveness. Apparently, Q-time involved these variables as well. The conceptual distance between the behaviors judges observed back in the dorm, and the behavior their judgments predicted, had to be bridged by these personality variables, and the resulting relationships in Table 15.2 between dorm behavior and lab behavior can only be described as "cross-situational consistency" of a profound sort. The informants somehow detected in the subjects' everyday behaviors a combination of traits so general in their significance that they ended up being predictive of a single measurement of such a strange variable as Q-time.

Of course, the fashion nowadays is to lament how each correlation in Table 15.2 is not 1.0. Some psychologists, just to be mean, will even square each of these r's so that they can derive a microscopic number to attach to the mysterious concept of "variance explained" (cf. Funder &

Ozer, 1983, O'Grady, 1982), but the correlations are good enough for me, at least for now. The volume of noise through which signals like Table 15.2 are detected implies that the ultimate sources of the signal must be extremely strong indeed. The two sources of signal are (1) the fundamental qualities of personality that are influential across such a broad range of situations and (2) the complex processes of observation and judgment that allow even a typical undergraduate informant to detect these qualities with some degree of accuracy.

Future Directions

Serious thought about results such as those in Tables 15.1 and 15.2 brings two research questions to mind. The first is, how do these informants do it? How do they go from the haphazard and idiosyncratic observations that they make of their friends' behaviors in various situations to general judgments of personality that are *valid,* according to the criteria of interjudge agreement and behavioral predictability?

A question like this ought to be, but seldom is, a central focus of research on social cognition (for a concurring view, see Neisser, 1980). Such research needs to do more than catalogue alleged biases of judgment, or conduct finely grained analyses of cognitive models that differ only slightly from each other, although these studies have their place. It should address directly the question of how people manage to extract complex *and valid* personality information from the ambiguous, incomplete and shifting array of social stimuli with which each acquaintance confronts them. Such research will have to take seriously the problem of cataloguing and analyzing the stimuli that people present, and of assessing the relationship between such stimuli and actual properties of people (cf. McArthur & Baron, 1983).

The second research question that comes to mind is, under what circumstances are individuals' judgments of each other more and less likely to be valid? Research to answer this question, like research on assessment more generally, is centrally concerned with construct validity (Cronbach & Meehl, 1955). The accuracy of a peer judgment, like the validity of a questionnaire, cannot be established in relation to any single criterion, but only through the lawfulness and coherence of the nomological net of relationships between the judgment and other sources of data about the target of judgment.

The two principal other sources of data are judgments provided by other informants, and direct measurements of behavior. I have just illustrated how each type of evidence can be used to support the essential validity of personality judgment. What we need to know next is, what kind of target, judge, relationship between judge and target, setting of interaction, or dimension of judgment makes accuracy most likely?

Research conducted within the error paradigm is absolutely no help in answering questions like those. The implicit, and sometimes explicit, assumption of error research is that we would be more accurate if we simply made fewer errors (see Dawes, 1988, and Nisbett & Ross, 1980). To my knowledge, however, the point has never been empirically established. Indeed, such research that does bear on the issue suggests that, if anything, the elimination of judgmental "error" will actually, often, *decrease* accuracy in realistic settings (Block & Funder, 1986; Bernardin & Pence, 1980).

What is needed, therefore, is more research that uses the two criteria just illustrated. The design of my own current program is outlined in Figure 15.1. Briefly, it entails the videotaping of the spontaneous behavior of each subject in three different situations, with two different partners. Each subject describes his or her own personality with the Q-sort and

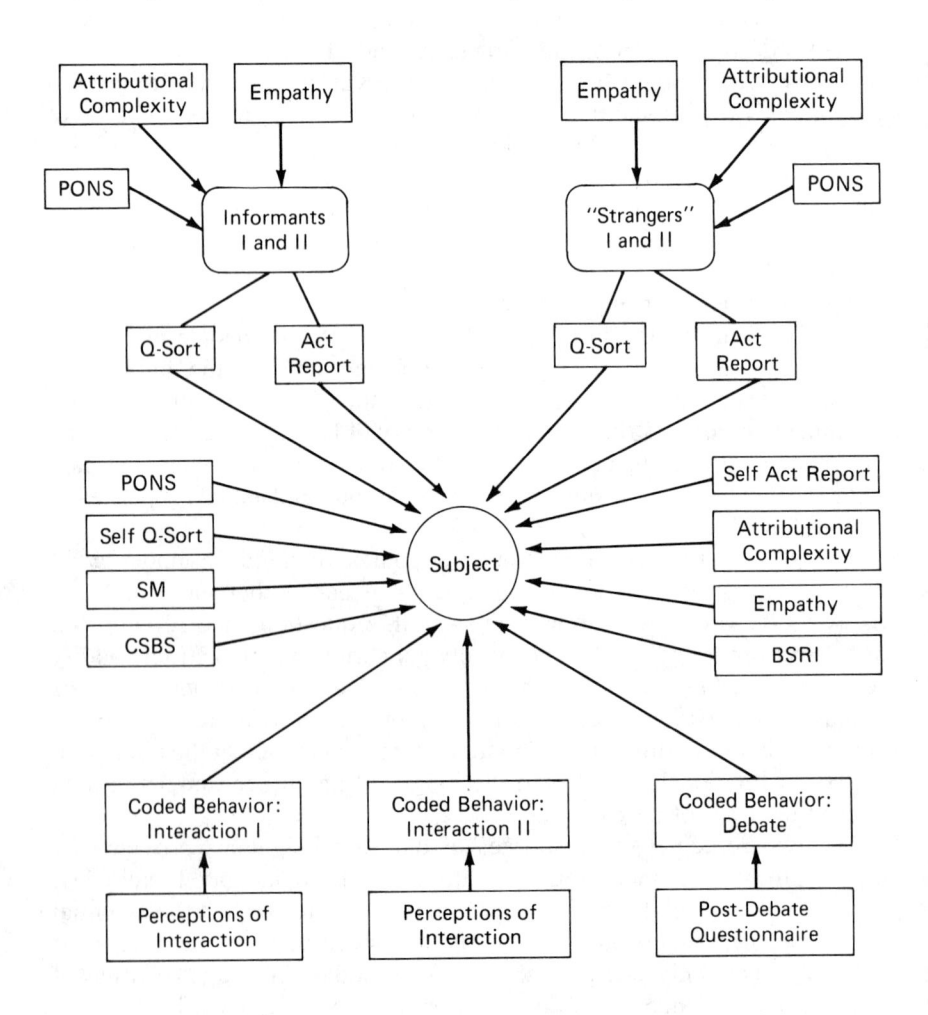

FIGURE 15.1

recruits two close acquaintances who also provide Q-sorts of the subject. Other measures of personality and ability are taken of subjects and informants. Finally, each informant views a five-minute videotape of a subject he or she does *not* know, and tries to construct a Q-sort of that individual's personality.

Analyses of this data set are allowing us to address many different questions relevant to judgmental accuracy. Under what kinds of circumstances are the convergences between these different sources of data maximized and minimized? For instance, is self-informant agreement better for some sorts of subjects, or informants, than others? Are some traits judged more accurately than others? Are some behaviors more predictable than others? It seems reasonable to expect that just as traits differ in visibility, so do behaviors. The implication might be that judgments made on the basis of more visible behaviors, as well as personality-based predictions of such behaviors, will tend to be relatively accurate. Our current research is examining this question, and others (Funder & Colvin, 1988; Funder & Dobroth, 1987; Funder & Harris, 1986).

The central aim of our research program is to assess the accuracy of judgments, *not* on the basis of their adherence to hypothetical, "normative" models, but on the basis of their fidelity with reality. "Reality," in this context, is something that I presume to be reflected through the agreement found between judgments and through the ability of judgments of personality to predict behavior. Other investigators are also beginning to pursue accuracy in this way (see Wright & Mischel, 1987; and Ickes, Tooke, Stinson, Baker & Bissonnette, 1988).

I believe that the thorough analysis of the circumstances under which personality judgments agree with each other and are predictive of behavior provides a research agenda that can lead to real progress in our ability to understand and improve social judgment. I also believe this research agenda yields enough questions, if I may take a long view, to keep us all productively busy for thousands of years.

Acknowledgments. The research reported in this chapter was supported by National Institute of Mental Health grants MH40808 and MH42427 to David Funder.

References

Andersen, S. (1984). Self-knowledge and social inference: II. The diagnosticity of cognitive/affective and behavioral data. *Journal of Personality and Social Psychology, 46,* 294–307.

Bem, D.J., & Funder, D.C. (1978). Predicting more of the people more of the time: Assessing the personality of situations. *Psychological Review, 85,* 485–501.

Bernardin, H.J., & Pence, E.C. (1980). Effects of rater training: Creating new response sets and decreasing accuracy. *Journal of Applied Psychology, 65,* 60–66.

Block, J. (1978). *The Q-sort method in personality assessment and psychiatric research.* Palo Alto, CA: Consulting Psychologists Press. (Original work published 1961).

Block, J., & Funder, D.C. (1986). Social roles and social perception: Individual differences in attribution and "error." *Journal of Personality and Social Psychology, 51,* 1200–1207.

Carlson, R. (1984). What's social about social psychology? Where's the person in personality research? *Journal of Personality and Social Psychology, 35,* 1055–1074.

Cheek, J.M. (1982). Aggregation, moderator variables, and the validity of personality tests: A peer-rating study. *Journal of Personality and Social Psychology, 43,* 1254–1269.

Cronbach, L.J., & Meehl, P.E. (1955). Construct validity in psychological tests. *Psychological Bulletin, 52,* 281–302.

Dawes, R. (1988). *Rational judgment in an uncertain world.* San Diego: Harcourt Brace.

Edwards, A.L., & Klockars, A.J. (1981). Significant others and self-evaluation: Relationships between perceived and actual evaluations. *Personality and Social Psychology Bulletin, 7,* 244–251.

Funder, D.C. (1980a). On seeing ourselves as others see us: Self-other agreement and discrepancy in personality ratings. *Journal of Personality, 48,* 473–493.

Funder, D.C. (1980b). The "trait" of ascribing traits: Individual differences in the tendency to trait ascription. *Journal of Research in Personality, 14,* 376–385.

Funder, D.C. (1982). On assessing social psychological theories through the study of individual differences: Template matching and forced compliance. *Journal of Personality and Social Psychology, 43,* 100–110.

Funder, D.C., & Block, J. (in press). The role of ego-control, ego-resiliency, and IQ in delay of gratification in adolescence. *Journal of Personality and Social Psychology.*

Funder, D.C., Bloc, J.H., & Block, J. (1983). Delay of gratification: Some longitudinal personality correlates. *Journal of Personality and Social Psychology, 44,* 1198–1213.

Funder, D.C., & Colvin, C.R. (1988). Friends and strangers: Acquaintanceship, agreement, and the accuracy of personality judgment. *Journal of Personality and Social psychology, 55,* 149–158.

Funder, D.C., & Dobroth, K.M. (1987). Differences between traits: Properties associated with interjudge agreement. *Journal of Personality and Social Psychology, 52,* 409–418.

Funder, D.C., & Harris, M.J. (1986). On the several facets of personality assessment: The case of social acuity. *Journal of Personality, 54,* 528–550.

Goldberg, L.R., Norman, W.T., & Schwartz, E. (1980). The comparative validity of questionnaire data (16PF scales) and objective test data (O-A) data in predicting five peer-rating criteria. *Applied Psychological Measurement, 4,* 183–194.

Hase, H.D. & Goldberg, L.R. (1967). Comparative validity of different strategies of constructing personality inventory scales. *Psychological Bulletin, 67,* 231–248.

Ickes, W., Tooke, W., Stinson, L., Baker, V.L., & Bissonnette, V. (1988). Naturalistic social cognition: Intersubjectivity in same-sex dyads. *Journal of Nonverbal Behavior, 12,* 58–84.

Jackson, D.N., Neill, J.A., & Bevan, A.R. (1973). An evaluation of forced-choice and true-false item formats in personality assessment. *Journal of Research in Personality, 7,* 21–30.

Kenrick, D.T. (1986). How strong is the case against contemporary social and personality psychology?: A response to Carlson. *Journal of Personality and Social Psychology, 50,* 839–844.

Kenrick, D.T., & Funder, D.C. (1988). Profiting from controversy; Lessons from the person-situation debate. *American Psychologist, 43,* 23–34.

Kenrick, D.T., & Stringfield, D.O. (1980). Personality traits and the eye of the beholder: Crossing some traditional philosophical boundaries in the search for consistency in all of the people. *Psychological Review, 87,* 88–104.

Kihlstrom, J.F. (Ed.). (1987). Integrating personality and social psychology. [Special issue]. *Journal of Personality and Social Psychology, 53.*

McArthur, L.Z., & Baron, R.M. (1983). Toward an ecological theory of social perception. *Psychological Review, 90,* 215–238.

McCrae, R.R. (1982). Consensual validation of personality traits: Evidence from self-reports and ratings. *Journal of Personality and Social Psychology, 43,* 293–303.

Monson, T.C., Tanke, E.D., & Lund, J. (1980). Determinants of social perception in a naturalistic setting. *Journal of Research in Personality, 14,* 104–120.

Neisser, U. (1980). On "social knowing." *Personality and Social Psychology Bulletin, 6,* 601–605.

Nisbett, R., & Ross, L. (1980). *Human inference: Strategies and shortcomings of social judgment.* Englewood Cliffs, NJ: Prentice-Hall.

Norman, W.T., & Goldberg, L.R. (1966). Raters, ratees, and randomness in personality structure. *Journal of Personality and Social Psychology, 4,* 681–691.

O'Grady, K.E. (1982). Measures of explained variance: Cautions and limitations. *Psychological Bulletin, 92,* 766–777.

Paunonen, S.V., & Jackson, D.N. (1985). Idiographic measurement strategies for personality and prediction: Some unredeemed promissory notes. *Psychological Review, 92,* 486–511.

Shrauger, J.S., & Schoeneman, T.J. (1979). Symbolic interactionist view of self-concept: Through the looking glass darkly. *Psychological Bulletin, 86,* 549–573.

Woodruffe, C. (1985). Consensual validation of personality traits: Additional evidence and individual differences. *Journal of Personality and Social Psychology, 48,* 1240–1252.

Wright, J.C., & Mischel, W. (1987). A conditional approach to dispositional constructs: The local predictability of social behavior. *Journal of Personality and Social Psychology, 53,* 1159–1177.

CHAPTER 16

Construct Validity in Personality Assessment

Daniel J. Ozer

In recent years, the conceptualization and assessment of validity in psychological measurement has been transformed. Where one could formerly denote various types of validity (i.e., construct, content, and criterion validity), there is a now widespread understanding that construct validity subsumes all that was previously seen as disparate (Guion, 1980; Messick, 1980). Where convergent and discriminant aspects of construct validity were inferred from inspection of a correlation matrix (Campbell & Fiske, 1959), there are now various quantitative procedures, including factor analytic (e.g., Jackson, 1975) and structural-equation models (e.g., Judd, Jessor, & Donovon, 1986) to aid in the interpretation of research outcomes.

These developments, which alter the meaning and assessment of validity in psychological measurement, can be understood as elaborations and extensions of the model of construct validity described by Campbell and Fiske (1959). While they have led to progress in several substantive areas (see Wainer & Braun, 1988 for various examples), one may question whether construct validation in personality assessment has been aided by the procedures suggested by Campbell and Fiske or any of the subsequent developments. Indeed, Campbell and O'Connell note the "disappointing results" (1982, p. 104) obtained in personality psychology through triangulation by multiple methods. Fiske (1986) is apparently pessimistic about the possibility of ever satisfactorily applying the method of construct validation to all but the most narrow and directly observable units of personality. How do the problems experienced in the application of construct validation methods in the domain of personality arise? Are there important defects in the formulation of construct validity, or do the difficulties originate within personality theory and the standard procedures of personality assessment? This essay will review aspects of the development of the current conceptualization of construct validity, and note how certain features of this conceptualization, together with the subject matter of personality psychology, combine to create the difficulties noted above. Some alterations in the way construct validity is understood, and in the way personality theory is articulated, will be suggested as possible escapes from the current predicament.

The "Received View" of Construct Validity

Cronbach (1988) describes two conflicting themes that coexist in various descriptions of the construct validation process. The historically older one, labelled the "weak program," emphasizes the examination of the relations between test scores and a multitude of external indicators. Gough (1965) provides the most detailed description of how one might proceed to determine the meaning of test scores through the application of this program. An alternative "strong program" first appeared in Cronbach and Meehl's (1955) pivotal contribution, was further elaborated by Loevinger (1957), and became established in the multi-trait multi-method matrix (MTMMM) procedure described by Campbell and Fiske (1959). Deriving specific predictions from theory and determining that the test data conform to predictions are the essentials of this second program. Such procedures are especially powerful when one may simultaneously reject plausible rival hypotheses derived from alternative theories.

These two programs set about determining the meaning of test scores from two different starting points. Phrased as questions, the weak program asks, What do these scores mean?, while the strong program asks, Do these scores have their intended meaning? A good answer to the former question requires a thorough exploration of the empirical relations between the test score and a wide-ranging set of external variables. The meaning of the scores is *inductively* derived through the examination of these relations. The latter question is answered through the *deduction* of specific hypotheses from theory, and the subsequent testing of the hypotheses. I have elsewhere (Ozer, 1986) referred to these strategies of construct validation as "inductive" and "deductive", and will use these labels here.

Cronbach, in granting "some merit" (1988, p.12) to the inductive strategy, offers a more even-handed evaluation than that which has become institutionalized in the *Standards for Educational and Psychological Testing* (AERA, APA, NCME, 1985). The *Standards* fully incorporate principles derived from the deductive approach, but generally ignore principles derived from inductive validational procedures. In contrast, the notion of construct validity, as introduced by Cronbach & Meehl (1955), explicitly discusses the utility of viewing "constructs as inductive summaries" (p. 292) of observed relations when there is little theory to provide more specific definition. Loevinger's (1957) characterization of construct validity moves towards a view emphasizing a deductive strategy. She suggests that the external correlates of test scores "be overdetermined" (p.687) by the construct's definition (i.e., ad hoc explanations accounting for discordant relations undermine the construct validation effort)——a view offering little role for "constructs as inductive summaries."

The kind of overdetermination needed to support a construct interpretation of test scores is considerably restricted by the MTMMM approach described by Campbell and Fiske (1959). An MTMMM is formed by including the test scores in a correlation matrix of additional traits, where each trait has been measured by several different methods. These additional traits should include content outside the domain of the trait of interest. Campbell and Fiske suggested several specific criteria that should be satisfied in such a matrix as part of the construct validation process. Convergent validity must be established by demonstrating that monotrait-heteromethod correlations (validity coefficients) are sufficiently large (i.e. the test scores under consideration should be similar to measures of the same trait obtained through different methods). Discriminant validity is established by showing that a test score's validity coefficient (a monotrait-heteromethod correlation) is larger than the test score's correlation with different traits measured either with the same (heterotrait-monomethod) or different (heterotrait-heteromethod) method used in obtaining the test score. While Campbell and Fiske do not elaborate, in detail, how one might proceed in choosing traits to include in an MTMMM, their discussion does indicate that these traits include both those that are suggested by theory to be similar to and different from the trait assessed by the test score under examination. Campbell (1960) also notes the desirability of including measures likely to be extraneous and unwanted influences on the test scores (e.g., measures of response bias and intelligence for assessing the validity of a personality scale).

The Campbell and Fiske recommendations form the basis of our current understanding of construct validity, and appear to be the primary inspiration for the current *Standards* (AERA, APA, & NCME, 1985). Three standards (1.8, 1.9, 1.10) pertain to the demonstration of construct validity, and their content is nearly isomorphic with the recommendations of Campbell and Fiske. The logic of convergent and discriminant validation as described by Campbell and Fiske has, therefore, become the institutionalized definition of construct validation.

Construct Validity: Criticisms and Correctives

If one were to regard the convergent and discriminant analyses of an MTMMM as but one means of construct validation, one especially useful for evaluating measures of constructs residing in well-developed and circumscribed theoretical contexts, then there would be little need for criticism. Campbell and Fiske argue, however, that their suggested procedures ". . . are intended to be as appropriate to the relatively atheoretical efforts typical of the tests and measurements field as to more theoretical efforts" (1959, p. 100), and the *Standards* are consistent with this argument.

Three reservations concerning the MTMMM procedure as a general scheme of construct validation will be described: (1) a failure to acknowledge construct validation through inductive procedures; (2) the interpretation of convergent and discriminant information; (3) the conceptualization of method variance. In each instance, alternatives to the canons of the "received view" will be suggested.

The Need for Inductive Procedures of Construct Validation

Psychological tests are developed for reasons other than measuring terms specified by psychological theory; practical considerations, not psychological theory, motivated early intelligence and psychodiagnostic tests (e.g., Binet's early efforts; the MMPI). Nevertheless, a measure cannot be developed for each inference required by practitioners; nor is there adequate theory to suggest constructs, which, if measured, would provide the needed information. Thus, neither construct validity nor criterion validity procedures can be counted on to serve current practical needs.

Even when theory does motivate the development of an instrument, the content of the theory may be insufficient for the demands of construct validation by deductive methods. In such circumstances, should personal hunches be treated as serious theoretical conjectures, or would it be preferable to admit ignorance and proceed to explore empirically as large a domain as possible? In the worst case scenario, blind empiricism seems more instructive, although more demanding, than testing uninformed speculation.

Gough (1965) offers a procedure for the inductive validation of test scores that is applicable in either of these two contexts. His procedure of conceptual analysis includes elements commonly associated with both criterion and content validity, and can utilize theory, if it exists, but does not depend on it. The development of the California Psychological Inventory (CPI) through the conceptual analysis method demonstrates that this procedure can generate theory as well. When first introduced (Gough, 1957), the scles of the CPI were a collection of "folk concept" measures. The current CPI (Gough, 1987) is informed by a well-articulated theoretical structure. While conceptual analysis is not an algorithm for theory creation, the history of the CPI clearly demonstrates its utility as an aid for theory construction.

Interpreting Convergent and Discriminant Information

In Campbell and Fiske's (1959) original discussion, convergent and discriminant validity appear to be given equal weight in the evaluation of construct validity, although later formulations (e.g., Cook & Campbell, 1979) recognize that evidence pertaining to convergent validity is useful even in the absence of discriminant validity. This disparity can be stated even more strongly:

1. Given evidence supporting the convergent validity of test scores, evidence pertaining to discriminant validity is useful for informing the interpretation of test scores, but is no more crucial than any other external correlate of the scale.

2. In the absence of evidence supporting convergent validity, evidence pertaining to discriminant validity is nearly useless.

This second proposition seems obviously true: knowing what test scores do *not* measure does not, by itself, provide much help in ascertaining what the test scores do measure. An example may clarify the first proposition. A classic failure to demonstrate discriminant validity is found in Thorndike's (1920) discussion of the "halo effect." Ratings of teachers' intelligence became suspect because of their correlation of .63 with ratings of voice quality. Suppose that the WAIS IQs of the teachers were available, and that the ratings of intelligence and the WAIS also had a correlation of .63. While the correlation between the ratings of intelligence and voice quality would seem an odd result, it would be inappropriate to dismiss the ratings of intelligence given the convergent validation. In many contexts, convergent evidence is of much greater utility for determining the meaning of a set of test scores than is discriminant evidence. Only when well-articulated theory leads to a provocative choice of alternative test interpretations will discriminant validity vitally inform the construct validation process by explicitly testing alternative formulations of the test scores.

Method Variance

When multiple measures of the same trait are employed in research, as suggested by an MTMMM approach to construct validation, almost invariably the correlations among these measures are less than perfect, even when corrected for attenuation due to measurement error. When measures of different traits share the same method of measurement, their correlation is often larger than that obtained when methods differ. Method variance is the systematic variability associated with measurement operations rather than the characteristic being measured, and is generally regarded as a distortion in measurement and irrelevant to the understanding of the construct being measured. Following Campbell and Fiske (1959), the systematic effect of method variance is most often understood as inflating the relations among traits sharing the same measurement operations. The logical alternative, suggested by Campbell and O'Connell (1967, 1982) is that method variance suppresses the relation among traits measured by different methods. In this rarely invoked second view, monomethod rather than heteromethod correlation matrices provide a more accurate picture of trait relations, although Campbell and O'Connell (1982) find little evidence to support this interpretation.

If neither interpretation of method variance can be successfully applied in personality measurement, there seem to be but two alternatives. Either there is nothing there (i.e., personality is a vacuous concept) or there is something *fundamentally* wrong with the way method variance is construed in the personality domain. Because there are at least some MTMMM's in the personality domain that are virtually picture-perfect (e.g., McCrae & Costa, 1987), the former possibility seems unduly nihilistic. There appears to be but one choice left; the conceptualization of method variance in personality assessment is fundamentally inadequate.

Common to both interpretations of method variance advanced to this point is the notion that measurement represents a "trait-method unit" (Campbell & Fiske, 1959, p. 81), and that it is possible to decompose this unit into constituent parts. The metaphor frequently offered as capturing the core of MTMMM procedures is triangulation—an object (i.e., a trait) viewed from several perspectives (i.e., methods) can be seen in ways that transcend the distortions or illusions inherent in a single viewpoint. As an alternative, one might suggest that the uncertainty principle of quantum physics translates neatly into psychological measurement such that the act of measurement itself alters the attributes of the object being measured, but this seems unnecessarily fanciful. I would suggest that chemistry provides a more useful metaphor for understanding compounds like trait-method units.

Thinking of trait-method units as analogous to chemical compounds suggests that two such units can have radically different properties even if one "element" is held in common (e.g., salt and hydrochloric acid have some very different properties despite the chlorine in each). In this view, the same trait can be paired with different methods, with different resulting characteristics. Various complications may be encompassed by a chemical metaphor. Isomers are compounds of atoms of identical kind and number but with different atomic arrangement and different chemical properties. The effect of question order in surveys (see Schuman and Kalton, 1985) suggests that metaphoric isomerism may exist in psychological measurement as well.

Construing trait-method units as analogous to chemical compounds must drastically alter the way we think about method. Properties of test scores are not distorted by the method through which they are obtained; rather, the test score can only be understood through a consideration of both the trait and the method. To accomplish this, the definition of a construct, or the theory in which it is embedded, must have implications for measurement; or alternatively, a psychological understanding of method is required. Each of these options deserves closer attention.

The Specification of Method Within Theory

The current *Standards* (AERA, APA, NCME, 1985) indicate that construct validation presumes a conceptual formulation of the construct. A careful formulation of a construct will often have methodological implications that should be made explicit. For example, suppose one sets out to measure "agreeableness" with a self-report scale. One could define "agreeableness" as a disposition to behave in certain (specified) ways, or as a consequence a person might intend their actions to have, or as a reaction others have to an individual's behavior. These three different definitions are not equivalent, and each has different implications for the construct validation process. If "agreeableness" is defined by the reaction of others, then construct validation requires that one demonstrate some convergence between the self-report test scores and observer evaluations. But, while one would certainly need to know whether the scale predicted "agreeable" behaviors in order to interpret the test scores, virtually any correlation between scale scores and behavioral measures would be acceptable. Within this theoretical context, there is no necessary convergence between behaving "agreeably" in a situational test and having a reputation for being "agreeable." Expecting convergence of measurement results across methods should be a theoretical prediction when it is warranted, not an unvarying methodological imperative.

Including methodological specifications in construct definitions may indicate not only that all traits cannot be measured by all methods (how would one assess field independence by self-report?), but perhaps more importantly, that some methods may have a prima facie claim for measuring particular traits. In assessing an individual's goals, self-report procedures have a certain kind of priority, just as observer ratings have a claim on interpersonal traits. If all of an individual's friends, family, and co-workers (the relevant and informed audience of the target) agree that person X is dominant, yet X scores low on a self-report scale and fails to exhibit dominant acts in a laboratory procedure, then it makes sense to conclude that X is dominant, unless we believe the audience members do not know what dominance means or are lying. Is it not more reasonable to ask why the person fails to report his or her dominance accurately and fails to behave as we expect a dominant person should than to ask how the relevant audience can collectively reject the "truth." Within the theoretical context implied here, the audience *defines* the "truth!"

Specifying constructs in methodologically implicative ways is not an unprecedented suggestion. Campbell & Fiske (1959) suggested that it may be appropriate to distinguish different trait-method units sharing a common trait (e.g., Trait A Method 1 and Trait A Method 2). Where this proposal differs from that offered by Campbell and Fiske (1959) is in explicitly suggesting that demonstrating convergence between two such units is *not* a required part of the construct validation process. Instead, some relation between these two units must be specified (virtually any kind of relation might be specified if there is theoretical justification); construct validation should provide an empirical test.

Method Variance as a Psychological Phenomenon

Developing psychological theories to explain method variance is hardly a new suggestion. Campbell and Fiske (1959) indicated that method variance should eventually be subsumed by psychological theory, and Fiske (1986) recently reiterated this call for a psychological understanding of method and instrument. Meehl notes that in more developed sciences, the methods, devices, and instruments of research ". . . are themselves legitimated by theory" (1978, p.819). For the past thirty years, however, the prevailing view has been that method variance is an unfortunate accompaniment to assessment and is irrelevant to theory. It is unlikely that substantive theories of procedures and instruments emerged by accident in the developed sciences, at least if the case of Enrico Fermi's discovery of the effects of slow neutron bombardment is a representative case. He seems to have viewed "method variance" as an unqualified scientific opportunity.

In 1934, Fermi noted that the radioactivity created by the neutron bombardment of silver seemed to vary, depending on whether the apparatus was placed on a wood or marble table. Confronted with a conceptually similar problem today, a psychologist might employ structural-equation models to statistically isolate and remove the "method variance" and, thereby, identify the true, "latent radioactivity" emitted. Had Fermi chosen a parallel course, he would have missed what he referred to as his most important discovery (see Rhodes, 1986, pp. 216-220 for a description of Fermi's experiments and citations to primary sources). Instead, Fermi began systematic experimentation, aimed at identifying what it was about wood and marble that created the difference, by filtering the neutron bombardment through various materials. He found that when the neutrons were filtered through a hydrogen-rich medium radiation increased, and hypothesized that when the neutrons collided with hydrogen (present in wood, paraffin, and water but absent in marble and lead) they slowed and were then more likely to be captured in the silver——radiation is emitted upon capture of a neutron.

Fermi's discovery of the efficacy of slow neutron bombardment for creating radiation was obtained by identifying a substantive interpretation of method variance.

Investigating method variance to inform substantive theory is possible in psychology as well. Mischel, Shoda, and Peake (1988) compared the discrepant results obtained in two different situational tests of delay of gratification, and hypothesized that particular elements in each led one to be more associated with J. H. Block and J. Block's (1980) construct of ego-resiliency, and the other with the Blocks' construct of ego-control. The mechanisms suggested by Mischel, Shoda, and Peake (1988) are clearly amenable to conceptual replication and verification. With further systematic experimentation, not only will we be less likely to err in interpreting measures of delay, and other tests of impulse regulation, but Block and Block's theory will be elaborated as well.

Of crucial importance in developing a psychological understanding of method effects is the identification of the relevant mechanism. In this way, research to identify the source of method effects is no different from the investigation of other psychological phenomena. Rather than viewing the development of substantive explanations of method variance as a task that requires more sophisticated psychological theory, it may be more appropriate to regard such research as a means by which such theory will be developed.

Conclusion

Personality assessment and research have not been well served by the current definition of construct validity. The deductive approach to construct validation, which presumes a reasonably well-developed theoretical context, may not always be appropriate in Personality Psychology. Inductive construct validation procedures may be better suited to personality assessment for the present, and may contribute to the empirical base needed for theory development. When specific, plausible, and rival interpretations to test scores are not investigated, discriminant validity considerations are markedly less important than convergent validity concerns. Personality theory is often incapable of providing suitable alternative interpretations, thereby trivializing tests of discriminant validity. Finally, interpretations of method variance as either suppressing heteromethod or inflating monomethod convergence are inadequate in the domain of personality; hence, the metaphor of "triangulation by multiple methods" may be in need of revision. Trait-method units may be thought of as analogous to chemical compounds, where the simple sharing of an element does not necessarily imply shared properties. In this view, convergence among test scores becomes a theoretical conjecture rather than a methodological injunction.

Why is it that Personality Psychology, rather than some other branch of the discipline, has been so adversely affected by the current conceptualization of construct validity? Some areas of measurement do not rely on construct validation procedures (e.g., content validation predominates in educational assessment), thereby avoiding many of the problems alluded to in this essay. In other areas, such as ability testing, considerable progress is being made in developing "theories of the instrument." Cognitive psychology has begun to elucidate the processes employed by individuals responding to intelligence items (e.g., Pellegrino, 1988), and is now defining mental abilities in ways that speak directly to measurement issues, and to the standards used to evaluate ability tests (Sternberg, 1988).

Finally, method variance poses a particular problem for Personality Psychology. As I have suggested elsewhere (Ozer, 1986, p.53), method variance is situational variance. The accumulated findings of personality research over the past two decades suggest that characteristics of persons and situations affect one another and behavior in subtle ways that defy easy formulation. Methodological imperatives demanding cross-method convergence beg the very question of cross-situational consistency of personality characteristics.

References

American Educational Research Association, American Psychological Association, & National Council on Measurement in Education. (1985). *Standards for Educational and Psychological Testing.* Washington, DC: Author.

Block, J.H. & Block, J. (1980). The role of ego-control and ego-resiliency in the organization of behavior. *The Minnesota symposia on child psychology, 13,* 39–101.

Campbell, D.T. (1960). Recommendations for APA test standards regarding construct, trait, or discriminant validity. *American Psychologist, 15,* 546–553.

Campbell, D.T. & Fiske, D.W. (1959). Convergent and discriminant validation by the multitrait-multimethod matrix. *Psychological Bulletin, 56,* 81–105.

Campbell, D.T. & O'Connell, E.J. (1967). Methods factors in multitrait-multimethod matrices: Multiplicative rather than additive? *Multivariate Behavioral Research, 2,* 490–426.

Campbell, D.T. & O'Connell, E.J. (1982). Methods as diluting trait relationships rather than adding irrelevant systematic variance. In D. Brinberg & L. Kidder (Eds.), *Forms of validity in research,* (pp.93–111). San Francisco: Jossey-Bass.

Cook, T.D. & Campbell, D.T. (1979). *Quasi-experimentation: Design and analysis issues for field settings.* Chicago: Rand McNally.

Cronbach, L.J. (1988). Five perspectives on the validity argument. In H. Wainer & H.I. Braun (Eds.), *Test validity* (pp. 3–17). Hillsdale, NJ: Erlbaum.

Cronbach, L.J. & Meehl, P.E. (1955). Construct validity in psychological tests. *Psychological Bulletin, 52,* 281–302.

Fiske, D.W. (1986). The trait concept and the personality questionnaire. In A. Angleitner & J.S. Wiggins (Eds.), *Personality assessment via questionnaires: Current issues in theory and measurement* (pp. 35–46). Berlin: Springer-Verlag.

Gough, H.G. (1957). *Manual for the California Psychological Inventory.* Palo Alto: Consulting Psychologists Press.

Gough, H.G. (1965). Conceptual analysis of psychological test scores and other diagnostic variables. *Journal of Abnormal Psychology, 70,* 294–302.

Gough, H.G. (1987). *The California Psychological Inventory adminsitrator's guide.* Palo Alto: Consulting Psychologists Press.

Guion, R.M. (1980). On trinitarian conceptions of validity. *Professional Psychology, 11,* 385–398.

Jackson, D.N. (1975). Multimethod factor analysis: A reformulation. *Multivariate Behavioral Research, 10,* 259–276.

Judd, C.M., Jessor, R., & Donovon, J.E. (1986). Structural equation models and personality research. *Journal of Personality, 54,* 149–198.

Loevinger, J. (1957). Objective tests as instruments of psychological theory. *Psychological Reports, 3,* (Suppl. 9), 635–694.

McCrae, R.R. & Costa, P.T., Jr. (1987). Validation of the five-factor model of personality across instruments and observers. *Journal of Personality and Social Psychology, 52,* 81–90.

Meehl, P.E. (1978). Theoretical risks and tabular asterisks: Sir Karl, Sir Ronald, and the slow progress of soft psychology. *Journal of Consulting and Clinical Psychology, 46,* 806–834.

Messick, S. (1980). Test validation and the ethics of assessment. *American Psychologist, 35,* 1012–1027.

Mischel, W., Shoda, Y., & Peake, P. K. (1988). The nature of adolescent competencies predicted by preschool delay of gratification. *Journal of Personality and Social Psychology, 54,* 687–696.

Ozer, D.J. (1986). *Consistency in personality: A methodological framework.* Berlin: Springer-Verlag.

Pellegrino, J.W. (1988). Mental models and mental tests. In H. Wainer & H.I. Braun (Eds.), *Test validity* (pp. 61–75). Hillsdale, NJ: Erlbaum.

Rhodes, R. (1986). *The making of the atomic bomb.* New York: Simon & Schuster.

Schuman H. & Kalton, G. (1985). Survey methods. In G. Lindzey & E. Aronson (Eds.), *Handbook of Social Psychology: Volume I. Theory and Method* (3rd ed.) (pp. 635–697). New York: Random House.

Sternberg, R.J. (1988). GENECES: A rationale for the construct validation of theories and tests of intelligence. In H. Wainer & H.I. Braun (Eds.), *Test validity* (pp. 61–75). Hillsdale, NJ: Erlbaum.

Thorndike, E.L. (1920). A constant error in psychological ratings. *Journal of Applied Psychology, 4,* 25–29.

Wainer, H. & Braun, H.I. (Eds.) (1988). *Test validity.* Hillsdale, NJ: Erlbaum.

Part IV
Advances in Identifying the Structure of Personality

CHAPTER 17

Why I Advocate the Five-Factor Model: Joint Factor Analyses of the NEO-PI with Other Instruments

Robert R. McCrae

Introduction

Although the five-factor model of personality originated in studies of natural language, recent research suggests that it can encompass dimensions of individual differences derived from many of the major schools of personality psychology. This chapter summarizes empirical evidence of the convergence of all these lines of theory and research on the five-factor model, and illustrates the validity of the factors across different instruments and observers and their stability over decades of adult life. These appear to be compelling reasons to adopt the model as a framework for the comprehensive description of personality.

Why I Advocate the Five-Factor Model: Joint Factor Analyses of the NEO-PI with Other Instruments

Over fifty years ago, Gordon Allport recognized that natural language trait terms—the words that have evolved over the centuries to describe socially significant individual differences in personality—could be used as the basis of more formal systems of personality. Research in this tradition (Goldberg, 1983; Norman, 1963; Tupes & Christal, 1961) has consistently identified five factors that appear to define the basic dimensions of the natural language of personality. In the past few years, my colleague, Paul Costa, and I have become convinced that these same dimensions are also basic to many other personality systems derived from quite different theoretical and measurement traditions. Once recognized, these five constructs appeared obvious, almost inevitable, offering insight into an extraordinarily wide range of personality concepts. My intent here is to present some of the empirical evidence that has made me an advocate of the five-factor model.

The NEO Personality Inventory (NEO-PI; Costa & McCrae, 1985b), which provides the basic measure of the five factors in the present article, can be traced indirectly to Allport and Odbert's (1936) list of English-language trait names. Cattell grouped these terms into synonyms, gathered ratings on the resulting clusters, and factored them as the first step in the development of the Sixteen Personality Factor Questionnaire (16PF; Cattell, Eber, & Tatsuoka, 1970). We in turn (Costa & McCrae, 1980) factored the 16PF scales and identified three broad dimensions or domains of personality: Neuroticism (N), Extraversion (E), and Openness to Experience (O). To operationalize our model, we developed facet scales to measure different aspects of each domain and confirmed the hypothesized three-dimensional structure in both self-reports and spouse ratings (McCrae & Costa, 1983). A few years later, however, we were persuaded by the work of Digman (Digman & Takemoto-Chock, 1981) and Goldberg (1983) that our model was incomplete, and we added scales to measure Agreeableness (A) and Conscientiousness (C) in the published version of the NEO-PI.

Most of our research on the five-factor model has been conducted on volunteer participants in the Baltimore Longitudinal Study of Aging (Shock et al., 1984) and their spouses, friends, and neighbors. The men and women in these studies ranged in age from twenty-one to ninety-six, and were generally healthy and well-educated. Data from various measures have been collected since 1959, although women were added to the study only in 1978. The number of subjects varies across studies; all available data are analyzed.

In 1986, we administered the NEO-PI to 983 adults and factored its scales; five principal components were rotated to maximize convergent and discriminant validity as assessed by external criteria (McCrae & Costa, 1989b). In the following analyses, these NEO-PI factors are used as markers of the Big Five. Joint factor analyses with other instruments from quite different traditions may give some idea of the scope and power of the five-factor model.

Joint factor analysis, of course, is neither the only, nor necessarily the best, way of examining relations between instruments. Depending on the nature of the instruments and theory they embody, additional analyses are generally required for a complete understanding. For example, statistical interactions need to be considered in evaluating the Myers-Briggs Type Indicator (MBTI; Myers & McCaulley, 1985), which purports to measure qualitatively distinct types. In most cases, such analyses have already been published. The factor analyses presented here simply summarize, in a convenient form, parallel analyses on a wide range of instruments. In each analysis, five (or six) factors are extracted, guided by theory rather than by eigenvalues or scree tests (the numbers of eigenvalues greater than 1.0 are given in the table notes). Varimax-rotated principal components are presented, reflected and reordered as necessary.

In each analysis, the questions are the same. Are the five factors clearly defined by the NEO-PI markers? Are any factors defined solely by scales from another instrument, suggesting a sixth dimension of personality? Are there scales unrelated to any of the Big Five, again suggesting the need for more factors? Do the factor definers from other instruments make theoretical sense? How do they illuminate the nature of the five factors? How adequately do other instruments measure the full range of personality traits, as defined by the five-factor model, and what is the nature of the omissions, if any? Within the space limitations of this chapter, I will only be able to point out highlights from these tables; my intent is to illustrate the breadth of applicability of the five-factor model.

Table 17.1 addresses the question of multi-method assessment. NEO-PI factors from self-reports, spouse ratings, and mean peer ratings were factored; each of the five factors is defined by the same trait dimension in all three methods of measurement, as the salient loadings (given in boldface) clearly show. Such findings demonstrate that personality traits are not cognitive fictions within the heads of raters, but are consensually-validated psychological facts. Having demonstrated this, we can return to self-reports, for which larger samples are available.

Table 17.2 demonstrates that the NEO-PI factors do indeed correspond to the natural language adjective factors that were first used to identify

TABLE 17.1. Joint factor analysis of NEO-PI factors in self-reports, spouse ratings, and mean peer ratings.

Variable	\multicolumn{5}{c}{Varimax-rotated principal components}
	N	E	O	A	C
Self-reports:					
Neuroticism	**80**	−06	−03	03	−03
Extraversion	04	**85**	−06	−01	−05
Openness	−12	02	**86**	07	−02
Agreeableness	06	06	00	**87**	10
Conscientiousness	−05	01	−02	11	**80**
Spouse ratings:					
Neuroticism	**81**	09	−03	−14	−05
Extraversion	35	**77**	14	03	07
Openness	05	−12	**79**	01	04
Agreeableness	−06	11	14	**82**	04
Conscientiousness	02	−18	08	06	**84**
Mean peer ratings:					
Neuroticism	**81**	18	−05	17	01
Extraversion	−10	**70**	−02	22	−23
Openness	−05	14	**81**	05	12
Agreeableness	06	02	00	**86**	−15
Conscientiousness	−03	−02	10	−19	**79**

Note: $N = 73$. Five eigenvalues were greater than 1.0. Data are taken from McCrae & Costa, in press-b.

TABLE 17.2. Joint factor analysis of NEO-PI factors and goldberg adjective scales.

Variable	Varimax-rotated principle components				
	N	E	O	A	C
NEO-PI factors					
Neuroticism	**90**	−03	−04	03	09
Extraversion	08	**90**	−07	15	−01
Openness	02	−07	**92**	00	−12
Agreeableness	07	−15	−04	**90**	−08
Conscientiousness	04	−06	16	03	**87**
Goldberg scales					
Surgency	−12	**83**	18	−19	19
Agreeableness	−31	21	08	**76**	25
Conscientiousness	−21	28	−15	06	**81**
Emotional Stability	**−85**	−01	10	18	26
Culture	−27	27	**71**	03	33

Note: N = 375. Five eigenvalues were greater than 1.0. Data are taken from McCrae & Costa, 1985b and in press-b.

the five-factor model. The adjective scales are taken from a forty-item instrument by Goldberg (1983). Despite some differences in labels, there are clear matches on each of the factors.

Both the Goldberg scales and the NEO-PI can be traced ultimately to natural language factors, so that agreement between them might be expected. Can the factors be found in independent systems? Block's (1961) California Q-Set represents one of the few attempts to provide a fully comprehensive assessment of personality that was not derived from analyses of trait adjectives. Instead, Block and his colleagues attempted to create a new language for the description of personality from a psychodynamic perspective. Five factors were recovered from an analysis of self-sorts on this instrument (McCrae, Costa, & Busch, 1986); they closely resembled the factors found in adjectives, and a joint analysis with the NEO-PI factors shows that each of the five joint factors is defined by the same-named trait from each instrument.

Table 17.3 makes a somewhat different point. Here the analysis has been repeated with the inclusion of measures of education and cognitive abilities. The five personality factors are in evidence again, joined by a factor of general intelligence—g. Although Openness to Experience does show modest correlations with cognitive ability measures—especially divergent thinking (McCrae, 1987)—Table 17.3 suggests that psychometrically measured intelligence is better regarded as a separate factor. This is one reason to prefer the term "Openness" to "Intellectance" (Hogan, 1983) or "Culture" (Goldberg, 1983) as the label for this dimension of personality.

Another fountainhead of individual difference variables was Jung's (1923/1971) *Psychological Types*. Introversion-Extraversion became a

TABLE 17.3. Joint factor analysis of NEO-PI factors, CQS factors, and intelligence tests.

	\multicolumn{6}{c}{Varimax-rotated principal components}					
Variable	N	E	O	A	C	G
NEO-PI factors:						
Neuroticism	**89**	−13	−04	11	−10	−03
Extraversion	−11	**90**	−02	−02	−02	−16
Openness	−01	04	**90**	−09	16	09
Agreeableness	−11	−23	07	**90**	−03	−02
Conscientiousness	−04	−06	−02	−22	**85**	07
CQS factors:						
Neuroticism	**87**	−08	−03	−16	−07	−14
Extraversion	−10	**90**	13	−07	03	00
Openness	−06	09	**79**	11	−05	37
Agreeableness	06	11	−07	**93**	−07	10
Conscientiousness	−13	07	14	12	**80**	22
Intelligence:						
WAIS Vocabulary	02	−24	25	10	00	**80**
Army Alpha Test	02	−16	09	09	13	**88**
Divergent Thinking	−13	03	05	−10	06	**86**
Education (Years)	−12	10	14	04	20	**73**

Note: N = 92 men. Six eigenvalues were greater than 1.0. Data are taken from McCrae, 1987, and McCrae & Costa, in press-b.

popular concept, and scales were soon created to measure it. Guilford (Guilford & Guilford, 1934) applied the newly-developed technique of factor analysis to show that Thinking Introversion was distinct from Social Introversion. He went on to develop other factored personality scales that became the Guilford-Zimmerman Temperament Survey (GZTS; Guilford, Zimmerman, & Guilford, 1976). Table 17.4 gives joint loadings with the GZTS in a sample of men only. N and E factors are clearly defined by variables from both instruments. Although GZTS Thoughtfulness and Restraint form a Thinking Introversion factor in analyses of the GZTS alone, the two break apart in this joint analysis. Thoughtfulness appears to measure O, Restraint to measure C. It is also noteworthy that the GZTS data in this table were gathered from eight to twenty-eight years prior to the NEO-PI data. Personality is sufficiently stable in adulthood to ensure that joint factors emerge despite the passage of two decades (Costa & McCrae, 1985a).

The MBTI attempts to measure not only Extraversion, but also the Jungian functions of Sensing versus Intuition and Thinking versus Feeling. Table 17.5 shows that the four scales in the MBTI appear to correspond well to E, O, A, and C. In other analyses, we found no evidence that the MBTI measures distinct types (McCrae & Costa, 1989a), so it is not clear that this instrument contributes anything unique to the measurement of personality.

TABLE 17.4 Joint factor analysis of NEO-PI factors and GZTS scales.

| | \multicolumn{5}{c}{Varimax-rotated principal components} |
Variable	N	E	O	A	C
NEO-PI factors					
Neuroticism	**76**	−15	−05	−04	02
Extraversion	−01	**83**	−04	01	−11
Openness	00	−02	**89**	−07	00
Agreeableness	−16	−09	10	**83**	−03
Conscientiousness	−06	08	05	−12	**88**
GZTS scales:					
General Activity	01	**62**	05	−50	20
Restraint	−23	−32	14	15	**72**
Ascendance	−22	**77**	19	−23	06
Sociability	−21	**81**	−07	12	−14
Emotional Stability	**−75**	18	−10	−05	09
Objectivity	**−86**	16	−08	04	08
Friendliness	**−62**	−28	−02	45	19
Thoughtfulness	25	14	**68**	28	33
Personal Relations	**−66**	10	−14	25	16
Masculinity	**−56**	−19	10	**−41**	−17

Note: N = 180 men. Four eigenvalues were greater than 1.0. Data are taken from Costa & McCrae, 1985a, and McCrae & Costa, in press-b.

Neuroticism is not measured in the MBTI, but it is included among the Eysenck scales, another set of instruments that also feature Extraversion (Eysenck & Eysenck, 1964, 1975). Joint factor analyses of Eysenck scales with NEO-PI factors show that both Sociability and Impulsivity are aspects of E, as Eysenck has hypthesized. Psychoticism has negative loadings on C and A (McCrae & Costa, 1985a), suggesting that it measures poor socialization. None of the Eysenck scales measures Openness.

TABLE 17.5. Joint factor analysis of NEO-PI factors and MBTI continuous scales.

| | \multicolumn{5}{c}{Varimax-rotated principal components} |
Variable	N	E	O	A	C
NEO-PI factors:					
Neuroticism	**96**	−09	03	06	−05
Extraversion	03	**93**	04	−01	−04
Openness	06	−04	**93**	−04	−01
Agreeableness	−13	−06	01	**92**	03
Conscientiousness	01	01	07	−03	**91**
MBTI scales:					
EI (Introversion)	12	**−91**	−04	−08	06
SN (Intuition)	−03	14	**89**	10	−15
TF (Feeling)	33	17	07	**79**	−17
JP (Perception)	11	14	36	09	**−75**

Note: N = 468. Four eigenvalues were greater than 1.0. Data are taken from McCrae & Costa, in press-a.

Murray's (1938) *Explorations in Personality* included a catalogue of needs that became the basis for many assessment devices, projective tests, and questionnaires; by psychometric standards, Jackson's (1984) Personality Research Form (PRF) is one of the best of these. A joint analysis of PRF scales with NEO-PI factors demonstrates that each of the five factors is represented in the PRF needs, and that all the needs load on at least one factor (Costa & McCrae, 1988). For example, the O factor is defined by needs for Understanding and Change; the C factor by needs for Achievement and Order. The structure is not simple, however, since many of the needs have loadings on two factors. Nurturance, for example, is both extraverted and agreeable.

The same phenomenon can be seen in some of the scales of Wiggin's (1979) Interpersonal Adjective Scales, which form a circumplex. The interpersonal circumplex, derived from the work of Bales, Sullivan, and Leary, can be viewed as a plane defined by the two dimensions of E and A (McCrae & Costa, 1989c). In this arrangement, Warmth is seen as an agreeable form of Extraversion, whereas Dominance is a disagreeable form.

We have previously examined the relations of the NEO-PI to item factors from the MMPI (Costa, Busch, Zonderman, & McCrae, 1986), and we are curerntly examining the Buss-Durkee (1957) Hostility Inventory and Gough's (1987) newly revised California Psychological Inventory. It appears that these instruments, too, can be understood within the framework of the five-factor model.

I believe these analyses show that Neuroticism, Extraversion, Openness, Agreeableness, and Conscientiousness are indeed basic dimensions of personality. They cross the boundaries of method and observer, endure across time, and are distinct from measures of cognitive ability. The five-factor model can provide the basis for a systematic analysis of proposed new scales and for the comprehensive assessment of individuals.

The same factors appear repeatedly, in whole or in part, in instruments derived from widely different theoretical sources: Murray's needs, Goldberg's adjectives, Block's psychodynamic descriptors. They can, therefore, be used as a common language through which findings from all these diverse approaches can be integrated. Each of the instruments examined has particular strengths and areas of emphasis, and each will continue to remain important in understanding personality. The five-factor model will not replace them, but it can provide a universal descriptive framework that complements their unique perspectives on personality.

References

Allport, G.W., & Odbert, H.S. (1936). Trait names: A psycho-lexical study. *Psychological Monographs, 47,* (1, Whole No. 211).

Block, J. (1961). *The Q-sort method in personality assessment and psychiatric research.* Springfield, IL: Thomas.

Buss, A.H., & Durkee, A. (1957). An inventory for assessing different kinds of hostility. *Journal of Consulting Psychology, 21,* 343–348.

Cattell, R.B., Eber, H.W., & Tatsuoka, M.M. (1970). *The handbook for the Sixteen Personality Factor Questionnaire.* Champaign, IL: Institute for Personality and Ability Testing.

Costa, P.T., Jr., Busch, C.M., Zonderman, A.B., & McCrae, R.R. (1986). Correlations of MMPI factor scales with measures of the five-factor model of personality. *Journal of Personality Assessment, 50,* 640–650.

Costa, P.T., Jr., & McCrae, R.R. (1980). Still stable after all these years: Personality as a key to some issues in adulthood and old age. In P.B. Baltes & O.G. Brim, Jr. (Eds.), *Life span development and behavior* (Vol. 3, pp. 65–102). New York: Academic Press.

Costa, P.T., Jr., & McCrae, R.R. (1985a). Concurrent validation after 20 years: Implications of personality stability for its assessment. *Advances in personality assessment, 4,* 31–54.

Costa, P.T., Jr., & McCrae, R.R. (1985b). *The NEO Personality Inventory manual.* Odessa, FL: Psychological Assessment Resources.

Costa, P.T., Jr., & McCrae, R.R. (1988). From catalog to classification: Murray's needs and the five-factor model. *Journal of Personality and Social Psychology, 55,* 258–265.

Digman, J.M., & Takemoto-Chock, N.K. (1981). Factors in the natural language of personality: Re-analysis, comparison, and interpretation of six major studies. *Multivariate Behavioral Research, 16,* 149–170.

Eysenck, H.J., & Eysenck, S.B.G.. (1964). *Manual of the Eysenck Personality Inventory.* London: University of London Press.

Eysenck, H.J., & Eysenck, S.B.G. (1975). *Manual of the Eysenck Personality Questionnaire.* San Diego: EdITS.

Goldberg, L.R. (1983, June). *The magical number five, plus or minus two: Some considerations on the dimensionality of personality descriptors.* Paper presented at a Research Seminar, Gerontology Research Center, Baltimore, MD.

Gough, H.G. (1987). *California Psychological Inventory administrator's guide.* Palo Alto, CA: Consulting Psychologists Press.

Guilford, J.P., & Guilford, R.B. (1934). An analysis of the factors in a typical test of introversion-extroversion. *Journal of Abnormal and Social Psychology, 28,* 377–399.

Guilford, J.S., Zimmerman, W.S., & Guilford, J.P. (1976). *The Guilford-Zimmerman Temperament Survey handbook: Twenty-five years of research and application.* San Diego: EdITS.

Hogan, R.T. (1983). Socioanalytic theory of personality. *Nebraska Symposium on Motivation, 1982,* 55–89.

Jackson, D.N. (1984). *Personality Research Form manual* (3rd. ed.). Port Huron, MI: Research Psychologists Press.

Jung, G.C. (1971). *Psychological types* (H.G. Baynes, Trans.). Princeton, NJ: Princeton University Press. (Original work published 1923)

McCrae, R.R. (1987). Creativity, divergent thinking, and openness to experience. *Journal of Personality and Social Psychology, 52,* 1258–1265.

McCrae, R.R., & Costa, P.T., Jr. (1983). Joint factors in self-reports and ratings: Neuroticism, Extraversion, and Openness to Experience. *Personality and Individual Differences, 4,* 245–255.

McCrae, R.R., & Costa, P.T., Jr. (1985a). Comparison of EPI and Psychoticism scales with measures of the five-factor model of personality. *Personality and Individual Differences, 6,* 587–597.

McCrae, R.R., & Costa, P.T., Jr. (1985b). Updating Norman's "adequate taxonomy": Intelligence and personality dimensions in natural language and in questionnaires. *Journal of Personality and Social Psychology, 49,* 710–721.

McCrae, R.R., & Costa, P.T., Jr. (1989a). Reinterpreting the Myers-Briggs Type Indicator from the perspective of the five-factor model of personality. *Journal of Personality, 57,* 17–40.

McCrae, R.R., & Costa, P.T., Jr. (1989b). Rotation to maximize the construct validity of factors in the NEO Personality Inventory. *Multivariate Behavioral Research, 24,* 107–124.

McCrae, R.R., & Costa, P.T., Jr. (1989c). The structure of interpersonal traits: Wiggins' circumplex and the five-factor model. *Journal of Personality and Social Psychology, 56,* 586–595.

McCrae, R.R., Costa, P.T., Jr., & Busch, C.M. (1986). Evaluating comprehensiveness in personality systems: The California Q-Set and the five-factor model. *Journal of Personality, 54,* 430–446.

Murray, H.A. (1938). *Explorations in personality.* New York: Oxford University Press.

Myers, I.B., & McCaulley, M.H. (1985). *Manual: A guide to the development and use of the Myers-Briggs Type Indicator.* Palo Alto, CA: Consulting Psychologists Press.

Norman, W.T. (1963). Toward an adequate taxonomy of personality attributes: Replicated factor structure in peer nomination personality ratings. *Journal of Abnormal and Social Psychology, 66,* 574–583.

Shock, N.W., Greulich, R.C., Andres, R., Arenberg, D., Costa, P.T., Jr., Lakatta, E.G., & Tobin, J.D. (1984). *Normal human aging: The Baltimore Longitudinal Study of Aging* (NIH Publication No. 84-2450). Bethesda, MD: National Institutes of Health.

Tupes, E.C., & Christal, R.E. (1961). *Recurrent personality factors based on trait ratings* (USAF ASD Technical Report No. 61-97). Lackland Air Force Base, TX: U. S. Air Force.

Wiggins, J.S. (1979). A psychological taxonomy of trait-descriptive terms: The interpersonal domain. *Journal of Personality and Social Psychology, 37,* 395–412.

CHAPTER 18

The Optimal Level of Measurement for Personality Constructs

Stephen R. Briggs

William McDougall once argued that tendencies are the indispensable postulates for all of psychology (1938). To the extent that his assertion is correct, the study of personality focuses on tendencies of two types: those common to the species and those specific to individuals (Murphy, 1966). In the first instance, students of personality explore the "nature of human nature", attempting to identify, understand, and integrate the qualities and tendencies that are central to our humanness. In the second instance, students of personality catalogue and measure personal tendencies: the actions, thoughts, feelings, perceptions, and motives that reliably distinguish individuals from one another. Thus, the study of personality encompasses two endeavors that are complementary, but quite distinct (Buss, 1984). One venture is directed toward the study of species-typical characteristics, the other toward individual differences. This difference in orientation is reflected in the name of the relevant section of the *Journal of Personality and Social Psychology*: Personality Processes and Individual Differences. It also emerges in the subject matter of textbooks that focus primarily on personality theory or personality measurement.

To some extent, this difference in orientation was also apparent in the scholarly interests of the researchers present at the "Conference on Emerging Issues in Personality" who are now represented in this volume of essays. The issues and trends that each of us points to as important, and our prophecies concerning the future, must always be examined in light of the type of tendency that is being studied. As Murphy put it, "Both of these conceptions of personality have to be used, but in every discussion of personality it makes considerable difference where the interest lies" (1966, p. 1).

Among researchers who are primarily interested in describing and systematizing human variability, there increasingly seems to be a consensus that the natural language for describing individual differences in personality can be summarized adequately in terms of five (plus or minus two) major dimensions. This finding emerged originally in factor analyses of trait attributions made by peer observers (e.g., Cattell, 1946; Fiske, 1949; Norman, 1963; Passini & Norman, 1966; Tupes & Christal, 1961). Subsequent replications have generally used peer or self-ratings on adjective scales (Conley, 1985; Digman & Takemoto-Chock, 1981; Goldberg, 1981), although more recent work suggests that these same factors can be extracted from self-reported and peer-rated personality inventories as well (Noller, Law, & Comrey, 1987; McCrae & Costa, 1988).

This apparently robust finding about how people think about and describe themselves and others qualifies as a significant advance for a variety of reasons. First, it provides us with a framework for building rating scales and omnibus inventories that will represent the domain of personality terms broadly and systematically; in other words, it serves to enhance the content validity of broad-gauged measures. Second, it allows us to locate the seemingly boundless supply of new constructs and measures within a known configuration. A well-defined structure clarifies the relations between what is new and what is established, and it exposes areas of needless redundancy. Third, it enables us to generate more specific hypotheses when attempting to relate personality variables to other constructs and criteria (physical and mental health, coping strategies, work productivity and dependability, etc.). Finally, it suggests that these basic dimensions should merit special attention in the continuing search for the mechanisms underlying individual differences in personality.

Reducing the enormous number of trait descriptors in the English language to a small number of workable factors is a monumental undertaking, and the identification of five (plus or minus two) reliable factors is a finding worth celebrating. But in our eagerness to accept and profit from this accomplishment, it would be foolish to assume that *an* answer—*this* answer—is *the* answer. The correctness of an answer depends on the question, and the utility of the five-factor structure of trait terms depends on the task at hand.

The five-factor solution emerged from a lexical approach to the study of trait taxonomy (Goldberg, 1982; John, Angleitner, & Ostendorf, 1988). This approach derives from a fundamental assumption: "*Those individual differences that are most significant in the daily transactions of persons with each other become encoded into their language.* The more important such a difference is, the more people will notice it and wish to talk of it, with the result that eventually they will invent a word for it" (Goldberg, 1982, p. 204). This assumption is sensible and provides a methodical way to tackle the larger task which is to develop a taxonomy of personality characteristics or enduring tendencies. Having discovered at least a preliminary answer based on the lexical strategy, we should not take for granted, however, that it will serve as an equally good solution for all needs and questions, nor should we let this accomplishment distract us from the larger task. Although the five-factor solution stands as the most robust taxonomy of trait descriptors currently available, we must use it judiciously and not allow it to become a procrustean bed.

In the next section, I specify some of the weaknesses that are apparent in the five-factor solution in order to buttress my call for restrained admiration and a contingent acceptance. In the final section, I argue for another approach that relies initially on the same data sources (self-reports and peer ratings) but that offers different advantages because it is not grounded on the analysis of adjective trait terms.

Five Reservations About the Five-Factor Solution

Imprecise Specification

Whereas the five-factor structure of trait descriptors is recognizable across samples and investigators (e.g., see Table 1 of Mershon & Gorsuch, 1988), the degree of correspondence has been less than ideal. Disagreements have emerged particularly with respect to Factor 5 (variously named Culture, Intellect, and Openness), but other factors also vary in their specifics from one study to the next. In a recent and comprehensive review of the lexical approach to trait taxonomic research, John et al. (1988) concluded that "the available taxonomies differ in numerous ways, such as in the instances included in the taxonomy, the kind of structure chosen to represent the domain under investigation, and the kinds of data from which they have been derived. . . . Norman, Goldberg, and Wiggins all started from essentially the same set of trait terms; yet their taxonomies are remarkably different, both in their general structure and in the specific details" (p. 198).

The lack of correspondence also emerges when the instances classified are items (or homogeneous groups of items) rather than adjectives. Although there are systems that are flagrantly at odds with the five-factor structure (e.g., Eysenck's three, Guilford's thirteen, Cattell's fifteen or sixteen, and Howarth's twenty), several studies have shown that a five-factor structure more or less reflects the independent variation measured by various self-report inventories (e.g., McCrae & Costa, 1987; Noller, Law, & Comrey, 1987). Nevertheless, the five factors do not emerge precisely in these studies, and it is sometimes necessary to rotate an additional factor or two. Moreover, the specific components of the five factors seem to vary as a function of the items included and the particular sample. Thus, whereas there is a general resemblance in the factors that replicate from sample to sample and investigator to investigator, the resemblance is more fraternal than identical. The five (plus or minus two) factors have yet to be defined by consensus with any degree of specificity.

Atheoretical Strategy

The unsettling lack of specificity in the definition of the five factors is due in part to the fact that they are empirically derived. The factors emerge reliably, but there is no theoretical reason why it should be these five rather than some other five. Thus, although reasonable, the lexical approach to the study of structure is essentially atheoretical. It assumes that language reflects social reality systematically, and it analyzes language (in the form of long lists of adjectives) in order to identify the basic dimensions of social observation. However, in the beginning it prompted no *a priori* predictions as to what factors should emerge, and a coherent and falsifiable explanation for the five factors has yet to be put forward. One could argue from an evolutionary viewpoint that these dimensions must have adaptive significance: "To the degree that social groups, and individuals within the groups, must do the same sorts of things to survive (e.g., acquire food, protect territory, raise and educate children, etc.), the presence and importance of the various trait terms in ordinary language will be lawful not random, and will mirror the relative importance of those traits in promoting individual and group survival" (Hogan, 1983, p. 59). To be scientifically useful, however, an account along these lines would have to generate testable hypotheses or be prey to charges of after-the-fact speculation.

In attempting to explain why the five-factor solution emerges even somewhat reliably, several facts seem certain. At the very least, this stable structure implies that people agree about the meaning of the individual adjectives (a requirement for language usage more generally) as well as the way in which various adjectives are related lexically or implicatively (see Wiggins, 1973, Chapter 8). The five-factor model functions as an "implicit personality theory" (Bruner & Tagiuri, 1954; Schneider, 1973). Observers will apply this implicit theory whether rating friends, strangers, or hypothetical people (Norman & Goldberg, 1966; Passini & Norman, 1966) or the similarity in meaning of trait terms (D'Andrade, 1965). However, the five-factor structure is not simply an institutionalized fiction that bears little or no correspondence to the individual being observed (cf., Jones & Nisbett, 1971; Schweder, 1975), because both interobserver agreement and self-other agreement increase as the level of acquaintanceship increases (Norman & Goldberg, 1966; Weiss, 1979).

Thus, it seems reasonable to conclude that individuals in a culture hold preexisting ideas about what types of attributes go together, and that the five-factor solution is a reflection of these culturally defined conceptual similarities. Although it is not yet clear how closely this particular implicit personality theory maps onto the regularities and covariations that characterize the raw flux of everyday action, recent work on the cognitive processing of social information suggests that people are indeed primed to detect and acquire covariations of this sort without any conscious awareness (Lewicki, 1986). Additional evidence is needed, however, before we can determine whether the lexical approach is correct in assuming that this particular implicit theory of personality exists because "the people in this language community have noticed in themselves or in others a characteristic that is salient in their daily transactions and relates, in systematic ways, to social outcomes they regard as important" (John et al, p. 198).

Indefinite Ontological Status

Just as the identification of regularities and covariations in the natural language of trait attributions may not correspond directly to social reality or attributes of the people being observed, so also the structure of trait attributions may not correspond straightforwardly to the deep structure or neurophysical basis of human tendencies. In fact, it seems improbable that language can reflect in any direct way the neurophysical mechanisms and processes that regulate behavioral, affective, and cognitive tendencies. Allport (1937) warned of "the deeper metaphysical problem concerning the relation of any name to the unit-structures of nature. . . . trait-names are symbols socially devised for the naming and evaluation of human qualities;" yet, "in denying perfect correspondence between names and traits," there is no reason to "deny the very existence of traits" (p. 310). One of the ironies of the emerging consensus regarding the structure of the trait descriptive language is the corresponding lack of formal consensus about the reality of traits as enduring tendencies or traits as neurophysical realities. If there are no such things as trait tendencies, this approach (the psychometric or individual differences approach) to the study of personality is precluded by definition. If, however, there are regularities of cognition, affect, or behavior that are characteristic of an individual, these tendencies must be represented or encoded in some real way in the brain—perhaps as a kind of procedural memory. As Murray succinctly put it, "No brain, no personality" (1951, p. 267).

Thus, my third reservation about the five-factor solution is that it might be viewed as the structure of personality trait dimensions rather than just the structure of the language of trait attributions. I assume that most personality researchers are interested ultimately in the structure of trait tendencies or even, more ambitiously, the underlying "neuropsychic entities" or "bona fide mental structures" and their organization (Briggs, 1985). It is premature to assume that the five-factor solution of trait attributions will reflect either the manifest tendencies or the latent structures—the surface or the depth of personality tendencies—and, therefore, it would be unfortunate to preclude alternate lines of inquiry. Trait attributions are convenient fictions by which we communicate; it remains to be seen how they relate to the reality of trait tendencies or the neurophysical substrate, although the progress in this area is encouraging (e.g., Gray, 1987; Strelau & Eysenck, 1987; Zuckerman, 1984).

Limited Predictive and Descriptive Utility

A primary goal of the lexical approach is to reduce the variability in trait attributions to a few major and independent factors. The relative stability of the five-factor model suggests that this goal has been initially realized. Identifying the major dimensions of trait attribution, however, does not mean that these five (plus or minus two) will optimize our ability to predict important criteria. In fact, Mershon & Gorsuch (1988) recently showed that the sixteen factors of the 16PF outperformed a six-factor solution of the 16PF consistently (88% of the studies) and substantially (the median increase in proportion of variance accounted for was 110%) in predicting occupational criteria. Along the same lines, it is interesting to note that two recent omnibus inventories, developed in line with the five (plus or minus two) factor model, also score a number of more homogeneous groups of items: the NEO-PI (Costa & McCrae, 1985) has eighteen additional facets, and the HPI (Hogan, 1986) has forty-three additional homogeneous item clusters (HICs).

In the same way, the limited descriptive utility of a five (plus or minus two) factor solution seems almost obvious. For example, both the NEO-PI and the HPI include subscales for anxiety and depression that contribute to the overall score on Neuroticism-Emotional Adjustment. Anxiety and depression are often related, and it makes sense to combine them when measuring overall adjustment. Nevertheless, the distinction between the two is also important and is likely to be of real descriptive value in clinical settings and of predictive utility in clinical research. In their review of the lexical approach, John et al. suggest at least two candidates for an extension of the five-factor model, but they go on to observe that "even a 'Big Five Plus Little Two' seems too limited to provide an adequately differentiated description of an individual" (1988, p. 190). Similarly, Buss & Craik (1985) argue that "formulations of personality based on arbitrarily or overly restricted criteria may explain or account for only fragments of everyday action" (p. 944). Thus, our success in reducing the trait language to its basic dimensions should not be taken to mean that these dimensions are optimal for description or prediction. Knowledge of phyla in the animal kingdom does not detract from the importance of distinguishing between species.

Limited Utility for Generating Hypotheses

Because the five (plus or minus two) factor model of trait attributions provides a description at the most general level, these broad dimensions gloss over the specific and subtle distinctions from which testable and interesting hypotheses often emerge. The distinctions between the concepts of neurotic and antagonistic hostility (Costa, McCrae, & Dembroski, 1989) and between shyness and sociability (Cheek & Buss, 1981; Briggs, 1988) can be linked to the five-factor model, but the hypotheses themselves are framed and tested at the level of more specific and homogeneous constructs and scales. I would contend that the distinctions among constructs subsumed by any one of the five factors are at least as important conceptually as the distinctions among the five (plus or minus two) factors themselves.

Summary

Several decades of painstaking effort by long-suffering investigators in the lexical tradition has produced a useful framework for describing the vocabulary of trait attributions. Although alluring, these broad brush strokes are simply the background for what eventually must be a more detailed portrait. Additional information is needed about the universality of these factors and how they are related to behavioral and biological variables. Here is a short list of what can be done to fill in some of the details that are currently missing.

1. We need to extend the work being done on the English language (in the U.S.A.) to other languages and cultures. Several projects of this sort are underway—e.g., see John et al.'s (1988) description of the Dutch and German projects. Additional work using nonGermanic language families is also needed (e.g., Chinese, Indo-Iranian, Semitic, and Slavic). In extending this work to other languages, a distinction should be made between replication and rediscovery of the five-factor model. It may be that five (plus or minus two) factors can be identified in other languages if these dimensions are imposed on the rating instruments (i.e., when current rating scales are translated into other languages). Replication of this sort, however, is neither as stringent nor as compelling as work that replicates the entire lexical strategy, beginning with the identification of the pool of trait descriptors in that language. For example, Yang and Bond (1989) recently examined the factor structure of trait ratings in a sample of Chinese students using both adjective markers for the five-factor model and a representative list of Chinese personality descriptors. The *imported* adjective markers did not reflect in any straightforward manner the *indigenous* factor structure derived from the Chinese trait terms. Future work in this area needs to attend closely to the systematic and representative sampling of trait terms (see Peabody, 1987; Tellegen & Waller, 1987).

2. Alternatively, it would be helpful to study the structure of trait attributions produced by monozygotic twins, comparing the matrix of correlations derived from twins as individuals with the matrix of cross-correlations derived from twins as pairs (see Rowe, 1982). Perhaps as part of this project, a variety of biological variables could be located in the space defined by the five-factor solution.

3. The construct validity of these factors needs to be established in laboratory and field settings. Each of the factors has acquired one or more labels, and these names suggest conceptual claims that need to be defined explicitly and examined. For example, Peabody and Goldberg (1988) have recently linked the five factors in a general way to the concepts of Power, Love, Work, Affect, and Intellect; this conceptualization suggests possible contextual factors (both situational and relational) that might help to clarify the meaning of the five factors. Perhaps the critical step in elucidating these concepts, however, is the specification of their exact nature: What are the elements or components of each factor? What is their relative contribution? How are they interrelated? This is the general issue to which I turn in the final section.

Top-Down or Bottom-Up?

Researchers pursuing the lexical strategy have sought to develop a systematic and adequate taxonomy of trait attributions. In doing so, their focus has been on the broad dimensions of personality. My thesis in this section is that we need an equally sharp focus on the elements or instances that comprise these broad factors. Focusing soley on broad constructs is analogous to focusing on the name of a scale but ignoring its items, never a prudent strategy. Whereas names make conceptual claims, items or instances operationalize a construct. In the same way, broad factors are operationalized by the components or subconstructs they subsume. Most conceptual analysis and hypothesis-testing occurs at the level of the components or subconstructs. A broad factor or concept is not adequately specified until its components are clearly identified and distinguished. There are two basic strategies by which these components can be elucidated: the top-down approach and the bottom-up approach.

The Top-Down Approach

This approach begins by identifying the broad constructs and then divides these higher-order factors into key components. The advantage of this approach is that it establishes the general layout of the terrain before filling in the individual details. For instance, this is the general strategy adopted by the empirical approach to test construction. Broad predictors are first identified, and subsequent analyses attempt to explicate how this predictor functions (Gough, 1965). Although reasonable, historically this strategy seems to have resulted in a lot of confusion and wasted time and effort, no matter whether the construct is one of the Big Five or a "middle-level" construct of moderate heterogeneity (e.g., Type A, empathy, hardiness, or self-monitoring).

For example, although Eysenck has conceptualized Extraversion as a higher-order factor consisting of various primary factors (see Eysenck & Eysenck, 1985, Figure 2, p. 15), these components are not clearly and systematically assessed in his various measures of Extraversion (Howarth, 1976). In part, this inexactness has generated considerable controversy about how the primary factors of impulsivity and sociability are related to each other, the higher-order factor, and theoretically relevant criteria.

More generally, there are two reasons that make it difficult to partition heterogeneous constructs into their homogeneous components. First, more often than not, the original theories have not specified the components rigorously enough. Consequently, these components are not represented systematically in the final item pool and, therefore, are unlikely to be assessed systematically in measures of the construct. When items are selected on the basis of their ability to predict specific criteria rather than because they appropriately operationalize a construct, it is important to push beyond this knowledge (of predictive validity) toward a conceptual understanding of how the scale works (construct validity). Scales of this sort often prove difficult to disentangle, however, because the parts or components were never built-in properly to begin with.

The second issue involves efficiency. Even when it is possible to identify what seem to be the "active ingredients" of a heterogeneous construct or measure, because the various elements are not assessed systematically, the original measure will need to be revised. Any significant revision, however, diminishes confidence in previous work with the scale, and raises the discouraging prospect of having to repeat previous validation studies using the newly derived components. Small wonder that heterogeneous and empirically derived scales are rarely revised.

The Bottom-Up Approach

Rather than attempting to dismantle a heterogeneous construct, this approach carefully specifies, from the outset, the components of a particular construct that would seem to be important on conceptual grounds; these components are then assessed methodically (Briggs & Cheek, 1986; Comrey, 1988). The bottom-up approach is more efficient than the top-down approach because it focuses on the building blocks from the beginning of the process rather than toward the middle or end. It requires analytical distinctions and clear conceptualization at inception, and thereby facilitates the process of generating and testing hypotheses; it both calls for and enables a sharp focus on the components of a construct, how they go together, and why. All along the way it is apparent which elements are working and which are not, and how the various parts are related. Therefore, revisions and reconceptualization occur early on.

A primary benefit of this approach is the emphasis on conceptualization and hypothesis-testing at the level of individual constructs rather than broad theories. A primary task for researchers adopting this strategy is to identify promising primary constructs, which then become the elements that are added together in the search for meaningful combinations. So what is a primary construct, and how do we decide which are the ones that matter?

Primary Factors. Eysenck and Eysenck (1985) describe primary factors as those "which are relatively pure and where it would be difficult to subdivide them again into subfactors" (p. 75). This description emphasizes item homogeneity and a resistance to partitioning. It is consistent with the contention that "a single scale ought to measure a single thing" (Briggs & Cheek, 1986, p. 109). Item homogeneity can be assessed in terms of the mean of the pairwise correlations among items. As a rule of thumb, I believe that the optimal average is in the range of .2 to .4; averages higher than this suggest excessive item redundancy, whereas lower averages imply that no single label will adequately represent the complexity of the items. Factor analytic techniques offer a method by which the dimensionality of scales can be evaluated more directly (e.g., see Comrey's 1988 discussion of factor analysis and factored homogeneous item dimensions—FHID's). However, the fact that a set of items can be partitioned reliably does not necessarily imply that an important distinction has been uncovered. The appropriate level of measurement and breadth of a construct is not an issue that can be wholly resolved statistically; it is an issue first and foremost of construct validity.

Factors that Matter. It is my contention that a primary factor worthy of its name will be empirically distinctive. Individual components of a scale are important to the extent that they are conceptually meaningful and empirically useful. Primary factors may correlate with one another— unlike the five (plus or minus two) broad factors which are presumably orthogonal—but they must also be differentially related to other factors. Examples of correlated primary factors that show distinctive patterns of correlations would include public and private self-consciousness (Carver & Scheier, 1987; Fenigstein, 1987), thrill-seeking and disinhibition (Zuckerman, 1979), and shyness and sociability (Cheek & Buss, 1981). One of the important avenues of research in the bottom-up approach is to examine the ways in which related factors differ as a function of motivational, contextual, or affective influences.

Identifying Primary Factors. Whereas the lexical approach to the study of trait attributions begins with a finite domain (and one that has been carefully defined by lexicographers), the universe of possible primary constructs is demarcated less plainly. The large literature that has accumulated on various constructs over the last half century, however, would provide an excellent source from which to generate an extensive list of candidates. Of course, it would be necessary to prune such a list carefully. Buss & Craik (1985) have suggested one set of criteria for identifying significant constructs based on the acts associated with a particular trait label; important constructs are those for which the act exemplars are numerous, distinctive, prototypical, stable, variable across individuals, and reasonably frequent.

The five-factor model would also be of benefit in culling the list of possible candidates, helping to expose redundancies and pointing to areas that have been missed or underrepresented (e.g., the domains of agreeableness or conscientiousness). Conversely, the psychological literature might yield interesting constructs that have not emerged from the lexical approach because the concepts are not well-represented by single adjective descriptors in the English language.

An approach that emphasizes primary factors seems essential if our understanding of the Big Five is to advance. The five-factor model originated in analyses of trait adjectives, but it is difficult to translate single adjectives into psychological constructs. It is necessary to identify the critical elements subsumed by the five (plus or minus two) factors, and then to measure these components in and of themselves. Interestingly, the few attempts to derive primary factors from the five-factor model have yielded widely divergent primary factors—compare Costa & McCrae's facets with Hogan's HICs. This divergence is inevitable, however, because there is nothing about the five-factor model that suggests what components matter the most. Thus, whereas the five-factor model is a noteworthy achievement because it provides a general framework for discussing and locating primary factors, we must resist any tendency to explain away a primary factor in terms of its location in the five-factor model. Knowing the location of a construct is not the same as understanding its nature or importance.

At the beginning of this essay, I argued that researchers in the field of personality study two types of tendencies: those that define people generally and those that define people specifically. I then discussed the optimal approach for describing and assessing individual differences in personality, contrasting broad, heterogeneous factors with narrow, homogeneous factors. Perhaps, in the way of a conclusion, I should point out that the search for common factors—whether they be broad or narrow—falls somewhere between the two endeavors of personality. The study of individual differences focuses on human variability and thus seems different from the study of human tendencies in general, but it also focuses on factors that are common to all people rather than tendencies that might characterize a single individual. Some critics would decry the study of individual *differences* as altogether irrelevant to an understanding of individual *tendencies* (Lamiell, 1987), but I prefer Allport's perspective. Although he pursued a nomothetic course of study and could reasonably be considered the father of the lexical approach, he also pointed out that "common traits are at best convenient approximations" (1937, p. 300). He always championed an adequate recognition of individual traits as essential to the entire field of personality. I close with his admonition: "The comparison of individuals is only *one* of the goals of the psychology of personality. Understanding the individual case and determining the laws of the individual's development are just as legitimate and even more important goals" (p. 303).

References

Allport, G.W. (1937). *Personality: A Psychological Interpretation*. New York: Holt, Rinehart & Winston.

Briggs, S.R. (1988). Shyness: Introversion or neuroticism? *Journal of Personality, 22,* 290–307.

Briggs, S.R. (1985). A trait account of social shyness. In P. Shaver (Ed.), *Review of Personality and Social Psychology,* Vol. 6. (pp. 35–64). Beverly Hills: Sage.

Briggs, S.R., & Cheek, J.M. (1986). The role of factor analysis in the development and evaluation of personality scales. *Journal of Personality, 54,* 106–148.

Bruner, J.S., & Tagiuri, R. (1954). The perception of people. In G. Lindzey (Ed.), *Handbook of Social Psychology: Vol. 2, Special Fields and Applications* (pp. 634–654). Cambridge, Massachusetts: Addison-Wesley.

Buss, D.M. (1984). Evolutionary biology and personality psychology: Toward a conception of human nature and individual differences. *American Psychologist, 39,* 1135–1147.

Buss, D.M., & Craik, K.H. (1985). Why *not* measure that trait? Alternative criteria for identifying important dispositions. *Journal of Personality and Social Psychology, 48,* 934–946.

Carver, C.S., & Scheier, M.F. (1987). The blind men and the elephant: Selective examination of the public-private literature gives rise to a faulty perception. *Journal of Personality, 55,* 525–541.

Cattell, R.B. (1946). *Description and measurement of personality*. New York: World Book.

Cheek, J.M. & Buss, A.H. (1981). Shyness and sociability. *Journal of Personality and Social Psychology, 41,* 330–339.

Comrey, A.L. (1988). Factor-analytic methods of scale development in personality and clinical psychology. *Journal of Consulting and Clinical Psychology, 56,* 754–761.

Conley, J.J. (1985). Longitudinal stability of personality traits: A multitrait-multimethod-multioccasion analysis. *Journal of Personality and Social Psychology, 49,* 1266–1282.

Costa, P.T., Jr., & McCrae, R.R. (1985). *The NEO Personality Inventory manual*. Odessa, Florida: Psychological Assessment Resources.

Costa, P.T., Jr., & McCrae, R.R. (1988). Personality in adulthood: A six-year longitudinal study of self-reports and spouse ratings on the NEO Personality Inventory. *Journal of Personality and Social Psychology, 54,* 853–863.

Costa, P.T., Jr., McCrae, R.R., & Dembroski, T.M. (1989). Agreeableness vs. antagonism: Explication of a potential risk factor for CHD. In A. Siegman & T.M. Dembroski (Eds.), *In search of coronary-prone behavior* 41–63. Hillsdale, New Jersey: Erlbaum.

D'Andrade, R.G. (1965). Trait psychology and componential analysis. *American Anthropologist, 67*, 215–28.

Digman, J.M., & Takemoto-Chock, N.K. (1981). Factors in the natural language of personality: Re-analysis and comparison of six major studies. *Multivariate Behavioral Research, 16*, 149–170.

Eysenck, H.J., & Eysenck, M.W. (1985). *Personality and individual differences: A natural science approach.* Plenum: New York.

Fenigstein, A. (1987). On the nature of public and private self-consciousness. *Journal of Personality, 55*, 543–554.

Fiske, D.W. (1949). Consistency of the factorial structures of personality ratings from different sources. *Journal of Abnormal and Social Psychology, 44*, 329–344.

Goldberg, L. (1981). Language and individual differences: The search for universals in personality lexicons. In Wheeler, L. (Ed.), *Review of Personality and Social Psychology,* Vol. 2. (pp. 141–165). Sage: Beverly Hills.

Goldberg, L. (1982). From Ace to Zombie: Some explorations in the language of personality. In Spielberger, C.D. & Butcher, J.N. (Eds.) *Advances in Personality Assessment,* Vol. 1 (pp. 203–234). Hillsdale, New Jersey: Erlbaum.

Gough, H.G. (1965). Conceptual analysis of psychological test scores and other diagnostic variables. *Journal of Abnormal Psychology, 70*, 294–302.

Gray, J.A. (1987). *The psychology of fear and stress.* New York: Cambridge University Press.

Hogan, R. (1983). A socioanalytic theory of personality. In M.M. Page (Ed.), *Nebraska Symposium on Motivation,* 1982 (pp. 55–89). Lincoln: University of Nebraska Press.

Hogan, R. (1986). *Manual for the Hogan Personality Inventory.* Minneapolis, MN: National Computer Systems.

Howarth, E. (1976). A psychometric investigation of Eysenck's Personality Inventory. *Journal of Personality Assessment, 40*, 173–185.

John, O.P., Angleitner, A., & Ostendorf, F. (1988). The lexical approach to personality: A historical review of trait taxonomic research. *European Journal of Personality, 2*, 171–203.

Jones, E.E., & Nisbett, R.E. (1971). The actor and the observer: Divergent perceptions of the causes of behavior. In E.E. Jones, et al (Eds.), *Attribution: Perceiving the causes of behavior* (pp. 78–94). Morristown, NJ: General Learning Press.

Lamiell, J.T. (1987). *The psychology of personality: An epistemological inquiry.* New York: Columbia University Press.

Lewicki, P. (1986). *Nonconscious social information processing.* New York: Academic Press.

McCrae, R.R., & Costa, P.T. (1987). Validation of the five-factor model of personality across instruments and observers. *Journal of Personality and Social Psychology, 52*, 81–90.

McDougall, W. (1938). Tendencies, as indispensable postulates of all psychology. In the *Proceedings of the XI International Congress on Psychology: 1937* (pp. 157–170). Paris: Alcan.

Mershon, B., & Gorsuch, R.L. (1988). Number of factors in the personality sphere: Does increase in factors increase predictability of real-life criteria? *Journal of Personality and Social Psychology, 55,* 675–680.

Murphy, G. (1966). *Personality: A biosocial approach to origins and structure.* New York: Basic Books.

Murray, H.A. (1951). Some basic psychological assumptions and conceptions. *Dialectica,* 1951, *5,* 266–292.

Noller, P., Law, H., & Comrey, A.L. (1987). Cattell, Comrey, and Eysenck personality factors compared: More evidence for the five robust factors? *Journal of Personality and Social Psychology, 53,* 775–782.

Norman, W.T. (1963). Toward an adequate taxonomy of personality attributes: Replicated factor structure in peer nomination personality ratings. *Journal of Abnormal and Social Psychology, 66,* 574–583.

Norman, W.T., & Goldberg, L. (1966). Raters, ratees, and randomness in personality structure. *Journal of Personality and Social Psychology, 4,* 681–691.

Passini, F.T., & Norman, W.T. (1966). A universal conception of personality structure?, *Journal of Personality and Social Psychology, 4,* 44–49.

Peabody, D. (1987). Selecting representative trait adjectives. *Journal of Personality and Social Psychology, 52,* 59–71.

Peabody, D., & Goldberg, L.R. (1988). *Variance and invariance in personality structures: Three determinants of the size and location of factors based on personality-trait adjectives.* Unpublished manuscript, Oregon Research Institute.

Rowe, D. (1982). Monozgotic twin cross-correlations as a validation of personality structure: A test of the semantic bias hypothesis. *Journal of Personality and Social Psychology, 43,* 1072–1079.

Schneider, D.J. (1973). Implicit personality theory: A review. *Psychological Bulletin, 79,* 294–309.

Shweder, R.A. (1975). How relevant is an individual difference theory of personality ratings: *Journal of Personality, 43,* 455–485.

Strelau, J., & Eysenck, H.J. (Eds.) (1987). *Personality dimensions and arousal.* New York: Plenum.

Tellegen, A., & Waller, N.G. (1987). *Re-examining basic dimensions of natural language trait descriptors.* Paper presented at the 95th Annual Convention of the American Psychological Association, New York, NY.

Tupes, E.C., & Christal, R.C. (1961). *Recurrent personality factors based on trait ratings.* USAF ASD Technical Report No. 61-97. Lackland Air Force Base, TX: U.S. Air Force.

Weiss, D. (1979). The effects of systematic variations in information on judge's descriptions of personality. *Journal of Personality and Social Psychology, 37,* 2121–2136.

Wiggins, J.S. (1973), *Personality and prediction: Principles of personality assessment.* Reading, MA: Addison-Wesley.

Yang, K.S., & Bond, M.H. (1989). *Exploring implicit personality theories with indigenous or imported constructs: The Chinese case*. Unpublished manuscript, Chinese University of Hong Kong.

Zuckerman, M. (1984). Sensation-seeking: A comparative approach to a human trait. *Behavioral and Brain Sciences, 7*, 413–471.

Zuckerman, M. (1979). *Sensation-seeking: Beyond the optimal level of arousal*. Hillsdale, NJ: Erlbaum.

CHAPTER 19

Towards a Taxonomy of Personality Descriptors

Oliver P. John

Personality psychology has not yet established a generally accepted, systematic framework for distinguishing, ordering, and naming individual differences in people's behavior and experience. Such a systematic framework is generally called a *taxonomy*. In biology, for example, the Linnean taxonomy established an orderly classification of plants and animals and a standard nomenclature. The availability of this initial taxonomy has been a tremendous asset for biologists: it has permitted researchers to study specified classes of instances instead of examining separately every individual instance, and it has served to facilitate the communication and accumulation of empirical findings about these classes and their instances.

Personality psychologists face a more difficult task than did the early biologists. Biologists classify individual exemplars according to their attributes; in personality taxonomies, the exemplars are the attributes themselves. Whereas exemplars of animals have a discrete physical existence and can thus be "found" by the researcher in the field, personality attributes can neither be seen nor found nor otherwise directly observed. Personality attributes are abstract concepts that have to be inferred, and the mere existence of personality attributes in people has been a matter of debate.

There is another important difference between personality attributes and natural objects. Although the number of animals, for example, is exceedingly large, it is, in principle, finite at any given time. In contrast, the number of ways in which people differ from each other is seemingly infinite, for one can always think of new attributes (e.g., computer literate, "nerdy") or subdivide previously known attributes into more specific ones. Given these difficulties, it should come as no surprise that personality psychologists have struggled for the past fifty years with the task of specifying, cataloguing, and ordering the domain of individual differences.

Some psychologists have turned to natural language as an initial source of personality attributes. Natural language provides a finite yet extensive set of terms that refer to differences among people. Historically, Allport and Odbert (1936) provided the basis for later taxonomic work by listing the personality-related terms found in an unabridged dictionary. By the early 1940s, Cattell had embarked on a major effort to select personality variables representative of the whole "personality sphere." Through a series of reduction steps, he derived, in 1947, thirty-five bipolar variables from the Allport and Odbert list (see John, Angleitner, & Ostendorf, 1988), analyses of which, in Cattell's own interpretation, suggested at least twelve factors. Other investigators (Fiske, 1949; Tupes & Christal, 1961; Norman, 1963; Borgatta, 1964; Digman & Takemoto-Chock, 1981) have demonstrated, however, that more common methods of analysis suggest only five replicable factors, which have become known as the Big Five. Similar five-dimensional structures based on variable sets different from Cattell's have been reported by Digman (1972), Goldberg (1980), John, Goldberg, and Angleitner (1984), Digman and Inouye (1986), McCrae and Costa (1985, 1987), Conley (1985), and Peabody and Goldberg (1988).

One Big Five—Or Many?

Although the Big Five structure has received much recent attention, it has not been universally accepted as a taxonomic superstructure in the field of personality. One of the problems, it seems, is the perception that there is no *one* Big Five, as is evident in questions such as "*which* Big Five" or "*whose* Big Five." In the upper section of Table 19.1, I have listed the various interpretative labels assigned to the five dimensions. Norman's (1963) labels, used most commonly in the literature, are highlighted. Although some general themes emerge from the factor names in Table 19.1, the labels do vary substantially. Indeed, Table 19.1 may look like bedlam. The third factor, for example, has variously been interpreted as Conscientousness, Dependability, Conformity, Prudence, Task Interest, and Will to Achieve. Factor V has been labeled Culture, Intellect, and Openness to experience. It appears as if each investigator has his or her "own" Big Five.

Some variation from study to study is to be expected with dimensions as broad and inclusive as the Big Five. Differences in factor solutions might arise because researchers differ in the variables they include, thus representing different parts of the factor's total range of meaning, or, they may use different labels for similar factor patterns. Nonetheless, there may be more commonality here than meets the eye; the fact that the labels differ does not necessarily mean that the factors are different too.

There is a very simple way to demonstrate that the factors which seem to provide such unacceptably heterogeneous definitions, actually share a common core of features across studies. Fuzzy and partially overlapping

TABLE 19.1. Five broad dimensions of personality and their interpretation over the past forty years.

Author	I	II	III	IV	V
Big Five variants					
Fiske	Confident Self-Expression	Social Adaptability	Conformity	Emotional Control	Inquiring Intellect
Tupes & Christal	Surgency	Agreeableness	Dependability	Emotional Stability	Culture
Borgatta	Assertiveness	Likeability	Task Interest	Emotionality	Intelligence
Norman	Surgency	Agreeableness	Conscientiousness	Emotional Stability	Culture
Digman	Extraversion	Friendly Compliance	Will to Achieve	Ego Strength (Anxiety)	Intellect
Hogan	Ambition and Sociability	Likeability	Prudence (Impulsivity)	Adjustment	Intellectance
McCrae & Costa	Extraversion	Agreeableness	Conscientiousness	Neuroticism	Openness
Peabody & Goldberg	Power	Love	Work	Affect	Intellect
Other structural models					
Block[1]	Undercontrol		Overcontrol		Resiliency
Buss & Plomin	Activity	Sociability	Impulsivity	Emotionality	
Cattell	Exvia	Cortertia	Superego Strength	Anxiety	
Eysenck[2]	Extraversion		Psychoticism	Neuroticism	
Gough[3]	Externality		Norm-Favoring		Self-Realization
Guilford	Social Activity	Paranoid Disposition	Thinking Introversion	Emotional Stability	
Leary, Wiggins	Dominance	Love			

[1]Resiliency is listed here under two columns because an ego-resilient individual is both intellectually resourceful and effective in controlling anxiety.
[2]Individuals scoring high on Psychoticism seem to be low in both Conscientiousness and Agreeableness (see McCrae, this volume).
[3]Self-realization, the third vector scale on the revised CPI, includes both Intellectual efficiency and Well-being.

definitions are typical of natural categories; these categories are still useful, however, because they can be defined by a range of prototypical exemplars. Similarly, the Big Five can be defined with prototypical exemplars that capture those elements that are common across studies. One way to integrate the various interpretations of the factors is to map the five dimensions conceptually into a common language. For this demonstration, I have used the attributes included in an instrument, the Adjective Checklist (Gough & Heilbrun, 1965), that was developed in the early 1950s, prior to Norman's (1963) publication of the Big-Five factor structure.

Conceptual Definition of the Big Five

As the first step, I reviewed, with a group of nine students, the factor solutions and interpretations of the most important articles of each investigator listed in Table 19.1. In the process, each member of the group formed an understanding of the five dimensions. The judges then independently sorted each of the 300 items in the *Adjective Checklist* (ACL) into one of the Big-Five domains or, if that was not possible, into a sixth category. There was substantial agreement among the judges; more than half of the 300 ACL items were sorted into one of the categories with at least 80% interjudge agreement, which suggests that the judges had formed a consensually shared understanding of the five categories.

Table 19.2 lists a subset of the items assigned to each of the five dimensions by 90% to 100% of the judges. The lists of trait terms generated by this task capture the most central core of each of the dimensions as it appeared across numerous and diverse studies. The list is conceptually derived, but the conceptual analysis is based on a series of empirical findings. Thus, Table 19.2 provides conceptual definitions of the Big-Five dimensions that are independent of the vagaries of the particular lists of variables included in specific studies. This approach is similar to that taken by Jack Block in the studies forming the basis for his book, *Lives through time* (Block, 1971). In that study, documents available about each child differed dramatically both across subjects and time. To integrate the vast amount of diverse information, Block used human judges as transducers, providing them with one standard descriptive language (i.e., the California Q-Set).

The range of items included under each factor attests to their extraordinary breadth. For example, Factor I includes active, ambitious, assertive, bossy, dominant, energetic, and enthusiastic. It is not surprising that different researchers have used heterogeneous labels for each dimension. Assuming that the items listed in Table 19.1 represent the core of the content covered by each of the factors, we can now examine their more specific components. The first factor combines attributes referring to Activity level (active, energetic), Dominance (assertive, bossy, forceful), Sociability (outgoing, sociable, talkative), Expressive undercontrol (outspoken, loud, noisy), Ambition and Postitive affect (enthusiastic).

This type of analysis can uncover relations between the Big Five and other structural models originating in different theoretical contexts and through different empirical procedures. The lower portion of Table 19.1 sketches some of those correspondences that might otherwise be overlooked. The similarities between Cattell's second-order factor Exvia, Eysenck's Extraversion, and Gough's new Vector scale, labeled Internality-Externality, have already been noted (see McCrae, this volume). The present analysis suggests that the concepts Activity, Dominance, Social activity, and maybe even Undercontrol each refer to components

TABLE 19.2. Conceptually derived definitions: Adjective Checklist items assigned to each of the Big Five by at least 90% of the judges.

Factor I		Factor II		Factor III		Factor IV		Factor V	
Low	High	Low	High	Low	High	Low	High	Low	High
Quiet	Active	Cold	Affectionate	Careless	Cautious	Anxious	Calm	Commonplace	Artistic
Reserved	Adventurous	Cruel	Appreciative	Disorderly	Conscientious	Despondent	Contented	Narrow Interests	Civilized
Retiring	Assertive	Fault-finding	Cooperative	Forgetful	Deliberate	Emotional	Stable	Shallow	Clever
Shy	Bossy	Hard-hearted	Forgiving	Frivolous	Dependable	Fearful	Unemotional	Simple	Curious
Silent	Dominant	Quarrelsome	Friendly	Irresponsible	Efficient	High-strung		Unintelligent	Dignified
Withdrawn	Energetic	Stern	Generous	Slipshod	Organized	Moody			Foresighted
	Enthusiastic	Stingy	Gentle	Undependable	Painstaking	Nervous			Imaginative
	Forceful	Thankless	Good-natured		Planful	Self-pitying			Ingenious
	Noisy	Unfriendly	Helpful		Practical	Self-punishing			Insightful
	Outgoing	Unkind	Kind		Precise	Temperamental			Intelligent
	Outspoken		Pleasant		Reliable	Tense			Inventive
	Show-off		Praising		Responsible	Touchy			Logical
	Spunky		Sensitive		Thorough	Unstable			Original
	Sociable		Soft-hearted			Worrying			Polished
	Talkative		Sympathetic						Resourceful
			Trusting						Sharp-witted
			Unselfish						Sophisticated
			Warm						Wide Interests
									Wise
									Witty

that together comprise Factor I. Conceptual definitions, like those presented in Table 19.1, may serve as a step towards achieving a canonical representation that integrates the findings in the personality literature. The next task is to specify, both conceptually and empirically, the hierarchical structure at levels *below* the Big Five.

Is the Big-Five Structure Too Parochial?

The above analysis has been addressed to the criticism that everyone has his or her own version of the Big Five. The opposite kind of criticism has also been voiced, namely, that the Big-Five structure is an artifact of a *particular* initial selection of variables. Much of the early factor-analytic work relied on relatively small sets of descriptors. In particular, there has been some concern that several of these analyses have employed a common set of variables—Cattell's—and that the selection of variables in other studies has been prestructured so as to yield the Big Five. More recent studies have overcome this limitation by using more extensive and systematically selected sets of descriptors (reviewed by John, in press).

Nonetheless, the reliance on experimenter-imposed variable sets to define the universe of descriptors may have unduly excluded important characteristics from consideration. To assess the importance of this limitation, studies are needed that select characteristics on the basis of new criteria. Given that the Big Five were intended to represent the major dimensions of natural-language personality descriptions, one option is to investigate the characteristics that people use most frequently in free descriptions of themselves and others. Would the Big Five replicate if the set of descriptors factored was based on the content of subjects' free descriptions rather than on those sets of terms selected by the taxonomers themselves?

Fortunately, for other purposes, William F. Chaplin and I had used a free-description methodology to elicit a large set of personality descriptors in a naturalistic setting. In one of our studies, we asked more than 300 college students to describe their own personalities and to generate terms for both their desirable *and* their undesirable characteristics. Here are the ten most frequently generated terms, with the percentage of subjects generating them in parentheses: friendly (34%), caring (25%), intelligent (22%), happy (20%), lazy (18%), moody (18%), shy (18%), outgoing (17%), selfish (16%), and kind (15%). Two aspects of this list are noteworthy and generally representative of our findings. First, subjects had little difficulty generating both positive and negative attributes when asked to do so; when not so instructed, they tended to generate mostly positive characteristics. Second, among the ten most frequent terms were at least one for each of the Big Five-domains: outgoing vs. shy (Factor I), kind and caring vs. selfish (II), lazy (low pole of III), happy vs. moody (IV), and intelligent (V).

To examine the content of these free descriptions further, we focused on sixty of the most frequently used descriptors and then factor analyzed self-ratings on these descriptors made by a *separate* sample of subjects. These analyses yielded five factors that closely resembled the conceptual definitions of the Big-Five presented here. The largest factor was marked by sincere, kind, and warm, which obviously corresponds to Agreeableness——Factor II of the Big Five. Talkative and energetic vs. quiet and shy had the highest loadings on the second largest factor, thus closely resembling Surgency (Factor I). The next factor seemed to resemble Emotional Stability (Factor IV), with high loadings from descriptors such as temperamental, possessive, moody, and high-strung. Finally, the two remaining factors, while substantially smaller than the other three, could, nonetheless, be identified by their highest loading variables: organized and responsible for Conscientiousness (Factor III), and intelligent and smart versus naive for Factor V, which included Intellect but not Culture or Openness to experience.

These initial analyses provide little evidence for the conjecture that the Big Five are a result of any particular sampling of descriptors. Rather, they indicate that individuals of college age find all five dimensions sufficiently important to include at least some reference to them in their free descriptions. The findings also indicate, however, that Agreeableness and Surgency, the two dimensions that figure prominently in the interpersonal circumplex (Wiggins, 1979), were of much more concern to this sample of college students than were the two dimensions related most closely to task or achievement behavior, Conscientiousness and Intellect.

Why Five?

Another objection to the Big Five is that five dimensions cannot possibly capture all of the variance exhibited in the personalities of the population. If a more detailed image is desired, however, one will have to shift to more differentiated constructs. The objection that five dimensions is too few overlooks the fact that the trait domain tends to be hierarchically structured (Hampson, John, & Goldberg, 1986). The advantage of categories as broad as the Big Five is their enormous bandwidth. Their disadvantage is their low fidelity. In any hierarchical representation, one always loses information as one moves up the hierarchical levels. (For example, the category "Poodles" contains more information than the category "dogs," which in turn contains more information than the category "animals.") In psychometric terms, one necessarily loses item information as one aggregates items into scales, and one loses scale information as one aggregates scales into factors.

Most of the work on the Big Five is expressly hierarchical (see John et al., 1988). The Big Five dimensions represent the broadest level of the hierarchy, and, in that sense, they are to personality what the categories "plant" and "animal" are to the world of natural objects—extremely useful for some initial rough distinctions but of less value for predicting specific behaviors of a particular object. At the broadest level, then, one would describe a person as extraverted (or surgent), at the next level as active, assertive, sociable, or expressive, or even more specifically as talkative or gossipy. The hierarchical level one selects will depend on one's predictive goals and preferences. That is, the number of attributes available for the description of an individual can be increased infinitely, limited only by one's objectives.

Nonetheless, there could be important trait dimensions of substantial breadth in addition to the Big Five. Costa and McCrae have embarked on an extensive program of research aimed at demonstrating that the Big-Five dimensions can be recovered from most comprehensive personality-assessment instruments currently in use (McCrae, this volume). This strategy, however, does not aim to uncover additional dimensions beyond the Big Five, and the type of conceptual analysis I applied to the ACL might be useful.

In that analysis, more than half of the items had been classified on one of the factors with interjudge agreement of at least 80%. Some of the items that did not receive clear classifications on any one of the Big Five are given in Table 19.3. These terms seemed to fall into five distinct clusters,

TABLE 19.3. Clusters of adjective checklist items not classified on one of the Big Five by a clear majority of the judges (and their Categorization by Norman, 1967).

(6) Individuation/Autonomy		(7) Traditional Values	
Independent	(1 -- prime trait)	Conservative	(3 -- quaint trait)
Individualistic	(3 -- quaint trait)	Conventional	(1 -- prime trait)
Rebellious	(3 -- quaint trait)	Prudish	(1 -- prime trait)
Suggestible	(1 -- prime trait)	Wholesome	(12 -- evaluation)
Peculiar	(12 -- evaluation)		
Queer	(14 -- ambiguous)		
(8) Maturity		(9) Gender Terms	
Mature	(14 -- ambiguous)	Effeminate	(1 -- prime trait)
Immature	(14 -- ambiguous)	Feminine	(1 -- prime trait)
Infantile	(1 -- prime trait)	Masculine	(1 -- prime trait)
(10) Physical Characteristics			
Attractive	(9 -- social effect)		
Good-looking	(13 -- physical)		
Handsome	(13 -- physical)		
Sexy	(13 -- physical)		
Healthy	(13 -- physical)		

Note. Norman's (1967) categorizations into 11 content domains (1-11) and four exclusion categories (12-15) are given in parentheses.

which may be labeled Individuation/Autonomy, Traditional values, Maturity, Gender, and Physical characteristics. The items for each of these clusters are listed in Table 19.3, along with their classifications into the domains of personality description used by Norman (1967).

Only three of these clusters contained *trait* terms, according to Norman's classification. The three terms referring to maturity are evaluations of people with respect to cultural age norms expressed metaphorically (e.g., *infantile* describes behavior seen as appropriate for an infant). The items referring to physical attractiveness, despite their evolutionary significance, are seldom considered proper *personality* traits. The three gender terms, although included by Norman in the trait category, seem rather complex syndromes that are largely dependent on current social roles and stereotypes. Individuation/Autonomy and Traditional Values appear to be the only possible candidates for further broad dimensions of personality. Indeed, variables related to these two clusters have been included by McCrae and Costa within Factor V, which they interpret as Openness to experience. In particular, the "open" individual should be one who values individuation and autonomy but rejects the constraints imposed by conventions and traditional values. However, the inclusion of these two clusters in a personality taxonomy raises issues about the differentiation between personality and attitudinal traits. An alternative position would be to consider these two domains as conceptually separate but closely related classes of individual differences.

In conclusion, the method of analysis used to classify the 300 ACL items did not lead to the discovery of any major dimensions of personality beyond those included in the Big Five, but suggested that attitudes, physical characteristics, and gender roles may need to be addressed outside the Big-Five framework.

Summary and Conclusions

A personality taxonomy should provide a systematic framework for distinguishing, ordering, and naming types and characteristics of individuals. Ideally, that taxonomy would be built around principles that are causal and dynamic, exist at multiple levels of abstraction or hierarchy, and offer a standard nomenclature for scientists working in the field of personality. The Big Five, however, are far from that ideal. In contrast to the biological taxonomies, they provide only a list of descriptive concepts, which, at this point, is specified solely at the highest level in the hierarchy, and a nomenclature that by no means has reached the status of a "standard." Still rooted in "vernacular" English, the theoretical context of the Big Five is the accumulated knowledge about personality as it has been laid down over the ages in natural language. Historical precedent suggests, however, that natural language is not necessarily a bad place to start a taxonomy. Even in animal taxonomy, as G.G. Simpson has pointed out, "the technical system evolved from the vernacular" (1961, pp. 12–13).

Acknowledgments. The preparation of this chapter was supported in part by Grant MH-39077 from the National Institute of Mental Health (United States Public Health Service) and by Biomedical Research Grants 87-20 and 88-24 (University of California). I wish to thank Harold Baize, Lewis R. Goldberg, Harrison G. Gough, Sarah E. Hampson, Robert R. McCrae, Richard Robins, Tina Rosolack and Marjorie Taylor for their help and support during the writing of this chapter, which I could not have completed single-armedly.

References

Allport, G.W., & Odbert, H.S. (1936). Trait-names: A psycho-lexical study. *Psychological Monographs, 47,* (1, Whole No. 211).

Block, J. (1961). *The Q-sort method in personality assessment and psychiatric research* (1978 Rpt. Edition). Palo Alto, CA: Consulting Psychologists Press.

Block, J. (1971). *Lives through time.* Berkeley, CA: Bancroft Books.

Borgatta, E.F. (1964). The structure of personality characteristics. *Behavioral Science, 9,* 8–17.

Buss, A.H., & Plomin, R. (1975). *A temperament theory of personality development.* New York: Wiley.

Cattell, R.B. (1947). Confirmation and clarification of primary personality factors. *Psychometrika, 12,* 197–220.

Conley, J.J. (1985). A personality theory of adulthood and aging. In R. Hogan and W.H. Jones (Eds.), *Perspectives in Personality* (Vol. 1, pp. 81–115). Greenwich, CN: JAI Press.

Digman, J.M. & Inouye, J. (1986). Further specification of the five robust factors of personality. *Journal of Personality and Social Psychology, 50,* 116–123.

Digman, J.M., & Takemoto-Chock, N.K. (1981). Factors in the natural language of personality: Re-analysis and comparison of six major studies. *Multivariate Behavioral Research, 16,* 149–170.

Fiske, D.W. (1949). Consistency of the factorial structures of personality ratings from different sources. *Journal of Abnormal and Social Psychology, 44,* 329–344.

Goldberg, L.R. (1980, May). *Some ruminations about the structure of individual differences: Developing a common lexicon for the major characteristics of human personality.* Paper presented at the annual convention of the Western Psychological Association, Honolulu, Hawaii.

Gough, H.G. & Heilbrun, A.B., Jr. (1965). *The Adjective Checklist manual.* Palo Alto, CA: Consulting Psychologists Press.

Gough, H.G. (1987). *California Psychological Inventory administrator's guide.* Palo Alto, CA: Consulting Psychologists Press.

Hampson, S.E., John, O.P., & Goldberg, L.R. (1986). Category breadth and hierarchical structure in personality: Studies of asymmetries in judgments of trait implications. *Journal of Personality and Social Psychology, 51,* 37–54.

Hogan, R. (1986). *Hogan Personality Inventory.* Minneapolis, MN: National Computer System.

John, O.P. (in press). Searching for the basic dimensions of personality: A review and critique. In P. McReynolds, J.C. Rosen, & G.J. Chelune (Eds.), *Advances in psychological assessment* (Vol. 7). New York: Plenum.

John, O.P., Goldberg, L.R., & Angleitner, A. (1984). Better than the alphabet: Taxonomies of personality-descriptive terms in English, Dutch, and German. In H.C.J. Bonarius, G.L.M. van Heck, & N.G. Smid (Eds.), *Personality psychology in Europe: Theoretical and empirical developments* (Vol. 1, pp. 83–100). Lisse: Swets and Zeitlinger.

John, O.P., Angleitner, A., & Ostendorf, F. (1988). The lexical approach to personality: A historical review of trait taxonomic research. *European Journal of Personality, 2,* 171–203.

McCrae, R.R., & Costa, P.T. (1985). Updating Norman's adequate taxonomy: Intelligence and personality dimensions in natural language and in questionnaires. *Journal of Personality and Social Psychology, 49,* 710–721.

McCrae, R.R., & Costa, P.T. (1987). Validation of the five-factor model of personality across instruments and observers. *Journal of Personality and Social Psychology, 52,* 81–90.

Norman, W.T. (1963). Toward an adequate taxonomy of personality attributes: Replicated factor structure in peer nomination personality ratings. *Journal of Abnormal and Social Psychology, 66,* 574–583.

Norman, T. (1967). *2,800 personality trait descriptors: Normative operating characteristics for a university population.* University of Michigan, Department of Psychology.

Peabody, D., & Goldberg, L.R. (in press). Some determinants of factor structures from personality-trait descriptors. *Journal of Personality and Social Psychology.*

Simpson, G.G. (1961). *Principles of animal taxonomy.* New York: Columbia University Press.

Tupes, E.C., & Christal, R.C. (1961). *Recurrent personality factors based on trait ratings.* (USAF ASD Technical Report No. 61-97). Lackland Air Force Base, TX: U.S. Air Force.

Wiggins, J.S. (1979). A psychological taxonomy of trait-descriptive terms: The interpersonal domain. *Journal of Personality and Social Psychology, 37,* 395–412.

Part V
Expansion of Levels of Explanation in Personality

Part A

CHAPTER 20

Identity Orientations and Self-Interpretation

Jonathan M. Cheek

The revival of the self as a popular topic among personality, social, and developmental psychologists in the 1980s has focused renewed attention on the psychology of identity. This is a positive development because Wylie (1974, 1979) concluded from her comprehensive review of earlier work that both the conceptualization and measurement of identity required considerable improvement. Recent work addresses a broad range of identity issues, such as Eriksonian identity achievement (Grotevant & Adams, 1984), identity crisis (Baumeister, 1986), identity narratives (McAdams, 1988), adult identity (Whitbourne, 1986), and the relationship between identity and social behavior (Schlenker, 1985). The purpose of this chapter is to review one particular program of research on the development and validation of a personality questionnaire assessing personal and social identity orientations.

Identity is the construct that defines who or what a particular person is. In 1890, William James described the fundamental distinction between the spiritual self, one's inner or subjective being and dispositions, and the social self, the recognition one receives from others. Psychologists and sociologists have been arguing ever since about whether the personal (internal) or social (external) aspects of identity are more important for understanding human behavior. Theorists such as Jung (1957) and Maslow (1961) assert that a person is most truly his/herself and closest to his or her authentic identity when experiencing a deep sense of personal uniqueness. On the other hand, social psychologists and sociologists such as Sarbin and Allen (1968) and Cooley (1902) define identity almost exclusively in social terms: "Identity is socially bestowed, socially sustained, and socially transformed" (Berger, 1963, p.98). It is clear, at least, that personal and social aspects of identity represent two central dimensions of the structure of identity (Caughey, 1980; Miller, 1963).

Regardless of disagreements among social scientists about the theoretical primacy of inner versus outer causes of behavior, it seems reasonable to expect that there are consequential individual differences in the relative importance or value placed on personal compared to social identity characteristics. Some people view their private, inner selves as being the most "true" and closest to their natural impulses, whereas others regard their social or institutionally defined selves as being the most significant part of their self-conceptions (Broughton, 1981; Insel, Reese, & Alexander, 1968; Turner & Gordon, 1981). Researchers have studied individual differences in identity by investigating the specific contents of people's self-descriptions (Gordon, 1968), their degree of commitment to particular social roles (Jackson, 1981), and the idiographic structure of identity features (Rosenberg & Gara, 1985). A different approach, first operationalized by Sampson (1978), focuses on a more abstract or global level by assessing the extent to which different individuals orient themselves towards their internal or external environment to define their identity.

Sampson (1978) constructed a list of twenty-two identity characteristics and had college students rate each one on a 20-point location scale ranging from internal ("it feels like part of me") to external ("it feels like part of my environment and my surroundings"). The five most internal characteristics (e.g., "my emotions and feelings") and the five most external (e.g., "memberships that I have in various groups") were used to form two location of identity measures. The response format for each item in these clusters of identity characteristics was a 5-point scale (0 = not at all important to my sense of who I am; 4 = extremely important to my sense of who I am). Notice that these identity characteristics do not refer to any specific emotion or internal state, nor to any particular membership or external role, but simply to categories of identity attributes that clearly have either an internal or an external location.

The assumption that individuals tend to orient themselves to *either* the internal *or* the external environment is implicit in Sampson's (1978) conceptualization and explicit in the way in which he analyzed and interpreted the relationships between his measures and other personality scales. Although Sampson (1978) did not report the correlation between these identity orientations, Cheek and Briggs (1982) found that importance rating scores on his Internal Location and External Location of Identity Scales had a slight positive correlation with each other ($r = .19$), rather than a bipolar relationship. This finding is consistent with several studies showing that measures of inner and outer orientation often form two relatively independent or orthogonal dimensions rather than a single, bipolar dimension (for a review, see Hogan & Cheek, 1983).

From a theoretical perspective, Erikson (1956) emphasized the importance of balancing and synthesizing the individual's personal needs with the opportunities and requirements of the social world in achieving a mature identity. Empirically, the measurement model presented in this chapter is based on the finding that personal and social identity orientations are two distinct dimensions. A person may score high on one or the other, or both or neither of these dimensions. Thus the personal and social aspects of identity may be viewed productively as *dialectical* rather than diametrical opposites. Moreover, the degree of balance or conflict between these two identity orientations may have a significant impact on the self-concept processes and social behavior of an individual.

The Aspects of Identity Questionnaire

The development of the Aspects of Identity Questionnaire began with the selection of items from Sampson's (1978) list of identity characteristics that were judged to represent the domains of personal and social identity (Cheek & Briggs, 1981, 1982). Subsequently, some items were reworded, others eliminated, and new items were developed to improve the reliability and content validity of the measures (Cheek, 1982a; Cheek & Hogan, 1981; Hogan & Cheek, 1983). Psychometric analyses indicated that certain items originally scored in the social identity category (e.g., "Being a part of the many generations of my family") were tending to cluster on a third factor representing communal or collective identity (cf. Abrams, 1988; Greenwald, 1988; Singer, 1982). A third scale for this domain is, therefore, currently under development. The final set of personal and social identity items is presented in Table 20.1.

To investigate the psychometric properties of the current versions of the scales, we administered the Aspects of Identity Questionnaire to a sample of 185 college students (Cheek, Underwood, & Cutler, 1985). As the columns of Table 20.1 reveal, there are two distinct factors—one each for personal and social aspects of identity. Every item loaded above .40 on its appropriate factor; the average interitem correlation was .34 for the Personal Identity Scale and .46 for the Social Identity Scale; the alpha coefficients were .84 and .86 respectively; the correlation between the two scales was .15. All of these results represent meaningful improvements compared to the earlier versions of the scales that were mentioned above.

Throughout the process of scale development, the average item mean has always been meaningfully higher for personal compared to social identity items (e.g., 3.99 versus 3.39 respectively for the sample reported in Table 20.1). From a cross-cultural perspective, it not only makes psychological sense that American college students have a high mean on personal identity items, but it is also clear that this outcome is *necessary* if the scale is to be useful for comparisons with other cultures (Munroe & Munroe, 1975, pp. 143–149).

A longitudinal study conducted in the early 1960s found that by the senior year in high school, females had developed a stronger social orientation, whereas males had developed a stronger personal orientation compared to members of the opposite sex (Carlson, 1965). In the present sample, there were no gender differences for social identity, and females tended to score slightly higher than males in personal identity, which is

TABLE 20.1. Factor analysis of personal and social identity items

Instructions: These items describe different aspects of identity. Please read each item carefully and consider how it applies to you. Fill in the blank next to each item by choosing a number from the scale below:

1 = Not important to my sense of who I am
2 = Slightly important to my sense of who I am
3 = Somewhat important to my sense of who I am
4 = Very important to my sense of who I am
5 = Extremely important to my sense of who I am

A priori scale assignment	Personal Identity[a]	Factor pattern loadings Personal	Social
My personal values and moral standards		.50	−.07
My dreams and imagination		.54	−.01
My personal goals and hopes for the future		.54	.26
My emotions and feelings		.70	.05
My thoughts and ideas		.69	−.04
The ways I deal with my fears and anxieties		.56	.10
My feeling of being a unique person, being distinct from others		.55	.13
Knowing that I continue to be essentially the same inside even though life involves many external changes		.45	.11
My self-knowledge, my ideas about what kind of person I really am		.68	.12
My personal self-evaluations, the private opinion I have of myself		.62	.12
	Social Identity[b]		
My popularity with other people		−.06	.63
The ways in which other people react to what I say and do		.13	.59
My physical appearance: my height, weight, and the shape of my body		.09	.66
My reputation, what others think of me		.12	.77
My attractiveness to other people		.10	.74
My gestures and mannerisms, the impression I make on others		.20	.70
My social behavior, such as the way I act when meeting people		.20	.61

n = 185

[a] The Personal Identity scale had a mean of 39.9, a standard deviation of 5.5, and an alpha coefficient of .84.
[b] The Social Identity scale had a mean of 23.7, a standard deviation of 4.9, and an alpha coefficient of .86.
The factor pattern correlation between these two factors was .12. The correlation between the Personal and Social Identity scales was .15.

consistent with contemporary work on other identity measures (Archer & Waterman, 1988). Previous research also suggests that older adults should show a tilt toward a social identity orientation and away from a personal identity orientation when compared to undergraduates (Insel et al., 1968). The one available study that permits such a comparison does indicate a trend in this direction (Leary, Wheeler, & Jenkins, 1986), but here again a cohort effect towards reduced differences might be expected (Seligman, 1988; Snow & Phillips, 1982).

Identity, Conformity, and Morality

Examination of the item content of the Personal and Social Identity Scales suggests that they measure orientations, where one looks to fulfill identity needs, rather than successful identity achievement. They appear to represent the denominator in William James' (1890) formula that self-esteem reflects a subjective ratio of one's successes to one's pretensions (i.e., aspirations or values). Neither scale has been found to correlate significantly with either self-ratings or peer-ratings of adjustment (Frantz, 1985; Miller & Thayer, 1988). Nevertheless, a recent study reported some weak to moderate correlations between the scales and Eriksonian identity status (Berzonsky, Trudeau, & Brennan, 1988). Personal identity correlated .25 with the achieved status and −.24 with the diffuse status. The only statistically significant correlation for social identity was .16 with the foreclosed identity status.

Stronger results have been obtained with a measure of the autonomy versus conformity dimension. Personal identity correlated positively with Barron's Independence of Judgement Scale, whereas the correlation for social identity was negative, and the multiple R employing both identity scales was .54 (Hogan & Cheek, 1983; replicated by Frantz, 1985, $R = .45$). Social identity has also been found to correlate positively with measures of concern for social appropriateness and an altruistic orientation, but personal identity is uncorrelated with those measures and positively correlated with achievement orientation and need for uniqueness (Cheek & Busch, 1982; Cutler, Lennox, & Wolfe, 1984).

The overall pattern of all these results suggests that people who are high in social and low in personal identity orientation will pursue a social strategy of trying to get along with others, and the contrasting group, high in personal and low in social identity orientation, will pursue an individualistic strategy of trying to get ahead (Hogan, Jones, & Cheek, 1985). Consistent with this speculation, social identity correlated .40 with susceptibility to shame, which was defined as concern with exposure of one's faults to others and failure to live up to public standards of moral behavior. Personal identity correlated .49 with susceptibility to guilt, which concerned one's own conscience and personal moral standards (Cheek & Hogan, 1983).

Identity, Self-Consciousness, and Self-Monitoring

Public self-consciousness is the dispositional tendency to be aware of one's appearance and to be concerned about making a good impression on others; private self-consciousness involves habitually focusing attention on the internal or covert elements of the self (Fenigstein, Scheier, & Buss,

1975). According to self-consciousness theory (Buss, 1980, p. 122), people high in private self-consciousness should emphasize personal aspects of their identities, whereas social aspects of identity should be especially important for those high in public self-consciousness. This expectation has been confirmed in a number of studies. Personal identity correlated between .29 and .39 with private self-consciousness, and social identity correlated between .30 and .58 with public self-consciousness (Cheek & Briggs, 1982; Cutler et al., 1984; Hogan & Cheek, 1983; Penner & Wymer, 1983).

The discriminant validity correlations (i.e., personal identity with public self-consciousness and social identity with private self-consciousness) have fallen between .00 and .20, although partial correlations controlling for the correlation between public and private self-consciousness have sometimes been necessary to clarify the relationships between identity and self-consciousness (Cheek & Briggs, 1982). These results, and the entire line of research on personal and social identity orientations, appear to undermine Wicklund and Gollwitzer's (1987) argument against the validity and utility of the public-private distinction in self-concept theory and research (Barnes, Mason, Leary, Laurent, Griebel, & Bergman, 1988).

Another popular and potentially relevant personality measure is Snyder's Self-Monitoring Scale. According to Snyder and Campbell (1982), high self-monitors should report a social identity orientation and low self-monitors a personal identity orientation. Self-monitoring does correlate around .30 with social identity, but the predicted negative correlation between self-monitoring and personal identity has never been obtained (Cheek & Briggs, 1981; Cheek & Busch, 1982; Miller & Thayer, 1988; Penner & Wymer, 1983; Sampson, 1978). The error in self-monitoring theory appears to be the assumption that personal and social identity orientations are bipolar opposites rather than two independent personality dimensions (Briggs & Cheek, 1988; Hogan & Cheek, 1983).

Reference Groups and Behavioral Preferences

Identity orientations should not only serve as an organizational structure for the person, but also direct purposive social behavior (Schlenker, 1985). In a study of memberships in adolescent social crowds, Johnson (1987) found that personal identity orientation was associated with memberships in the groups he labeled Brains, Freaks, and Politicos (i.e., primarily Holland's Artistic and Investigative types). Social identity orientation correlated with membership in the Socialites crowd, equivalent to Holland's Social type.

A pair of studies investigated the relationship between identity orientations and various occupational and recreational choices (Leary et al.,

1986). Compared to low scorers, students high in personal identity expressed a preference for jobs permitting self-fulfillment and creativity. Social identity was related to job characteristics involving good relationships with co-workers, high income, and prestige. In the area of recreational choices, personal identity was associated with self-satisfaction and personal health concerns as reasons for engaging in sports. High scorers in social identity emphasized group activities, concerns about appearance, and wanting others to know that they were physically active. The pattern of results described in this section suggests that longitudinal research on the impact of identity orientations on role selection could be worthwhile.

Identity Orientations as Moderator Variables

Personal identity and other measures of inward orientation tend to moderate the relationships between self-ratings and peer-ratings of personality traits and attitude-behavior consistency, with high scorers showing increased congruence (Cheek, 1982b; Wymer & Penner, 1985). Cheek and Hogan (1983) introduced the term *self-interpretation* to argue that debates about self-verification versus self-presentation should be reconceptualized as an issue of individual differences. During social interactions, people high in personal identity, especially those who are socially confident, should rely on their stable, internal values and dispositions as a guide for social behavior. People high in social identity, especially those who are socially anxious, should be responsive to the press of the immediate social situation. From this perspective, social behavior is the product of a transactional process of identity negotiation (Cheek & Hogan, 1983; Swann, 1987).

A recent laboratory study examined the moderating effects of identity orientations on the experience of public and private threats to self-images (Barnes et al., 1988). Subjects with high scores in social identity reacted more strongly to threats to their social esteem compared to those low in social identity, and a high personal identity orientation seemed to buffer subjects against threats to social esteem.

Individual items on the Aspects of Identity Questionnaire may also be useful as moderators of relationships among dimensions of self-esteem. For example, Liebman and Cheek (1983) found that importance ratings on the physical appearance item (see Table 20.1) moderated the relationship between shyness and self-evaluations of physical attractiveness. This relationship was significantly negative ($r = -.69$) only for subjects who rated physical appearance to be a very or extremely important aspect of their identity. The promising results obtained to date indicate that further work should be conducted in the controversial research area of moderator variables.

Future Directions

I hope that during the 1990s researchers will be able to integrate various lines of work on self-awareness, self-definition, and self-evaluation into a comprehensive model of self-concept structure and dynamics. Developmental speculations about the origins of personal and social identity orientations certainly need to be tested and refined (Greenwald, 1988; Hogan & Cheek, 1983; Hogan et al., 1985). As I have argued elsewhere (Cheek, 1985; Cheek & Melchior, in press), I believe that the psychology of the self will play an essential role in the emerging development of new personality theories.

References

Abrams, D. (1988). Self-consciousness scales for adults and children: Reliability, validity, and theoretical significance. *European Journal of Personality, 2,* 11–37.

Archer, S.L., & Waterman, A.S. (1988). Psychological individualism: Gender differences or gender neutrality? *Human Development, 31,* 65–81.

Barnes, B.D., Mason, E., Leary, M.R., Laurent, J., Griebel, C., & Bergman, A. (1988). Reactions to social vs self-evaluation: Moderating effects of personal and social identity orientations. *Journal of Research in Personality, 22,* 513–524.

Baumeister, R.F. (1986). *Identity: Cultural change and the struggle for self.* New York: Oxford University Press.

Berger, P.L. (1963). *Invitation to sociology.* Garden City, NY: Doubleday.

Berzonsky, M.D., Trudeau, J.V., & Brennan, F.X. (1988, March). *Social-cognitive correlates of identity status.* Paper presented at the meeting of the Society for Research on Adolescence, Alexandria, VA.

Briggs, S.R., & Cheek, J.M. (1988). On the nature of self-monitoring: Problems with assessment, problems with validity. *Journal of Personality and Social Psychology, 54,* 663–678.

Broughton, J.M. (1981). The divided self in adolescence. *Human Development, 24,* 13–32.

Buss, A.H. (1980). *Self-consciousness and social anxiety.* San Francisco: Freeman.

Carlson, R. (1965). Stability and change in the adolescent's self-image. *Child Development, 36,* 659–666.

Caughey, J.L. (1980). Personal identity and social organization. *Ethos, 8,* 173–203.

Cheek, J.M. (1982a). *The Aspects of Identity Questionnaire: Revised scales assessing personal and social identity.* Unpublished manuscript, Wellesley College.

Cheek, J.M. (1982b). Aggregation, moderator variables, and the validity of personality tests: A peer-rating study. *Journal of Personality and Social Psyhology, 43,* 1254–1269.

Cheek, J.M. (1985). Toward a more inclusive integration of evolutionary biology and personality psychology [Comment]. *American Psychologist, 40,* 1269–1270.

Cheek, J.M., & Briggs, S.R. (1981, August). *Self-consciousness, self-monitoring, and aspects of identity.* Paper presented at the meeting of the American Psychological Association, Los Angeles, CA.

Cheek, J.M. & Briggs, S.R. (1982). Self-consciousness and aspects of identity. *Journal of Research in Personality, 16,* 401–408.

Cheek, J.M., & Busch, C.M. (1982, April). *Self-monitoring and the inner-outer metaphor: Principled versus pragmatic self?* Paper presented at the meeting of the Eastern Psychological Association, Baltimore, MD.

Cheek, J.M., & Hogan, R. (1981). *The structure of identity: Personal and social aspects.* Paper presented at the meeting of the American Psychological Association, Los Angeles, CA.

Cheek, J.M., & Hogan, R. (1983). Self-concepts, self-presentations, and moral judgments. In J. Suls & A.G. Greenwald (Eds.), *Psychological perspectives on the self* (Vol. 2, pp. 249–273). Hillsdale, NJ: Erlbaum.

Cheek, J.M., & Melchior, L.A. (in press). Shyness, self-esteem, and self-consciousness. In H. Leitenberg (Ed.), *Handbook of social anxiety.* New York: Plenum.

Cheek, J.M., Underwood, M.K., & Cutler, B.L. (1985). *The Aspects of Identity Questionnaire (III).* Unpublished manuscript, Wellesley College.

Cooley, C.H. (1902). *Human nature and the social order.* New York: Scribner

Cutler, B.L., Lennox, R.D., & Wolfe, R.N. (1984, August). *Reliability and construct validity of the Aspects of Identity Questionnaire.* Paper presented at the meeting of the American Psychological Association, Toronto, Canada.

Erikson, E.H. (1956). The problem of ego identity. *The Journal of the American Psychoanalytic Association, 4,* 56–121.

Fenigstein, A., Scheier, M.F., & Buss, A.H. (1975). Public and private self-consciousness: Assessment and theory. *Journal of Consulting and Clinical Psychology, 43,* 522–527.

Frantz, R.P. (1985). *Self-actualization and social interest.* Unpublished B.A. Honors thesis, Wellesley College.

Gordon, C. (1968). Self-conceptions: Configurations of content. In C. Gordon & K. Gergen (Eds.), *The self in social interaction* (pp. 115–136). New York: Wiley.

Greenwald, A.G. (1988). A social-cognitive account of the self's development. In D.K. Lapsley & F.C. Power (Eds.), *Self, ego, and, identity* (pp. 30–42). New York: Springer-Verlag.

Grotevant, H.D., & Adams, G.R. (1984). Development of an objective measure to assess ego identity in adolescence: Validation and replication. *Journal of Youth and Adolescence, 13,* 419–438.

Hogan, R. & Cheek, J.M. (1983). Identity, authenticity, and maturity. In T.R. Sarbin & K.E. Scheibe (Eds.), *Studies in social identity* (pp. 339–357). New York: Praeger.

Hogan, R., Jones, W.H., & Cheek, J.M. (1985). Socioanalytic theory: An alternative to armadillo psychology. In B.R. Schlenker (Ed.), *The self and social life* (pp. 175–198). New York: McGraw-Hill.

Insel, S.A., Reese, C.S., & Alexander, B.B. (1968). Self-presentations in relation to internal and external referents. *Journal of Consulting and Clinical Psychology, 32,* 389–395.

Jackson, S.E. (1981). Measurement of commitment to role identities. *Journal of Personality and Social Psychology, 40,* 138–146.

James, W. (1890). *The principles of psychology* (Vol. 1). New York: Holt.

Johnson, J.A. (1987). Influence of adolescent social crowds on the development of vocational identity. *Journal of Vocational Behavior, 31,* 182–199.

Jung, C.G. (1957). *The undiscovered self.* New York: New American Library.

Leary, M.R., Wheeler, D.S., & Jenkins, T.B. (1986). Aspects of identity and behavioral preference: Studies of occupational and recreational choice. *Social Psychology Quarterly, 49,* 11–18.

Liebman, W.E., & Cheek, J.M. (1983, August). Shyness and body image. In J.M. Cheek (Chair), *Progress in research on shyness.* Symposium conducted at the meeting of the American Psychological Association, Anaheim, CA.

Maslow, A.H. (1961). Peak-experiences as acute identity-experiences. *American Journal of Psychoanalysis, 21,* 254–260.

McAdams, D.P. (1988). *Power, intimacy, and the life story: Personological inquiries into identity.* New York: Guilford.

Miller, D.R. (1963). The study of social relationships: Situation, identity, and social interaction. In S. Koch (Ed.), *Psychology: A study of a science* (Vol. 5). New York: McGraw-Hill.

Miller, M.L., & Thayer, J.F. (1988). On the nature of self-monitoring: Relationships with adjustment and identity. *Personality and Social Psychology Bulletin, 14,* 544–553.

Munroe, R.L., & Munroe, R.H. (1975). *Cross-cultural human development.* Monterey, CA: Brooks/Cole.

Penner, L.A., & Wymer, W.E. (1983). The moderator variable approach to behavioral predictability: Some of the variables some of the time. *Journal of Research in Personality, 17,* 339–353.

Rosenberg, S., & Gara, M.A. (1985). The multiplicity of personal identity. *Review of personality and social psychology, 6,* 87–114.

Sampson, E.E. (1978). Personality and the location of identity. *Journal of Personality, 46,* 552–568.

Sarbin, T.R., & Allen, V.L. (1968). Role theory. In G. Lindzey and E. Aronson (Eds.), *The handbook of social psychology.* Reading, MA: Addison-Wesley.

Schlenker, B.R. (1985). Identity and self-identification. In B.R. Schlenker (Ed.), *The self and social life* (pp. 65–99). New York: McGraw-Hill.

Seligman, M.E.P. (1988). Boomer blues. *Psychology Today, 22* (10), 50–55.

Singer, M. (1982). Personal and social identity in dialogue. In B. Lee (Ed.), *Psychosocial theories of the self* (pp. 129–177). New York: Plenum.

Snow, D.A., & Phillips, C.L. (1982). The changing self-orientations of college students: From institution to impulse. *Social Science Quarterly, 63,* 462–476.

Snyder, M., & Campbell, B.H. (1982). Self-monitoring: The self in action. In J. Suls (Ed.), *Psychological perspectives on the self* (Vol. 1, pp. 185–207). Hillsdale, NJ: Erlbaum.

Swann, W.B., Jr. (1987). Identity negotiation: Where two roads meet. *Journal of Personality and Social Psychology, 53,* 1038–1051.

Turner, R.H., & Gordon, S. (1981). The boundaries of the self: The relationship of authenticity in the self-conception. In M.D. Lynch, A.A. Norem-Hebeisen, & K.J. Gergen (Eds.), *Self-concept: Advances in theory and research* (pp. 39–57). Cambridge, MA: Ballinger.

Whitbourne, S.K. (1986). *The me I know: A study of adult identity.* New York: Springer.

Wicklund, R.A., & Gollwitzer, P.M. (1987). The fallacy of the private-public self-focus distinction. *Journal of Personality, 55,* 491–523.

Wylie, R.C. (1974). *The self-concept* (rev. ed., Vol. 1). Lincoln: University of Nebrasks Press.

Wylie, R.C. (1979). *The self-concept* (rev. ed., Vol. 2). Lincoln: University of Nebraska Press.

Wymer, W.E. & Penner, L.A. (1985). Moderator variables and different types of predictability: Do you have a match? *Journal of Personality and Social Psychology, 49,* 1002–1015.

CHAPTER 21

Using Traits to Construct Personality

Sarah E. Hampson

This chapter is about the way traits are used in personality descriptions. My research is concerned with what traits mean, both in isolation and in combination. It is grounded in a constructivist view of personality, which is an example of the broader social-constructivist movement in psychology (Gergen, 1985; Landman & Manis, 1983). According to this view, socially constructed concepts (e.g., "madness," "childhood," and "aging") are composed of attributes in the real world and the social significance attached to them. Personality may also be thought of as a social creation based on behaviors and the social meanings attached to them (Hampson, 1988).

When one thinks about the process of personality construction, it is useful to assign the participants in a social interaction the roles of *actor* and *observer* (Goffman, 1959). The actor possesses certain resources that may be broadly defined as social intelligence (Cantor & Kihlstrom, 1987), accumulated past experience, and inherited biological characteristics, and these resources interact with situational variables to produce behavior. This behavior is interpreted by the observer with the aid of the observer's comparable resources of social intelligence, past experience, and biological characteristics. In this way, the actor's behavior is made meaningful by the observer and can be used to construct the actor's personality, which is composed of both the actor's behaviors and the observer's constructions of those behaviors. Much of personality psychology is concerned with the resources of the actor that result in the actor's unique behavior patterns, whereas social cognition is the study of the observer's resources that result in the observer's unique constructions. Constructed personality focuses on the interface between the two.

There are many ways to study this interface. One approach, identity negotiation, emphasizes the dimension of self-awareness. According to this approach, actors strive to verify their self-views (Swann, 1987), whereas observers strive to validate their expectancies (Snyder, 1984). Identity negotiation focuses on the dynamic aspects of personality construction, emphasizing the way personality is molded by the forces of impression management. An alternative to this macroconstructionism is the kind of microanalysis I shall be describing. Instead of studying actual occurrences of personality construction, I have chosen to examine the basic tool used by all parties to the process: the language of personality description.

In particular, I study *traits,* which are shorthand terms for behaviors plus their ascribed social significance. Traits may be viewed as semantic categories (Rosch, Mervis, Gray, Johnson, & Boyes-Braem, 1976) applied to behaviors whose association with a given category is determined by family resemblance (Buss & Craik, 1983; Hampson, 1982). Uninterpreted behavior is ambiguous with respect to category membership. For example, the behavior of shaking hands could be "friendly," "ingratiating," "dutiful," or "precocious," depending on a host of attributes not specified by the behavior alone (e.g., the participants' relative social standing, their ages, or the situation). These more abstract attributes are supplied by the observer's social knowledge and motivations, and it is by combining the abstract attributes and the "raw" behavior that categorization with the appropriate trait concept is possible.

In the work to be described, trait meaning has been examined primarily from the observer's perspective. As interactions unfold, however, observers and actors change roles. The knowledge that the erstwhile observers applied to construct the actors' personalities is now applied in determining their own behavior. The same beliefs about the relations between behaviors and traits are used in both the message-sending and the message-receiving aspects of personality construction. Consequently, the more we understand about the way the observer constructs personality, the more we also learn about the determinants of the actor's personality-related behavior. In the following sections, I shall discuss two lines of research on trait meaning. The first looks at people's understandings of traits as single descriptors of personality, whereas the second looks at the meanings of combinations of traits.

The Meaning of Traits Used Singly

Trait meaning may be divided into two constituents—the descriptive and evaluative aspects of meaning (Peabody, 1967). The descriptive aspect refers to the content of the behaviors implied by the trait, whereas the evaluative aspect refers to the social desirability of those behaviors. For example, descriptively, "a creative person" is someone who thinks in novel ways, and, evaluatively, "a creative person" is socially desirable.

We have studied the descriptive content of trait categories by developing a measure of category breadth that indicates the diversity of behaviors to which the trait refers (Hampson, John, & Goldberg, 1986; Hampson, Goldberg, & John, 1987). Broad trait categories subsume a wider and more diverse range of behavioral instances than do narrow ones. For example, there are many different ways of being *extraverted* (broad), but only a limited range of similar behaviors may be categorized as *talkative* (narrow). We have developed separate U.S. and British normative category-breadth values for a sample of 573 commonly used personality terms by asking subjects to rate these words on the category-breadth dimension.

The British and U.S. category-breadth ratings correlated .75 (.89 when corrected for attenuation), indicating substantial agreement. There were, however, interesting cross-national differences on some of the terms. For example, the British ratings were substantially broader than the U.S. ratings for *natural, pleasant, merry, mannerly,* and *spirited,* whereas the U.S. ratings were substantially broader than the British ones for *dominant, cynical, ethical,* and *honest*. These findings could reflect cultural differences in the diversity of behaviors that are believed to be categorized by a particular trait. For example, there may be more culturally recognized ways of being *natural* in Britain than in the United States, but more culturally recognized ways of being *dominant* in the United States than in Britain.

Social-desirability ratings were collected from the British judges for the same set of 573 terms. These contemporary British social-desirability ratings correlated .96 with those obtained by Norman over twenty years ago, and .97 with Anderson's (1968) likableness ratings, suggesting that the evaluative aspect of trait meaning is virtually immune to the differences between these two countries.

We have also examined the relation between the descriptive and evaluative components of trait meaning. Category breadth and social desirability were modestly positively correlated in the British ratings ($r = .39$), replicating an earlier finding with U.S. judges (Hampson et al., 1986). That is, desirable terms are somewhat broader than undesirable ones. Apparently, the English language affords us finer distinctions (narrower terms) for undesirable than for desirable person characteristics, so that when describing a "bad" person, it is possible to be more precise than when describing a "good" person. The correlation is modest enough, however, to confirm that category breadth and social desirability are correctly viewed as distinct aspects of trait meaning.

Some traits varying in category breadth form hierarchical structures (Hampson et al., 1986) in which the same type of behavior can be described by any of the traits in the hierarchy. These traits are related by class inclusion such that all the behaviors categorized by the narrower trait are also included in the meaning of the broader term. For example, *extraverted* and *talkative* are hierarchically related: behaviors categorized as *talkative* may also be categorized as *extraverted*.

Given that traits at alternative levels are available, what determines the level chosen for personality descriptions? We have studied the preferred level of personality description by asking subjects to choose one trait from two- and three-tiered trait hierarchies when describing a variety of targets (John, Hampson, & Goldberg, 1989). So far, we have found a consistent tendency for subjects to prefer the broadest traits offered to them. It would appear that in this type of personality-description task, subjects are more interested in achieving broad bandwidth than they are in achieving high fidelity (Cronbach & Gleser, 1957).

Although the tendency to prefer broad traits was not modified by the familiarity of the targets being described, we have observed an interaction between target likability and the social desirability and category breadth of the trait. When subjects described targets they liked, they tended to use broad desirable traits and narrow undesirable traits. On the other hand, when they described disliked targets, they tended to use narrow desirable traits and broad undesirable traits. The task required subjects to select undesirable traits for liked targets and desirable traits for disliked targets, but subjects took advantage of the category-breadth differences to emphasize their evaluations.

Together, these studies of the meaning of traits used singly in personality descriptions suggest a considerable complexity underlying the apparent simplicity of the task. Selecting a trait to describe a person involves not only getting the descriptive aspect right, but also conveying the appropriate evaluation and paying attention to the possible interaction between these two components of meaning. The observer selects a trait based on the actor's behavior and its perceived social significance from the observer's point of view. In this way, the observer constructs an aspect of the actor's personality when making his or her trait choice. The preference for broad traits suggests that in the process of social construction the specifics of behavior, including inconsistencies, are lost in favor of a more general and coherent impression. The process of social construction may also lead to more polarized impressions on the desirability dimension, as our finding of an interaction between target likability, category breadth and desirability suggests. The construction process may, at least for the time being, end with the observer's construction (e.g., when making a trait ascription in a letter of recommendation). Alternatively, the trait label may be renegotiated by the actor and observer during a subsequent interaction (e.g., Snyder & Swann, 1978).

In the next section, I shall describe some work on the meaning of traits used in pairs. Personality impressions can be conveyed by combinations of traits as well as one or more single-trait descriptors. Therefore, an understanding of the language of personality description as the medium of personality construction would be incomplete without an examination of trait combinations.

The Meaning of Traits Used in Combination

In everyday life, we are able to maintain coherent impressions of others despite inconsistencies in their behavior. Personality construction takes place at the trait level, so one way of investigating how personality is constructed from inconsistent behaviors is to examine how impressions are formed from conflicting traits. Although this approach does not mimic the reality of being confronted by inconsistent *behaviors,* it does substitute for the everyday situation of receiving conflicting trait descriptions of the same person from different sources. A number of studies have demonstrated that, when asked nicely, subjects are able to reconcile almost any conflicting trait information (Asch & Zukier, 1984; Cohen, 1973; Gergen, Hepburn, & Comer Fisher, 1986), but no study has examined the factors affecting the relative ease or difficulty with which it is done. Perhaps by understanding how the lay person (the observer) constructs a coherent personality for the target (actor) from seemingly contradictory traits, we may gain some valuable insights into the nature of so-called personality inconsistency.

Working with Patricia Casselden, I have begun to investigate the meaning of congruent and incongruent trait combinations. We defined congruence in terms of Peabody's (1967) two aspects of trait meaning. In our first study, congruent trait pairs were those in which the constituent traits were both descriptively and evaluatively consistent (i.e., they both described the same domain of personality, in either a socially desirable or undesirable way). Incongruent trait pairs were those in which the constituent traits were taken from the same domain of personality but were descriptively and evaluatively inconsistent. For example, *dependable* and *organized* formed a congruent pair, whereas *kind* and *cold* formed an incongruent pair. Subjects were presented with a series of targets described with congruent or incongruent trait combinations and they were asked to rate how difficult it was to imagine these targets. Other subjects were asked to rate the same trait pairs for semantic similarity. We found that imaginability was affected substantially by congruence: although subjects could imagine the targets described with incongruent trait pairs, they found this more difficult than imagining the congruent targets. Congruent pairs were also rated as semantically more similar than incongruent pairs, and imaginability and semantic similarity correlated highly ($r = .91$).

These findings may be explained by the view of traits as semantic categories for behaviors. Congruent pairs (e.g., *dependable* and *organized*) invoke consistent acts that need no effort to reconcile, whereas incongruent pairs (e.g., *kind* and *cold*) invoke inconsistent acts that require explanation. In terms of Borkenau's (1986; Borkenau & Ostendorf, 1987) act-overlap account of trait categories, congruent pairs are characterized by act overlap whereas incongruent pairs are characterized by act contradiction.

In a second study, we separated the descriptive and evaluative components of trait meaning. Descriptively, the pairs were taken either from the same domain of personality description (as in the first study) or from different domains. Evaluatively, the pairs were either consistent or inconsistent. There were four kinds of trait pairs: consistent, same domain (e.g., *unsociable* and *unfriendly*); consistent, different domain (e.g., *tolerant* and *inventive*); inconsistent, same domain (e.g., *scornful* and *tactful*); and inconsistent, different domain (e.g., *reliable* and *nagging*). As predicted, we found that domain interacted with evaluation to affect imaginability. Consistent, same domain targets were more easily imagined than consistent, different domain targets, because the former benefited from act overlap, whereas the latter were handicapped by act independence. In contrast, inconsistent, same domain targets were even more difficult to imagine than inconsistent, different domain targets, because the former were seriously disadvantaged by act contradiction, whereas the latter were rendered only somewhat incongruous by act independence. The same pattern of results was obtained with the frequency of perceived cooccurrence and the semantic similarity ratings, and all three kinds of ratings were highly intercorrelated (imaginability and frequency, $r = .94$; imaginability and semantic similarity, $r = .84$; semantic similarity and frequency, $r = .84$).

Together, these studies indicate how the descriptive and evaluative aspects of trait meaning affect the ease with which two traits can be reconciled to form a coherent impression. The findings fit a semantic-category account of traits in which it is easiest to imagine targets described by trait pairs from the same domain that share many overlapping acts, whereas it is most difficult to imagine targets described by trait pairs from the same domain that invoke contradictory acts. Where the acts are independent because the traits are drawn from different domains, then evaluatively inconsistent pairs are only somewhat less imaginable than evaluatively consistent pairs.

In order to examine the ecological validity of these studies, we asked the subjects in our first investigation to describe a recent incident in which they had to resolve the discordant characteristics of another person. Forty-seven of the fifty subjects did so with ease. Typically, subjects wrote about incidents in which their broad, positive, default view of a person was challenged by a salient item of specific and negative information. Of the 115 different traits generated, category-breadth values were available for eighty-one, and indicated that the traits used in the first part of the account were broader than those in the second. The conflicting evidence in the second part typically involved an interaction with the target in a different situation, which questions Mischel and Peake's (1982) speculation that people are unaware of cross-situational inconsistency. These accounts of actual incidents of trait reconciliation indicate that incongruent traits are a familiar hazard in the everyday construction of personality.

Future Directions

This chapter has described two lines of research into the meaning of traits as they are used singly and in combination to describe personality. Our studies of single traits have investigated both a descriptive aspect and an evaluative aspect of trait meaning, and our studies of trait combinations have led us to explore the effects of descriptive and evaluative incongruence on impressions. This work could now be extended to more realistic personality descriptions involving several traits, personality-descriptive nouns, and nouns qualified by adjectives, thus incorporating varying degrees of consistency and inconsistency among these elements.

Cohen (1973) made the interesting observation that as the inconsistency between given personality information increases, so does the intersubject disagreement about the resulting impression. The disambiguation of personality information should be a task capable of revealing a subject's personality construction processes. By examining how people make sense of conflicting information, we may gain insights into how they do this more routinely for consistent information. As well as studying how people comprehend complex trait descriptions, the constructivist approach calls for the study of how people (observers) ascribe a combination of more or less congruent traits to an actor. Both the comprehension and the creation of personality descriptions are constructive processes, and both are conducted with the tool of personality construction: the language of personality description.

Acknowledgments The preparation of this chapter was supported by Grant MH-39077 from the National Institute of Mental Health, U.S. Public Health Service. I would like to thank Patricia A. Casselden, Lewis R. Goldberg, and Tina Rosolack for their comments on an earlier draft.

References

Anderson, N.H. (1968). Likeableness ratings of 555 personality-trait words. *Journal of Personality and Social Psychology, 9*, 272–279.

Asch, S.E., & Zukier, H. (1984). Thinking about persons. *Journal of Personality and Social Psychology, 46*, 1230–1240.

Borkenau, P. (1986). Toward an understanding of trait interrelations: Acts as instances for several traits. *Journal of Personality and Social Psychology, 51*, 371–381.

Borkenau, P., & Ostendorf, F. (1987). Retrospective estimates of act frequencies: How accurately do they reflect reality? *Journal of Personality and Social Psychology, 52,* 626–638.

Buss, D.M., & Craik, K.H. (1983). The act of frequency approach to personality. *Psychological Review, 90,* 105–26.

Cantor, N., & Kihlstrom, J.K. (1987). *Personality and social intelligence.* Englewood Cliffs, NJ: Prentice-Hall.

Cohen, R. (1973). *Patterns of personality judgment.* New York: Academic Press.

Cornbach, L.J., & Gleser, G.C. (1957). *Psychological tests and personnel decisions.* Urbana, IL: University of Illinois.

Gergen, K.J. (1985). The social constructionist movement in modern psychology. *American Psychologist, 40,* 266–275.

Gergen, K.L., Hepburn, A., & Comer Fisher, D. (1986). Hermeneutics of personality description. *Journal of Personality and Social Psychology, 50,* 1261–1270.

Goffman, E. (1959). *The Presentation of Self in Everyday Life.* New York: Doubleday.

Hampson, S.E. (1982). Person memory: A semantic category model of personality traits. *British Journal of Psychology, 73,* 1–11.

Hampson, S.E. (1988). *The Construction of Personality: An Introduction* (2nd ed.). London: Routledge & Kegan Paul.

Hampson, S.E., Goldberg, L.R., & John, O.P. (1987). Category breadth and social desirability values for 573 personality terms. *European Journal of Personality Psychology, 1,* 241–258.

Hampson, S.E., John, O.P., & Goldberg, L.R. (1986). Category breadth and hierarchical structure in personality: Studies of asymmetries in judgments of trait implications. *Journal of Personality and Social Psychology, 51,* 37–54.

John, O.P., Hampson, S.E., & Goldberg, L.R. (1989). Is there a basic level of personality description? Unpublished manuscript, Oregon Research Institute.

Landman, J., & Manis, M. (1983). Social cognition: Some historical and theoretical perspectives. In L. Berkowitz (Ed.) *Advances in Experimental Social Psychology* (Vol. 16, pp. 49–123). New York: Academic Press.

Mischel, W., & Peake, P.K. (1982). Beyond deja vu in the search for cross-situational consistency. *Psychological Review, 89,* 730–755.

Peabody, D., (1967). Trait inferences: Evaluative and descriptive aspects. *Journal of Personality and Social Psychology Monograph, 7* (4, Whole No. 644).

Rosch, E., Mervis, C.B., Gray, W.D., Johnson, D., & Boyes-Braem, P. (1976). Basic objects in natural categories. *Cognitive Psychology, 8,* 382–439.

Snyder, M., & Swann, W.B., Jr. (1978). Hypothesis-testing processes in social interaction. *Journal of Personality and Social Psychology, 36,* 1202–1212.

Snyder, M. (1984). When beliefs create reality. In L. Berkowitz (Ed.), *Advances in Experimental Social Psychology* (Vol. 18, pp. 247–305). New York: Academic Press.

Swann, W.B. (1987). Identity negotiation: Where two roads meet. *Journal of Personality and Social Psychology, 53,* 1038–1051.

CHAPTER 22

Personality Theory and Behavioral Genetics: Contributions and Issues

David C. Rowe

Introduction

Personality psychologists can work in comfortable ignorance of behavioral genetics; without knowledge of this field, they can devise trait measures, validate them and show their practical utility, and the more ambitious can develop general theories of personality that identify fundamental traits. What then is the usefulness of behavioral genetic methods and results for the personality psychologist? I find not one answer to this question, but several. In the first place, behavioral genetics is useful because it provides a comprehensive theory of personality traits. The theory of genetics can explain facts about the maintenance of traits, their interrelatedness, and their survival in a population. In addition, behavioral genetics offers methods for the investigation of some persisting problems in personality theory.

The field of behavioral genetics has made advances in knowledge (Hay, 1985; Plomin, 1986). In the first section, this chapter briefly describes the behavioral genetic approach and answers the question, "what do we know about personality?" The chapter next presents three issues that can be investigated by a behavioral genetic approach: (1) what is the structure of personality?; (2) what maintains personality constancy as people grow older?; (3) what are some of the "heterotypic" continuities in personality? The purpose of this chapter is to entice personality theorists to take advantage of methods and concepts in the behavioral genetic tradition and to turn them to advantage in their own research.

Behavioral Genetic Methods

The concept of personality presupposes variation within a population: not all people are alike. One goal of our research is to understand the "ultimate" origin of this variation: that is, whether personality differences arise because of differences in *genotypes* (i.e., genetic make-up);

differences in family environments; or differences in unique experiences. The source of genetic variation is well-understood. Some genes occur in multiple forms, with each type of gene having slightly different effects. The simplest case is a two-gene system, where three genotypes are possible depending on which combination of two genes was inherited. These "genotypes"—AA, Aa, and aa—give rise to either two (when A is dominant) or three traits. Variation in behavioral traits, however, usually results from "polygenic" variation—the action of many genes, each one of which has a small effect. In a population, polygenic variation reflects the existence of "normal" genetic alternatives, rather than the existence of any particular "defective" genetic material.

The *heritability* coefficient is a number that serves to estimate the degree of "polygenic" influence on a trait. It equals the ratio of V_g/V_p, where V_g is genetic variation produced by the inheritance of different gene combinations and V_p is phenotypic (i.e., observed trait) variation. The heritability coefficient refers to the effects of genetic variation within a particular population at a particular time. For example, the heritability of height would be greater in a population in which everyone received adequate calories than in one in which some people received excellent nutrition and others were malnourished. As with any statistic, its value will vary from one personality trait to another depending on ordinary sampling variation in a particular study as well as on differences in the true degree of genetic determination among traits.

Although these limitations are often noted by critics of behavioral genetic research, they can apply with equal force to any statistic serving to estimate environmental effects. More assurance of generality will come as we begin to understand the particular mechanisms by which genes affect behavior. The same logic applies to environmental effects. We want to go beyond statistical effect sizes to an understanding of the mechanisms producing these effects (an important goal, but one that may exceed current knowledge).

In addition to estimating heritability, behavioral geneticists distinguish, in their research designs, two types of environmental effects. The shared or "common" component of environmental variation refers to all environmental influences that operate to make family members alike. Specific influences that stay constant from one family member to another contribute to this component; for example, except when siblings are disparate in age, familial social class is probably a "shared" influence. Analogously with the heritability coefficient, one can compute a coefficient of shared environmental effect, V_s/V_p, where V_s is the shared environmental component of variation. By contrast, the "nonshared" (or specific) environment component refers to influences that operate with unique effects for each individual. Unless some statistical correction is done, this component also contains measurement error. A self-evident example of a nonshared type of influence is birth order. Because birth order varies among siblings, any influence with an association to birth order will operate to make them unalike.

Quasi-experimental research designs can be employed to separate genetic and environmental effects. These designs take data from *pairs* of relatives of two or more family types and use, as the unit of analysis, the phenotypic similarities of these pairs (e.g., brothers should resemble one another more than uncle-nephews). Twin and adoption studies are most frequently employed for separating environment and hereditary effects. The *twin* study method involves the comparison of one-egg (MZ; monozygotic) twins with two egg (DZ; dizygotic) twins. As the former possess twice the genetic similarity of the latter, they should show about double the behavioral resemblance for a given genetically determined trait. Equality of age also may equate twins for many of the environmental influences on which nontwins differ. Environmental effects that are approximately equal for the two kinds of twins will cancel one another in the comparison process.

If the environments of MZ twins were more alike than those of DZ twins, however, then the twin method assumption of "equal" twin environments has been violated. Critics often challenge twin study results on these grounds. This assumption need be true only for environments *relevant* to a particular trait, however, not for all environments. Recent tests have supported this assumption for personality traits (Plomin, Willerman, & Loehlin, 1976; Loehlin & Nichols, 1976; Scarr & Carter-Saltzman, 1979). For instance, Loehlin and Nichols found that greater treatment similarity of some MZ twin pairs failed to make them more alike than other MZ twin pairs given less similar treatments. Thus, although MZ twins were treated more alike than DZ twins in some respects (for example, in sleeping arrangements), these particular treatments failed to be influential on the kind of traits assessed by Loehlin and Nichols.

The adoption study method is a natural analogue of a true experimental design, because adoptive placement can separate genetic and environmental influences. In the case of genetically influenced traits, adoptive children should resemble their biological parents, with whom they share only heredity. (Note that adoptive child and adoptive parent will share some genetic similarities by chance—but none that will contribute to a genetic correlation over many adoptive parent/child pairs.) For enviromentally influenced traits, adoptive children should resemble their adoptive parents, who provide the environmental context. For the purpose of research, adoptive placements should be nearly random with respect to the characteristics of biological parents. Because some adoption agencies attempt to match biological parent to adoptive parent for particular characteristics (e.g., income), this assumption may be violated in a particular study. Punitive effects of selective placement can be controlled statistically, however (Carey, 1986); for personality traits other than I.Q., selective placement is usually not a problem.

More and more, behavioral genetic studies have moved beyond the basic twin or adoption design. In current studies, statistical models are formed using structural equations that express the phenotypic correlations (or related statistics) for pairs of relatives in terms of general genetic and environmental parameters (Eaves, Last, Young, & Martin, 1978; Rao, Morton, & Yee, 1974). These equations then provide a means for combining, into a single study, any set of familial relationships; for example, a study can combine twins and adoptees.

Another new approach uses family pedigrees (Morton & MacLean, 1974). A typical study involves a small number of fairly extensive pedigrees (e.g., including several children, parents, an uncle, and a grandparent). The pedigrees may differ in structure (e.g., one with grandparents, another without). Using maximum likelihood methods, the observed trait value for each person in each pedigree is checked for degree of fit to a value predicted from genetic/environmental models making different assumptions. Although the pedigree approach is not ideal for separating family environmental from genetic variation, it offers a method of detecting single-gene influence, even against a background of polygenic and environmental variation.

Other advances include linkage analysis using biological markers made available by the new molecular genetic technologies, sibling effects analysis, and multivariate methods. The personality researcher should learn about these new methods as well as about the simpler but reliable twin and adoption approaches.

What We Know

Behavioral genetic studies have led to a counter-intuitive discovery: the absence of *shared* environmental influences. Rowe (1987) identified three lines of evidence leading to this conclusion. First, adoptive children raised in the same family are hardly more alike in personality than children raised in different families. Although this conclusion holds most strongly for nonintellectual traits, it also held for I.Q. in two replications using adolescent or older adoptees (Plomin, 1986). Secondly, in general, structural-equation models can be fitted to statistics from pairs of relatives without assuming shared environmental influence. Thirdly, family "environment" measures are themselves embedded with genetic variation.

Does this mean that behavioral genetic methods are flawed? Probably not, because the socializing or learning influence of the shared environment can be detected. One example (to please many a parent) is the apparent value of music lessons. Dividing a twin sample into groups with and without music lessons, Coon and Carey (1989) found that when twins received music lessons (always, both twins went), MZ twins were not more alike than DZ twins in musical performance abilities. In the untutored sample, however, MZ twin resemblance in musical performance exceeded that of DZ twins. The simplest interpretation is that, for twins provided with lessons, the length and quality of the lessons determined their level of musical performance. The spontaneous desire of untutored twins to pursue musical interests may have been genetically influenced.

If "shared" environmental influences do not (in general) affect personality, then what environmental influences do? In terms of their theoretical mode of operation, these influences must be of the *nonshared* variety. That is, they are influences that operate uniquely on each individual. Because the MZ twin correlations for a personality-trait measure are usually less than its reliability, some nonshared influences must make an indelible mark on personality. Rowe and Plomin (1981) identified different categories of nonshared influences: perinatal traumas, (nonmutual) sibling interaction effects, differential parental treatments, and extrafamilial influences (peer groups, teachers, TV). From a process viewpoint, these environmental factors must be ones that operate with respect to each child's unique learning history and temperament. That is, do not expect family environmental influences to be doled out in the "unit" of the family. Rather, these effects will be specific to each child and may often represent gene × environment interactions, where the exposure of one child to an influence will have little or no effect; the same exposure may, however, have a large effect on another child, depending on differences in his or her (geneticallybased) temperament and personality traits. A further discussion of the issues surrounding shared versus nonshared influences can be found in Plomin and Daniels (1987).

The other main finding from behavioral genetic studies is that most personality traits are heritable (Loehlin, Willerman, & Horn, 1988). In general, I.Q. appears to be somewhat more heritable than nonintellectual personality traits (I.Q., 50-70%; nonintellectual traits, 40-50%). For nonintellectual traits, estimates of heritability tend to be lower (20-40%) for nontwins than for twins, possibly a result of genetic "non-additivity." That is, inheritance of personality may depend more on the interactions of genes at different chromosomal positions than does I.Q. Clearly, much remains to be learned, but behavioral genetic studies have laid a foundation for understanding the origin of personality differences. In the next section, we consider three future directions for applying behavioral genetics to issues of interest to the personality researcher.

Personality Structure

Personality researchers have sought a periodic table for personality: a list of the most elemental traits. At least in the domain of factor-analyzed personality ratings, a consensus has emerged that five traits adequately cover all aspects of personality. They are agreeableness, conscientiousness, neuroticism, extraversion, and openness to experience (McCrae & Costa, 1987). Eysenck's (1981) "big-three"——extraversion, neuroticism, and psychoticism——offer a reduction of lower-level traits in the domain of factor-analyzed self-reports. Nevertheless, less certainty exists over these lists than over the periodic table's ordering of chemical compounds. Indeed, factor-analysis itself is viewed, by critical scientists, as being no better than an alchemy that serves up the organization of what is entered into analysis, but does not reveal anything about nature's own categories. The ways of describing personality seem as variable as personality psychologists themselves, and new trait categories are invented with some regularity (e.g., self-monitoring, Snyder, 1979).

It would be wrong to expect a behavioral genetic approach, more than than any other method, to identify the most fundamental entities of personality. If however, the goal is to seek a set of personality traits that may map onto neurophysiology, then the behavioral genetic criterion of genetic inheritance is certainly a good one. Buss and Plomin (1975) pioneered this idea by offering heritability as a defining criterion of temperament traits. According to their literature review, four traits satisfied these criteria: sociability, activity, emotionality, and impulsivity. In a later revision, impulsivity was dropped on the grounds of insufficient evidence for its heritability and early appearance in childhood (Buss & Plomin, 1984).

If any problem exists in using the criterion of heritability, it is that most personality traits show some heritability (Buss, 1983, p. 55). The problem is especially acute because traits that, on the surface, should reflect purely environmental family transmission may, instead, be about as genetically influenced as other traits. For instance, twin data suggest that social attitudes may obey a simple pattern of genetic inheritance (Martin, Eaves, Heath, Jardine, Feingold, & Eysenck, 1986). A universal finding of heritability would fail to identify more or less "fundamental" traits. Different degrees of optimism concerning the demonstration of differential trait heritability exists among behavioral geneticists (Loehlin, 1978; 1982).

Until recently, the search for the "genetic core" of personality focused on each trait independently. Multivariate methods, however, permit the parceling of covariation among traits to environmental and genetic components. For example, Figure 22.1 illustrates how the correlation of traits X and Y can be apportioned to a genetic pathway ($h_x h_y r_g$) and a nonshared environmental pathway ($e_x e_y r_e$), where h and e are regression coefficients for genetic and environmental effects respectively; r_g represents the traits' genetic correlation; and r_e represents the traits' environmental correlation.

How can we estimate the values of these pathways? In the twin design, one can form a correlation matrix of twin correlations. The matrix includes the correlation of the same trait across both twins and also

$$r_{xy} = h_x h_y r_g + e_x e_y r_e$$

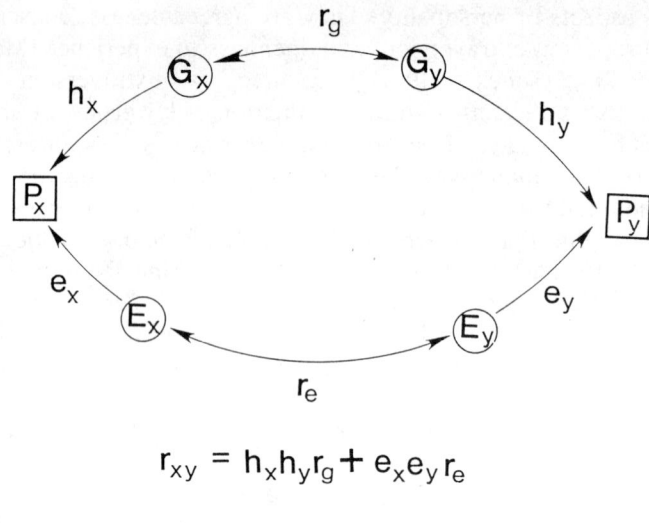

FIGURE 22.1

different traits. For example, height in one MZ twin can be correlated with weight in the other. Suppose this MZ twin correlation equals .70, and suppose further that the same twin "cross-trait" correlation equals .35 for DZ twins. An estimate of genetic influence on the *correlation* of height and weight is twice the difference of these two correlations (.70 − .35 = .35*2 = .70). This indicates that the association of height and weight is highly heritable. Naturally, they share a common cause in genetically determined body size. This genetic pathway can be compared to the "in" individuals correlation of height and weight. If they correlate .75 within persons, then only .05 of this ordinary correlation is due to nongenetic influences.

More formally, the diagonal of the "twin" correlation matrix consists of the twin intraclass correlations for a particular trait. The off-diagonal elements are the correlation of trait A in one twin with trait B in the other. If such matrices are computed for MZ and DZ twins respectively, then twice the difference of the two matrices represents the "genetic" part of trait interrelationships (i.e., $G = 2(M_{MZ} - M_{DZ})$). More specifically, the diagonal elements of this matrix consist of heritabilities; the off-diagonal elements consist of each pair of traits' genetic correlation times the square roots of their respective heritabilities. The interpretation of these elements is illustrated by "genetic effects" in Figure 22.2. Subtracting the MZ twin matrix from the corresponding matrix of correlations *within* individuals yields a matrix of purely environmental intertrait associations (see Figure 22.2). That is, any source of covariation *not* shared by MZ twins must be the result of an environmental influence that acted on each

Matrices:

Within Person

$$\begin{array}{c} X \\ Y \end{array} \begin{bmatrix} e_x^2 + h_x^2 & \\ r_{xy} & e_y^2 + h_y^2 \end{bmatrix}$$

Genetic Effects

$$\begin{array}{c} X \\ Y \end{array} \begin{bmatrix} h_x^2 & \\ h_x h_y r_g & h_y^2 \end{bmatrix}$$

Environmental Effects

$$\begin{array}{c} X \\ Y \end{array} \begin{bmatrix} e_x^2 & \\ e_x e_y r_e & e_y^2 \end{bmatrix}$$

FIGURE 22.2

person independently. For example, perinatal injuries may induce a correlation of vocabulary and spatial I.Q.s, but such injuries may be random with respect to which twin in a pair is affected.

The tools of the factor analyst can be applied to matrices of statistical environmental and genetic relationships. Hence, more fundamental units of personality may emerge from analyzing the structure of such matrices than from analyzing the structure of the typical "in individuals" matrix. The factor-structure of the "genetic" matrix may reveal which traits are influenced by a common set of genes and, therefore, share common physiological pathways. Carey (1988) cautions, however, that the analysis of genetic correlations is support for pleiotropy (i.e., one set of genes influencing several traits), but that such statistical evidence is not fully conclusive unless verified by identifying the participating genes (a feat beyond current technology). Factor analysis of the "environmental" matrix can reveal traits correlated for sharing environmental determinants.

This type of multivariate approach may reveal which categories of personality are most biologically fundamental. Martin, Jardine, and Eaves (1984) applied multivariate analysis to the subtests of the National Merit Qualifying Test. Their analysis suggested that one genetic factor loads on all subtests, but that genetic factors other than this first component contribute to mathematics and to three verbally demanding tests (vocabulary, social studies, and English). Nonshared environmental influences made small contributions to ability covariation. A multivariate analysis of speed of information-processing tests and general I.Q. revealed a genetic correlation between them (Ho, Baker, & Decker, 1988); both of these examples came from the abilities domain. Few studies have applied the multivariate approach to the analysis of nonintellectual traits. Moreover, if the earlier results on the absence of shared environmental influences prove correct, as I believe they will, then the use of rare twin pairs may be unnecessary. The same kind of analysis can be accomplished by intercorrelating traits across nontwin siblings, where the object of factor analysis is the matrix of intercorrelations of trait A measured on sibling 1 with trait B measured on sibling 2. This approach may yield new insights into personality structures originating in genetic influences——as, perhaps, the Big-Five factors of rating data do——and personality psychologists should consider whether it may be used to answer their own research questions.

What Maintains Personality Constancy

Since the initiation of longitudinal studies extending into adulthood, impressive evidence has been obtained for the constancy of personality during long periods of the life span. Even after individuals have left home, graduated from college, established a family, and practiced a profession, their personalities remain strikingly similar to their young adult traits. Over the span of thirty years, correlations on the order of .3–.4 are evidence of personality stability in the face of the many unpredictable environmental events separating youth from adulthood. How can we explain personality stability? Longitudinal twin or adoption studies permit an exploration of the processes underlying personality constancy. Eaves and his colleagues, in a creative series of papers, advanced a structural-equation approach to distinguishing two hypotheses about development (Eaves, Long, & Heath, 1986; Hewitt, Eaves, Neale, & Meyer, 1988). One hypothesis is that development occurs by a process of transmission, whereby influences on development entering at one age affects later ages. Another hypothesis is that it occurs by nontransmitted common influences in the organism, or in the environment, that act in the same way throughout development (i.e., they always exist). In this chapter, only a brief exposition of these ideas is possible.

To illustrate a "transmission" process, suppose children were put in either good- or poor-quality classrooms. At each age, their classroom assignment either helps or hurts their vocabulary acquisition. Their knowledge of vocabulary at one age is transmitted to the next (but not perfectly, because forgetting occurs along with learning). Over time, the test-retest correlation for vocabulary tends to increase, thus reflecting the greater variance in vocabulary because of the increasing difference between advantaged and disadvantaged children.

22. Personality and Behavior Genetics

To illustrate a common influence, suppose genotypes determine how easily individuals are angered. Short-tempered and placid individuals will react in basically the same way at different ages. Temporary events may affect anger, but these effects are not lasting ones that would permanently change the rank order of individuals on the dimension of temper. In this example, "genotype" is a common influence at all ages.

More complex models of development can be constructed. A genetic model of vocabulary might include both genetic influences on rapidity of acquisition, which are common to all ages, and genetic influences, which are transmitted from one age to the next. The latter could reflect a genetically influenced organization and retention of vocabulary. New genetic influence could enter at different ages, however, as developmentally timed genes are activated and inactivated in their expression.

Eaves' developmental model raises a challenging issue for psychology: do environments have lasting effects? If environments do have lasting effects, then twins who are exposed to different environments over time should gradually become unlike. Thus, the average MZ twin correlation for twins aged twenty years should be greater than that for twins aged fifty years, because each twin should have been exposed to many unique experiences during adulthood. If the effects of these experiences are lasting, then the twins will gradually take a "random walk," becoming less and less similar.

In fact, however, the few data available do not suggest such a process. In a study of the California Psychological Inventory, the average MZ twin correlations for older (in the fifties) and younger (in the teens and early twenties) were quite similar in magnitude (Horn, Plomin, & Rosenman, 1976). Moreover, the *heritability* of old versus young twins' IQ scores was quite similar (i.e., the MZ-DZ difference did not change with age). This kind of result supports a developmental model in which genetic effects are constant at all ages, but environmental effects are relatively temporary. That is, new environmental effects entering at each age may be developmentally transmitted, so that adjacent ages share more resemblance than distant ages. This model does not, however, permit environmental transmission to be combined with a *constant* environmental influence. Such a constant environment can represent permanent effects of "learning." If such effects were operating, the twin correlations would decline over time. On the other hand, a constant heritability supports *constant* genetic influences. Heredity may be active in the same way at each age. Test-retest correlations will fall with age as new environmental (and possibly genetic) influences enter, but the test-retest correlation would not fall much below the MZ twin correlation.

The complexities of the foregoing "thought experiment" may baffle some readers. Developmental genetic models are new; the actual data are few; their true evaluation requires a quantitative, rather than verbal, statement of hypotheses. Nonetheless, it should be clear that the marked similarities of adult twins——whether raised together or apart——is a true develomental puzzle (Pedersen, Plomin, McClearn, & Friberg, 1988; Plomin, Pedersen, McClearn, Nesselroade, & Bergeman, 1988).

The implication that the effects of socialization or learning may be impermanent is a foreign notion to psychological theories that emphasize the lasting importance of one type of early experience (for instance, "unconditional" parental love). Yet, in *Early Experience: Myth and Evidence,* fascinating case histories have documented the ability of humans to overcome early emotional deprivations (Clarke & Clarke, 1976). One wonders why early experiences should be permanent. The more individuals rely on early learning to shape later behavior, the less their behavior is adaptive to new environmental circumstances. Indeed, implicit in social-learning theory is the idea that behavior is adaptive to current conditions of expected reward and punishment (although there is also an inertia because some self-concepts change slowly). We may want to choose, as a concept of personality, being atuned to different kinds of nonshared environmental influences that change as individuals enter into new life circumstances. Behavioral geneticists, with their sometimes major focus on quantitative models and results, may have neglected the broader meaning of their findings—hence, a need exists for personality psychologists to join in this endeavor.

Heterotypic Continuities

In the study of development, a difficult problem is that behaviors representing a latent trait at one age may differ from those representing the same latent trait at an earlier age. Aggression in a four year-old is not displayed in the same way as that in a teenager or adult. Ill-tempered children experience, as adults, greater marital instability, erratic work lives, and lower occupational attainment (Caspi, Bem, & Elder, 1988). To discover these consequences of ill-temperedness, one would need ordinarily to conduct a longitudinal study spanning several decades.

Similarly, the measurement of I.Q. before the age of one or two years is difficult. In longitudinal studies, early infant tests correlate weakly with later I.Q., although a new measure of habituation to novelty is proving to be more predictive (Fagan, 1985). Again, to evaluate a new measure of infant I.Q., a longitudinal study is required.

If, however, the latent trait is believed to be genetically transmissible, then a short-cut method using the family-study method to screen for heterotypic continuities is possible. Mid-parent scores for various behaviors can be correlated against the child's behaviors. If adult and child behaviors tap into the same latent trait, then they will show intergenerational continuity. In this way, adult behavioral correlates that differ in content from child behaviors may be discovered. Longitudinal studies could be used to confirm that these behaviors were the adult manifestations of the same latent trait.

Furthermore, heterotypic continuities may be discovered using familial correlations across opposite-sex individuals. Females, for example, tend to display less overt physical aggression than males. This apparent sex difference, however, does not preclude the latent trait of aggression as having some other manifestation in females, yet to be discovered. The rich network of possible correlations across *brother-sister* pairs has been barely explored——a problem aggravated by the failure to include opposite-sex twins in most twin studies. Clearly, scientists interested in the sex-moderated expression of personality can gain by taking advantage of such behavioral genetic methods.

Conclusions

I ask that personality psychologists consider using the family-study method, and other behavioral genetic methods, in their own research on personality structure and development. Adding siblings to studies of personality is not a very expensive undertaking——even college sophomores, psychology's perennial subject, often have accessible brothers and sisters. Personality psychologists should attempt to place the challenging results of this field into a broader theoretical context. What does the lack of *shared* environmental influences mean for simple "exposure" concepts of family influence, which are often resorted to in sociology and psychology. If there is no "developmental memory" for early childhood experiences, is their meaning then only one of promoting either proximal distress or happiness? Why do children in the same family develop so differently? In closing, I hope that once personality researchers have had a first taste of these behavioral genetic methods, they will decide that the appetizer was good and will ask for the main course.

References

Buss, A.H., & Plomin, R. (1975). *A temperament theory of personality development*. New York: Wiley.

Buss, A.H., & Plomin, R. (1984). *Temperament: Early, developing personality traits*. Hillsdale, NJ: Erlbaum.

Buss, D.M. (1983). Evolutionary biology and personality psychology: Implications of genetic variability. *Personality and Individual Differences, 4,* 51–63.

Carey, G. (1986). A general multivariate approach to linear modeling in human genetics. *American Journal of Human Genetics, 39,* 775–786.

Carey, G. (1988). Inference about genetic correlation. *Behavior Genetics, 18,* 329–338.

Caspi, A., Bem, D.J., & Elder, G.H. (in press). Continuities and consequences of interaction styles across the life course. *Journal of Personality*.

Clarke, A.M., & Clarke, A.D.B. (1976). *Early experience: Myth and evidence*. New York: Free Press.

Coon, H., & Carey, G. (1989) *Genetic and environmental determinants of musical ability in twins, 19,* 183–193.

Eaves, L.J., Last, K.A., Young, P.A., & Martin, N.G. (1978). Model-fitting approaches to the analysis of human behavior. *Heredity, 41,* 249–320.

Eaves, L.J., Long, J., & Heath, A.C. (1986). A theory of develpmental change in quantitative phenotypes applied to cognitive development. *Behavior Genetics, 16,* 143–162.

Eysenck, H.J. (1981). *A model for personality.* Berlin: Springer.

Fagan, J.F., III. (1985). A new look at infant intelligence. In D. Detterman (Ed.), *Current topics in human intelligence: Research methodology* (pp. 223–246). Norwood, NJ: Ablex.

Hay, D.A. (1985). *Essentials of behavior genetics.* Oxford: Blackwell.

Hewitt, J.K., Eaves, L.J., Neale, M.C., & Meyer, J.M. (1988). Resolving the causes of developmental continuity or "tracking:" I. Longitudinal twin studies during growth. *Behavior Genetics, 18,* 133–151.

Ho, H., Baker, L., & Decker, S.N. (1988). Covariation between intelligence and speed of cognitive processing: Genetic and environmental influences. *Behavior Genetics, 18,* 247–261.

Horn, J.M., Plomin, R., & Roseman, R. (1976). Heritability of personality in adult male twin pairs. *Behavior Genetics, 6,* 17–30.

Loehlin, J.C. (1978). Are CPI scales differentially heritable: How good is the evidence? *Behavior Genetics, 8,* 381–382.

Loehlin, J.C. (1982). Are personality traits differentially heritable? *Behavior Genetics, 12,* 417–428.

Loehlin, J.C., & Nichols, R.C. (1976). *Heredity, environment, and personality: A study of 850 sets of twins.* Austin, Texas: University of Texas Press.

Loehlin, J.C., Willerman, L., & Horn, J.M. (1988). Human behavior genetics. *Annual Review of Psychology, 39,* 101–133.

Martin, N.G., Eaves, L.J., Heath, A.C., Jardine, R., Feingold, L.M., & Eysenck, H.J. (1986). Transmission of social attitudes. *Proceedings of the National Academy of Sciences, 83,* 4364–4368.

Martin, N.G., Jardine, R., & Eaves, L.J. (1984). Is there only one set of genes for different abilities? A reanalysis of the National Merit Scholarship Qualifying Test (NMSQT) data. *Behavior Genetics, 14,* 355–370.

McCrae, R.R., & Costa, P.T., Jr. (1987). Validation of the five-factor model of personality across instruments and observers. *Journal of Personality and Social Psychology, 52,* 81–90.

Morton, N.E., & McLean, C.J. (1974). Analysis of family resemblance: III. Complex segregation analysis of quantitative traits. *American Journal of Human Genetics, 26,* 489–503.

Pedersen, N.L., Plomin, R., McClearn, G.E., & Friberg, L. (1988). Neuroticism, extraversion, and related traits in adult twins reared apart and together. *Journal of Personality and Social Psychology, 55,* 950–957.

Plomin, R. (1986). *Development, genetics, and psychology.* Hillsdale, NJ: Erlbaum.

Plomin, R., & Daniels, D. (1987). Why are children in the same family so different from one another? *Behavior and Brain Sciences, 10,* 1–16.

Plomin, R., Pedersen, N.L., McClearn, G.E., Nesselroade, J.R., & Bergeman, C.S. (1988). EAS temperaments during the last half of the life span: Twins reared apart and twins reared together. *Psychology and Aging, 3,* 43–50.

Plomin, R., Willerman, L., & Loehlin, J.C. (1985). Resemblance in appearance and the equal environments assumption in twin studies of personality traits. *Behavior Genetics, 6,* 43–52.

Rao, D.C., Morton, N.E., & Yee, S. (1974). Analysis of family resemblance: II. A linear model for familial correlation. *American Journal of Human Genetics, 26,* 331–359.

Rowe, D.C. (1987). Resolving the person-situation debate: Invitation to an interdisciplinary dialogue. *American Psychologist, 42,* 218–227.

Rowe, D.C., & Plomin, R. (1981). The importance of nonshared (E_1) environmental influences in behavioral development. *Development Psychology, 17,* 517–531.

Scarr, S., & Carter-Saltzman, L. (1979). Twin method: Defense of a critical assumption. *Behavior Genetics, 9,* 527–542.

Snyder, M. (1979). Self-monitoring processes. In L. Berkowitz (Ed.), *Advances in experimental social psychology* (Vol. 12). New York: Academic Press.

CHAPTER 23

A Biosocial Perspective on Mates and Traits: Reuniting Personality and Social Psychology

Douglas T. Kenrick

Ethnocentrism is a pervasive human characteristic. Even though two hunter/gatherer groups may have originally split from the same family lines, they forget their common ancestry before long and may come to regard their cousins as aliens (e.g., Chagnon, 1968). Social and personality psychologists are, in many ways, like other primitive human groups —quick to forget common ancestors. However, an acknowledgement of our common family roots could provide a means of reuniting the two tribes. If we only had the good sense to recognize Charles Darwin as the father of modern personality and social psychology, in fact, the family might not have broken up.

Of the two subdisciplines, personality has probably been the less guilty of denying its lineage. Darwin's theory was focally concerned with the way natural selection operates on individual differences, and many of the great personality theorists have grounded their ideas in evolutionary theory. Freud was certainly heavily influenced by Darwin and based his ideas about life instincts and the primal horde on the work of the great naturalist. The evolutionary tradition has been, to some extent, maintained over the last century. As two recent examples, Robert Hogan's *Nebraska Symposium* paper (1982), and Lewis Goldberg's paper in the *Review of Personality & Social Psychology* (1981) explained the Big five (or six) personality factors in explicitly Darwinian terms. Similarly, Arnold Buss and Robert Plomin (1975) couched their discussion of inherited temperament in evolutionary terms.

All of these approaches implicitly or explicitly connect personality to social interaction. Hogan and Goldberg both assume that the central personality factors are cognitive structures that evolved in our ancestors to help them code important social behaviors. Freud believed that all the important issues in the ontogenesis of life instincts involved social interactions. When William McDougall wrote his classic, *Social Psychology,* in 1908, he also assumed an intimate connection among evolution, traits, and social interactions. Social psychologists have, however, scorned McDougall like a senile old uncle, and have focused aggressively on proximate explanations of behavior. The rejection of biologically based traits has widened the gap between social psychology and personality, and although social cognition researchers have shown some interest in reintegrating personality and social psychology, they have tended to ignore the ultimate picture—how social thoughts and social learning are constrained by phylogenetic and ontogenetic biological factors.

Elsewhere, I have argued that a modern biosocial model can connect social learning, social cognition, and sociobiology (Kenrick, 1987; Kenrick, Montello, & McFarlane, 1985), and in so doing reunite the personality and social subdisciplines (Kenrick, 1986). In this paper, I will summarize some of my own evolution-based research that connects gender differences in personality to social processes.

Sexual Selection and Differential Parental Investment

Charles Darwin assumed an intimate association between social processes and the different traits of males and females; he made the connection via the mechanism of *sexual selection*. Darwin argued that males and females of many animal species "differ in structure, colour, or ornament" because individual males had, over many generations, slight advantages over other males "in their weapons, means of defence, or charms" (Darwin, 1859, p. 95). Males who possessed those advantageous features were more successful at mating, and passed those characteristics on to their own male offspring. Although Darwin thought the process applied more to the selection of male characteristics, he did not rule out the possibility that sexual selection could also lead to the preferential adaptiveness of certain features of females.

Sexual selection can occur either because some members of one sex compete more successfully with their own sex, or because some members of one sex have characteristics that appeal directly to the tastes of the opposite sex (Wilson, 1975). Evolutionary biologists use this concept of sexual selection to help explain cross-cultural universalities in gender-linked personality traits (e.g., Williams & Best, 1982). For instance, males across cultures show more of the trait of dominance because, according to the model, dominance was appealing to our female ancestors (Sadalla, Kenrick, & Vershure, 1987). In line with this reasoning, Buss (1989) found evidence that traits related to dominance were more valued in a husband than in a wife across thirty-seven cultures. On the other hand, an evolutionary model would predict that males would prefer to mate with females with physical characteristics signalling fertility, and social traits signalling nurturance (Buss, 1989; Kenrick & Keefe, 1989; Symons, 1979).

Modern evolutionary biologists follow Darwin in assuming that females are more choosy than males about their mate's traits (Daly & Wilson,

1983; Hinde, 1984; Symons, 1979; Trivers, 1985). Evolutionary theorists explain this presumed difference in terms of *differential parental investment* (Trivers, 1972; Williams, 1966). Since females have an initial high investment in each individual offspring, and more to lose from a careless mating choice, they are assumed to be more discriminating about their partner's characteristics. According to this model, males are less invested in any given offspring, and have more to gain by multiple, and less discriminating, sexual liasons. There are a number of human sex differences that fit with this model (Daly & Wilson, 1983; Kenrick & Trost, 1987; Symons, 1979; Trivers, 1985). To give an example from my own research, Sara Gutierres, Laurie Goldberg, and I found that males exposed to beautiful female centerfolds decreased their felt commitment and attraction to their female companions. Although females were susceptible to similar "contrast effects," and found male centerfolds highly attractive and erotic, exposure to those attractive males had no effect on their commitment to or attraction towards their partners (Kenrick, Gutierres, & Goldberg, 1989). In another study, we found that males were more likely to volunteer to put themselves in sexually arousing situations in the first place (Kenrick, Stringfield, Wagenhals, Dahl, & Ransdell, 1980).

Ed Sadalla, Beth Vershure, and I found strong support for applying such a model to human mate choice. In line with Darwin's reasoning, we found that nonverbal dominance increased the attractiveness of male targets, but had no effect on female attractiveness. Our effects were clear and unambiguous, showing up across four studies and three different operationalizations. Buss and Barnes (1986) also applied an evolutionary model to human mate choice. They found some differences in line with the model. For instance, females ranked earning capacity and college graduation as relatively more important in potential mates, whereas males ranked physical attractiveness as relatively important. However, Buss and Barnes also found that seven of the top ten ranked characteristics were exactly the same for males and females. These authors explain the many similarities in male and female choice by noting that monogamous species commonly show few gender differences, because males and females in such species have more comparable levels of parental investment.

It may seem problematic to use an evolutionary explanation when we do find sex differences, and also when we do not. To avoid tautologies, we need to specify when humans will act like monogamous species, with males and females similar in choosiness, and when humans will act like more typical mammals, with females being more discriminating. The social psychological literature on relationships may provide the essential clue here. Studies of human relationships commonly make a distinction between different stages of the relationship, on the assumption that selection criteria change with the course of relationships. Melanie Trost and I have reviewed that literature elsewhere (Kenrick & Trost, 1989), but the essential point is that very different processes seem to operate in first attraction, dating, and long-term commitment. With this in mind, my colleagues and I (Kenrick, Sadalla, Groth, and Trost, in press) noted that the Sadalla et al. (1987) and the Buss and Barnes (1986) studies differed crucially on the type of relationship they were investigating. Buss and Barnes, who found many similarities between males and females, focused on the ideal characteristics of a long-term mate. On the other hand, Sadalla and his colleagues focused on the sexual attractiveness of a stranger. In line with the parental-investment model, however, it makes sense that males and females will differ most at the level of sexual relations, and least when considering a long-term mate. Since a causal sexual opportunity leaves females with relatively more to lose, they should be more selective at that level. In choosing a long-term mate, however, the sexes make similar investments, and should be more similar in requirements.

Another crucial distinction may have to do with the type of trait under consideration. As indicated in our earlier quote, Darwin reasoned that traits related to dominance should be more relevant to males. More recent evolutionary models support Darwin's reasoning, and, as we indicated above, suggest that females should be selected for traits related to fertility (like physical attractiveness; Buss, 1989; Symons, 1979). The relatively clear sex differences found by Sadalla et al. (1987), therefore, could also be due to the fact that they focused on the trait of dominance.

To address this discrepancy, we asked college students about the characteristics desired at four levels of courtship: date, sexual relations, dating steadily, and marriage (Kenrick, Sadalla, Groth, and Trost, 1989). In line with a *relationship qualified parental investment model,* we found most sex differences at the level of sexual relations. In some cases, males actually demanded less in a sexual partner than they asked for in a date. For example, females required progressively more intelligence as they progressed through the levels of date, sexual relations, steady dating, and marriage. Males demanded almost exactly the same intelligence levels as the females, except at the level of sexual relations, where their IQ requirements took an abrupt drop. That is, males indicated a willingness to have sexual relations with someone who did not meet their minimum intelligence criteria for a date. In other cases, as in the variable "kind and understanding," males simply did not increase demands when moving from date to sexual relations, while females jumped radically. For several variables, particularly those related to dominance and social status, females were more selective at all levels. Males were generally more selective than females for only one variable—physical attractiveness.

These findings suggest the fruitfulness of applying the differential parental investment and sexual selection principles to human behavior, and they suggest when and how the principles will apply. By considering a distinction from the social psychological literature on relationships, we were able to specify more precisely when sex differences in mate requirements would be found.

Schematic Processing

The study I have just described was an attempt to bridge the gap between evolutionary biology and psychology. It also bridged a gap that sometimes seems like a canyon—that between the different sections of the *Journal of Personality & Social Psychology*. That study made a connection between the kind of studies typically found in the personality and relationships sections. Our field requires not a simple bridge, however, but one like New York's TriBoro—with footings in three different neighborhoods—personality, interpersonal relations, and social cognition (how each area corresponds to Manhattan, the Bronx and Queens I leave to the reader's own imagination).

Let me turn to a study that uses an evolutionary framework to make a preliminary three-way bridge. Social cognition researchers study the processes used to select, encode, and recall information about other people. One of the popular ideas in this area is that social thinking is "schematic" (Fiske & Taylor, 1984). The term *schema* is used in several ways, but I want to focus on its use as a filter that guides the selection of stimuli for attention, and the selection of information for encoding into and retrieval from memory. Cognition researchers note that it would be impossible to attend to every stimulus in our environment, impossible to remember everything we attend to, and impossible to relate every new thought to every detail in our long-term memory. Instead, we use mental schemas or templates to assist in the process. For instance, you could process the speakers at a conference in terms of how eloquent they are in delivering their talks, which would lead you to focus on and remember different features than if you were considering how liberal each one is, which in turn leads to different processing than if you were trying to determine how rich each one is, and so on. These schemas simplify the task of sorting through the vast complexity of information in the environment.

Social psychologists have examined how schematic processing influences our attention to, interpretation of, and memory for other people's facial characteristics (Rothbart & Birrell, 1977), and personality traits (Hastie & Park, 1986), our reactions to attitude change attempts (Ross, McFarland, & Fletcher, 1981), and so on (Fiske & Taylor, 1984). Most studies in this area have attempted to artificially manipulate people's processing. There has been little investigation of default schemas. What do people pay attention to and remember from social situations when they are operating on automatic, and have not been specifically primed by the experimenter?

An evolutionary theorist would assume that we automatically process for information that is relevant to survival and reproduction. Before processing whether someone is dressed like an artist or a dirt farmer, or even whether that person seems more like a personality than a social psychologist, we should notice what gender that person is, how sexually attractive they are, and whether they pose a potential threat or a mating opportunity for us. In line with the differential parental investment hypothesis, which sees females as buyers in a buyers' market, males should be more likely to actively process information about potential mates.

What little evidence there is indicates support for this sort of reasoning. For instance, in a recent paper examining the way people process personality information, Hastie and Park (1986) report an unpredicted finding that subjects automatically processed even a list of neutral trait adjectives in terms of gender. Similar findings come from studies of dichotic listening, which strain people's attentional capacities by asking them to repeat back a complex message delivered through one earphone while a completely different message is delivered to the other ear. Usually, subjects notice very little about the nonattended message. People do not process changes in language, or even changes from English into nonsense syllables on the nonattended ear. They do, however, note changes in the gender of the voice (Cherry, 1953). Other research has shown that subjects are tremendously sensitive to small variations in facial symmetry, even though they are unable to verbally describe the underlying processes (Hill & Lewicki, in press). Finally, some very recent research tested an evolutionary model of attention and found that people can detect an angry face in a rapidly flashed crowd more quickly and more accurately than they detect other facial expressions (Hansen & Hansen, 1988). In short, there is some, mostly indirect, support for the notion that people automatically attend to simuli in terms of dimensions relevant to survival and reproduction.

Lidia Dengelegi and I examined "default processing" in a free recall study in which we asked subjects to look at a series of yearbook photos (Kenrick & Dengelegi, 1988). Afterwards we asked them to bring any one of the faces to mind, and then to go back through the book and locate the first two faces they brought to mind. We also collected information about whether the subjects were currently single, dating one person steadily, or married.

The first finding of interest involves the physical attractiveness of the photographs. If a subject recalled someone of the opposite sex, that person tended to be more physically attractive than when the subject remembered someone of the same sex. That finding itself is consistent with the idea that people "automatically" select mating-relevant stimuli to pay attention to. Another aspect of the data is more interesting, however, and fits nicely with the differential parental investment hypothesis. Females were about equally likely to bring a male as a female to mind, whether they were attached or not. Males, on the other hand, were more likely to recall a female. Being attached tended to reduce that tendency, but even attached males were still more likely than females to attend selectively to the opposite sex.

Those findings suggest three things, then. First, they support the idea that people automatically attend to features of others that relate to potential mating opportunities. Second, they indicate that the tendency is stronger in males. Third, they suggest that being attached lessens males' tendency to scan for attractive females, but that even attached males still have their antennae tuned to the opposite sex. The latter two tendencies fit nicely with the differential parental investment model.

Conclusion

To summarize, I have been arguing that Charles Darwin is the legitimate father of personality and social psychology, and that we ought to reunite the family. By focusing on ultimate causes—on the roots of human behavior—an evolutionary approach allows us to see the kinship between personality traits, relationships, and social cognition. At one time, it may have been possible to dismiss an evolutionary approach as untestable and tautological. There is, however, increasing evidence that an evolutionary approach provides not simply an interesting post-hoc perspective on many psychological findings, but also a powerful heuristic tool capable of making a priori predictions that do not follow from existing proximate psychological models (c.f. Kenrick & Trost, 1989). Although a radical environmentalism may once have been revolutionary, it is now reactionary.

In describing sex differences in psychological traits, the evolutionary perspective can explain many findings that simply do not fit with existing psychological models (c.f. Kenrick, 1987; Kenrick & Trost, 1987, 1989). For instance, an evolutionary approach easily deals with findings linking the hormone testosterone to "stereotypically" masculine behaviors (e.g. Dabbs, Frady, Carr, & Besch, 1987; Rose, Holaday, & Bernstein, 1971), as well as findings of cross-cultural similarities in sex-typed characteristics (Williams & Best, 1982). Although one can frequently come with post-hoc normative explanations of many individual findings, an evolutionary perspective can parsimoniously explain the totality of findings.

One common complaint about evolutionary approaches is that they offer explanations at the wrong level of analysis for psychology. Evolutionary theory is concerned with "ultimate" explanations that stress historically

EVOLUTIONARY HISTORY

(Ultimate)

BEHAVIOR GENETICS

INDIVIDUAL LEARNING HISTORY

CONSCIOUS AND NON-CONSCIOUS INFO. PROCESSING

BIOCHEMICAL AND NEUROLOGICAL PROCESSES

(Proximate)

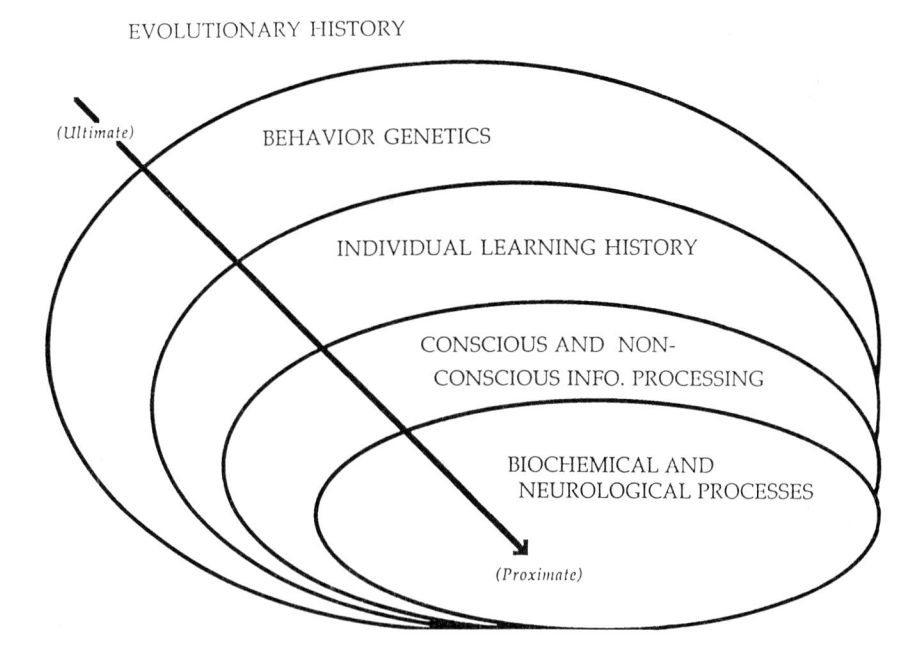

FIGURE 23.1. *The proximate/ultimate continuum.* Ultimate explanations deal with more historically remote causes of behavior, whereas relatively more proximate explanations stress more immediate causes. Each level of explanation is constrained by those that encircle it.

distant causes, whereas psychologists tend to be more interested in "proximate" explanations that stress more contemporaneous events. Figure 23.1 depicts the "proximate/ultimate" continuum.

Although one could reasonably argue with the completeness of this figure, it should serve to demonstrate the point I wish to make here. Note that inner circles involve proximate, or immediate, explanatory levels, whereas outer circles apply progressively to more ultimate, historically distant levels of analysis. Social cognition approaches to personality tend to operate at the level of conscious and nonconscious information processing, often stressing the ways in which immediate attentional and encoding processes are connected to structures from individual learning history. They are not usually concerned with evolutionary history, behavior genetics, or ongoing biochemical processes. Behavior genetic approaches are concerned with how individual differences are passed from one generation to another. Behavior geneticists may or may not be concerned with the evolutionary significance of those individual differences, and they may or not be concerned with how those individual characteristics relate to individual learning-history, but they are unlikely to be concerned with ongoing information processing (see Rushton, 1984, for an interesting discussion of these issues). The level of analysis argument suggests that this division of labor is as it should be, and implies that it is useless to jump more than one step in this diagram. The suggestion that we should deal with the local Caesar only in the local currency may, however, be short-sighted. For one thing, each level in this diagram is constrained by all those encircling it. Evolutionary selection acts on the individual differences studied by behavior geneticists; genetically based individual differences constrain one's learning experiences as well as what one learns from those experiences. Learning-history determines ongoing attention and encoding processes, and those ongoing processes influence acute biological states. To some extent, the arrow could also be reversed. Immediate physiological state (testosterone level or adrenaline level, for instance) influences attention and encoding; ongoing information processing influences what is learned for the future, and although learning experiences do not change genes, they can produce important changes in chronic physiological mechanisms originally constructed by those genes (see Kenrick, 1987; Kenrick et al., 1985; Lumsden & Wilson, 1981, for a fuller discussion of these issues). By maintaining some awareness of the evolutionary context of human behavior, we are in a better position to answer a number of questions about proximate process and structure. Why are certain personality characteristics, like ascendance and likability, so important to our species? Why are humans prone to learn certain things, like phobic responses to snakes, so much more easily than others, like phobic responses to the kitchen cookware (despite the fact that many more people are burned in the kitchen than are bitten by a snake)? Why do we remember some things more readily than others? Why do we pay attention to certain things more than others, as in the research discussed above? Without an ultimate perspective on our work, we are sometimes bemused by findings that, once we take a step backward from the immediate present, make eminent sense.

Another mistaken complaint about evolutionary approaches is that they ignore the environment. Evolutionary analyses assume that personality and social behaviors in modern humans result, at least in part, from naturally selected genetic mechanisms. Those genetic tendencies do not operate in a vacuum. They evolved in interaction with the environment, and only unfold in interaction with environmental factors. Exactly how genes interact with the pressures of the socializing environment is an important question, arguably the most important one that now faces the field of psychology. With regard to gender differences in mating behavior, several preliminary answers can be advanced. At a very simple level, genes program physical differences among us. Size and shape differences lead to different life experiences—large muscular people are more likely to be reinforced for attempts to bully others, for instance. At a less obvious level, males produce more of the hormone testosterone, and this hormone is implicated in enhanced libido and dominance behaviors, in exactly the way predicted by the differential investment model. Neurophysiological data now suggest that the human brain is not a tabula rasa, but is specialized to perceive certain stimuli and not others, to think about certain things and not others, and to generate certain responses (e.g., facial expressions) and not others (Gazzaniga, 1985). Humans are not programmed with much in the way of rigid instincts, but neither are we quite so malleable as we sometimes like to believe (Lumsden & Wilson, 1981).

Many gender differences in experience thus follow directly from differences in the way male and female brains and bodies are architectured, and from differences in the hormones that flow through male and female bloodstreams. However, many of these gene/environment influences are indirect. Ours has always been a social species, and socialization can act to oppose, or to underline, existing sex differences. Except under unusual circumstances, I suspect that nurture serves to reinforce what nature has wrought. Also, the developing individual is not simply passively exposed to the same life experiences. The different proclivities of males and females cause them to choose different courses of socialization, and to have different effects on the same social environment (see Kenrick, 1987, for a fuller discussion of these interactional issues).

It should be clear that I am not suggesting that social and personality psychologists abandon their current business and learn gene-mapping techniques, or head for the nearst cave to dig bones. In fact, I think that the interesting advances in the coming years may come via the methods of psychology. Many forms of human adaptation are undoubtedly mediated by ongoing cognition and learning-history, and psychologists are best equipped to study those proximate processes. Personality and social psychologists have already gathered a wealth of findings that could enrich the existing evolutionary literature (see Kenrick & Trost, 1987, for a preliminary attempt in this direction). Thus, we stand in a unique place to contribute to the revolutionary developments in evolutionary biology and to connect them to the other revolution in cognitive science. The buried family tree is, after all, one that leads back to intellectual royalty.

References

Barash, D.P. (1977). *Sociobiology and behavior*, New York: Elsevier.

Buss, A.H., & Plomin, R. (1975). *A temperament theory of personality development*. New York: Wiley/Interscience.

Buss, D.M. (1989). Sex differences in human mate preference: Evolutionary hypothesis tested in 37 cultures. *Behavioral and Brain Sciences, 12,* 1–49.

Buss, D.M., & Barnes, M. (1986). Preferences in human mate selection. *Journal of Personality and Social Psychology, 50,* 559–570.

Chagnon, N.A. (1968). *Yanomamo: The fierce people.* New York: Holt, Rinehart, & Winston.

Cherry, E.C. (1953). Some experiments upon the recognition of speech, with one and with two ears. *Journal of the Acoustical Society of America, 25,* 975–979.

Dabbs, J.M., Frady, R.L., Carr, T.S., Besch, N.F. (1987). Saliva testosterone and criminal violence in young adult prison inmates. *Psychosomatic Medicine, 49,* 174–182.

Daly, M., & Wilson, M. (1983). *Sex, evolution, and behavior.* Boston, MA: Willard Grant.

Darwin, C. (1958). *The origin of species* (6th ed.). New York: New American Library. (Original work published 1859)

Fiske, S.T., & Taylor, S.E. (1984). *Social cognition.* Reading, MA: Addison-Wesley.

Gazzaniga, M.S. (1985). *The social brain.* New York: Basic Books.

Hansen, C.H., & Hansen, R.D. (in press). Finding faces in the crowd: The anger superiority effect. *Journal of Personality and Social Psychology.*

Hastie, R., & Park, B. (1986). The relationship between memory and judgment depends on whether the judgment task is memory based or on-line. *Psychological Review, 93,* 258–268.

Hill, T., & Lewicki, P. (in press). Personality and the unconscious. In V.J. Derelega, B.A. Winstead, & W.H. Jones (Eds.) *Introduction to contempoarry research in personality.* Chicago, IL: Nelson/Hall.

Hinde, R.A. (1984). Why do the sexes behave differently in close relationships? *Journal of Social and Personality Relationships, 1,* 471–501.

Hogan, R. (1983). A socioanalytic theory of personality. *Nebraska Symposium on Motivation 1982, 55*–89.

Kenrick, D.T. (1986). How strong is the case against contemporary social and personality psychology? A response to Carlson. *Journal of Personality and Social Psychology, 50,* 839–844.

Kenrick, D.T. (1987). Gender, genes, and the social environment: A biosocial interactionist perspective. *Review of personality and social psychology, 7,* 14–43.

Kenrick, D.T. & Dengeligi, L. (in preparation). Gender differences in spontaneous recall of faces: Default processing fits a reproductive fitness model.

Kenrick, D.T., Gutierres, S.E., & Goldberg, L. (1989). Influence of erotica on judgment of strangers and mates. *Journal of Experimental Social Psychology, 25,* 159–167.

Kenrick, D.T., & Keefe, R.C. (1989). Time to integrate social psychology and evolutionary biology. *Behavioral and Brain Sciences, 12,* 24–26.

Kenrick, D.T., Montello, D., & MacFarlane, S. (1985). Personality: Social learning, social cognition, or sociobiology? In R. Hogan & W. Jones (Eds.), *Perspectives in personality* (Vol. 1, pp. 201–234). Greenwich, CT:JAI.

Kenrick, D.T., Stringfield, D.O., Wagenhals, W.L., Dahl, R.H., & Ransdell, H.J. (1980). Sex differences, androgyny, and approach responses to erotica: A new variation on the old volunteer problem. *Journal of Personality and Social Psychology, 38,* 517–524.

Kenrick, D.T., Sadalla, E.K., Groth, G., & Trost, M.R. (in press). Traits and mates: Evolutionary theory as a bridge between personality and social psychology. *Journal of Personality.*

Kenrick, D.T., & Trost, M.R. (1987). A biosocial theory of heterosexual relationships. In K. Kelley (Ed.), *Females, males, and sexuality: Theories and research* (pp. 59–100). Albany, NY: State University of New York Press.

Kenrick, D.T., & Trost, M.R. (1989). A reproductive exchange model of heterosexual relationships: Putting proximate economics in ultimate perspective. *Review of Personality & Social Psychology, 10,* 92–118.

Lumsden, C.J., & Wilson, E.O. (1981). *Genes, mind, and culture: The coevolutionary process.* Cambridge, MA: Harvard University Press.

McDougall, W. (1908). *Social psychology: An introduction.* London: Methuen.

Rose, R.M., Holaday, J.W., & Bernstein, I.S. (1971). Plasma testosterone, dominance rank, and aggressive behavior in male rhesus monkeys. *Nature, 231,* 366–368.

Ross, M., McFarland, C., & Fletcher, G.J.O. (1981). The effect of attitude on the recall of personal histories. *Journal of Personality and Social Psychology, 40,* 627–634.

Rothbart, M., & Birrell, P. (1977). Attitude and the perception of faces. *Journal of Research in Personality, 11,* 209–215.

Rusthon, J.P. (1984). Sociobiology: Toward a theory of individual and group differences in personality and social behavior. In J.R. Royce & L.P. Moss (Eds.) *Annals of Theoretical Psychology* (Vol. 2, pp. 1–81). New York: Plenum.

Sadalla, E.K., Kenrick, D.T., & Vershure, B. (1987). Dominance and heterosexual attraction. *Journal of Personality and Social Psychology, 52,* 730–738.

Symons, D. (1979). *Evolution of human sexuality.* New York: Oxford University Press.

Trivers, R.L. (1972). Parental investment and sexual selection. In B. Campbell (Ed.), *Sexual selection and the descent of man* (pp. 136–179). Chicago, IL: Aldine.

Trivers, R. (1985). *Social evolution.* Menlo Park, CA: Benjamin/Cummings.

Williams, G.C. (1966). Natural selection, the costs of reproduction, and a refinement of Lack's principle. *American Naturalist, 100,* 687–690.

Williams, J.E., & Best, D.L. (1982). *Measuring sex stereotypes.* Beverly Hills, CA: Sage.

Wilson, E.O. (1975). *Sociobiology.* Cambridge, MA: Harvard University Press.

CHAPTER 24

The Evolutionary History of Genetic Variation: An Emerging Issue in the Behavioral Genetic Study of Personality

Steven W. Gangestad

Over the past twenty years, research in behavioral genetics has established that genetic factors play an important role in personality development. Although no one study can be regarded as conclusive, the literature taken as a whole leaves little doubt that genetic factors account for a substantial amount of the variance in important personality traits. The recent Minnesota twins reared apart study (Tellegen, Lykken, Bouchard, Wilcox, Segal, & Rich, 1988), for example, illustrates typical findings. Across eleven different traits assessed by the Multidimensional Personality Questionnaire (Tellegen, 1982), hertiabilities were estimated to range between 39-55%. Intraclass correlations for MZ twins reared apart ranged from .29 to .61; correlations of zero would be expected if no genetic influence existed (see Henderson, 1982, and Loehlin, Willerman, & Horn, 1988, for reviews of other studies).

What do these heritabilities tell us? They tell us that genetic factors are correlated with behavior; that is their narrow interpretation, but do they tell us anything else? Unfortunately, very little. In particular, they neither tell us *why* genetic factors are correlated with behavior, nor *how* they become that way. For that reason, some researchers have claimed that an estimate of heritability represents a fairly low-level achievement, especially if our goal is to develop theoretical understandings of behavior (e.g., Lewontin, 1974). Heritability estimates can tell us that genetic factors play *some* role in the development of a trait. They don't say *what* role.

In the last decade or so, we have seen behavioral geneticists trying to move beyond the mere task of estimating heritabilities and attempt to *specify* the causal processes that mediate the gene-behavior relation. In this regard, sophisticated thinking about the gene-behavior relationship has emerged, and this may represent one of the significant achievements in the area. Thus, although behavior geneticists have, for a long time, recognized that the social environment may mediate the gene-behavior relation, we now have explicit models of how environmental mediation may occur. Scarr and McCartney (1983), for instance, describe the ways in which different genotypes may elicit or select different environments and suggest how they may vary in importance across developmental periods. These processes may sort different genotypes into different environments, such that, to the extent that the different environments have an effect on behavior, correlation between genotypes and behavior results.

Other issues that have been addressed under the general rubric of "causal specification" are: "During what period of life do genetic effects become manifest?" and "To what extent are genetic effects moderated by environmental conditions? That is, to what extent are there important genotype-environment interactions?" Furthermore, given that genes are physical units, there continues to be interest in identifying the physiological substrate that mediates genetic effects.

Recognition of these issues has led to the development of quantitative methods and research designs that were not available a decade ago (e.g., Plomin, 1986). Some might say we have answers to many of the theoretical questions—a point that is arguable. In any case, what is important is that conceptual frameworks that allow us to talk about genetic effects in sophisticated ways have been developed, and that efforts have been made to establish methods that can address the difficult issues of causal process. This is a trend that is generally welcomed and, I hope, is one that we can count on to continue.

I want to devote the remainder of my comments, however, to another trend that is perhaps emerging, but which has not yet received much attention. This involves the attempt to specify ultimate explanations of genetic differences—that is, to construct evolutionary histories of genetic variation. A nonzero heritability on a trait implies, of course, that there exists genetic variability in the population under study. Genetic variability, in turn, is subject to evolutionary pressures such as selection, drift, and mutation pressure. Therefore, much of the genetic variation currently associated with behavior is the result of pressures that existed in our evolutionary past. What were the evolutionary pressures that produced this genetic variability? That is, what is the evolutionary history of this genetic variation?

As noted, with few exceptions (e.g., Theissen, 1972), interest in this issue is just now emerging. Why has its emergence been slow? At least two reasons may be tentatively offered. First, there may be a widespread belief that specification of ultimate causality is not the business of psychologists. Psychology, after all, deals with relatively *proximate* causes of behavior. Addressing ultimate causality may add to our understanding of natural history. It may, furthermore, inform evolutionary biology, but what does evolutionary history tell us about the proximate mechanisms which constitute the subject matter of psychology?

Secondly, many researchers are skeptical about the testability of evolutionary explanations of human behavior. The evolutionary forces that formed the nature of the human psyche exerted their effects long ago and in environments much different from those we inhabit today. How can we possibly test theories about those forces? Certainly, we can speculate about what forces could possibly have resulted in behavioral forms we observe today, but given the flexibility of evolutionary biology to explain, post hoc, adaptive behavior, how can we know our constructions are not merely "just so" stories that have no empirical test (e.g., Gould & Lewontin, 1979)? Even many biologically oriented psychologists hold this view. For instance, Zuckerman (1983), after having filled two pages with various speculations about the evolutionary origins of sensation seeking, admitted: "Sociobiology is great intellectual fun, but like psychoanalysis it is basically unverifiable when limited to post hoc types of retrospective interpretation" (p. 39).

Surely, evolutionary biology is limited in what it can tell us about human behavior. Furthermore, some evolutionary speculation is purely post hoc and untestable. Nonetheless, it would be wrong to conclude, on the basis of these limitations, that evolutionary considerations have nothing to offer in the way of psychological understanding. In fact, constructing evolutionary histories of genetic variation in personality may offer much to personality psychology and, at times, lead to testable predictions (see also Buss, 1984). I will try to make this point through illustration. Specifically, I wish to describe some of my own efforts to construct an evolutionary history of one particular source of genetic variability. After describing this research, I will turn to what this sort of effort might potentially offer personality psychology. (See Rushton, 1985, and Tooby & Cosmides, in press, for other examples.)

Individual Differences in Sociosexuality

In the past couple of years, Jeffry Simpson and I have been trying to understand the evolutionary history behind genetic variation in a trait we refer to as *sociosexuality*. As we conceive it, this trait refers to individual differences in one's implicit prerequisites to entering a sexual relationship (Simpson & Gangestad, 1988b). Individuals at one extreme require relatively more time and stronger attachment to, commitment to, and closeness with their romantic partners before they are willing to enter a sexual relationship with them. People who have these attributes are said to possess *restricted sociosexuality*. People at the other end of the dimension, those who possess *unrestricted sociosexuality*, require relatively less time and weaker attachment to, commitment to, and closeness with their partners before engaging in sex with them. The measure of sociosexuality we have developed consists of both attitudinal indices (e.g., having respondents indicate how comfortable they are with casual sex or sex without commitment) and behavior self-report indices (e.g., having respondents report the number of partners they have had sex with in the past year, the number of "one-night stands" they have engaged in, the length of time they dated their most recent sexual partner before having sex with him/her, etc.). These behavioral and attitudinal indices covary highly with one another. Moreover, they can be distinguished from general interest in sex; there is virtually no correlation between scores on sociosexuality and self- or other-reported frequency of sex when in a stable relationship. Finally, they have been validated by independent reports provided by dating partners (Simpson & Gangestad, 1988b).

Direct and indirect evidence indicates that there is substantial genetic variation in both male and female sociosexuality. The direct evidence is a British twin study of sexual attitudes reported by Eysenck (1976), which indicated that perhaps 30 to 50% of the variance in indicators similar to our own is genetic variance. The indirect evidence consists of twin studies indicating that a number of different personality traits that correlate substantially with sociosexuality genetically covary. The pattern of genetic covariance is such that the covariance of these measures with sociosexuality is almost certain to be genetic in nature as well (Gangestad & Simpson, 1988b). This genetic variance must be the result of evolutionary forces such as mutation, migration, and selection. What is its evolutionary history?

Before concerning ourselves with this specific question, let us consider more generally why genetic variation may exist in a population.

Population Genetic Models

There is no one reason why genetic variation exists. A number of different processes contribute to the flux and maintenance of genetic variation in a population. The field of population genetics is concerned with understanding these processes and the conditions under which they may operate. Broadly speaking, two major categories of variance-maintenance mechanisms exist: nonselectionist and selectionist.

Nonselectionist Mechanisms

Ultimately, variation in a population derives from two sources: mutation of genetic alleles and the introduction of genes into the pool due to migration of individuals. According to the classical theory of population genetics, these nonselectionist phenomena are among the major forces that maintain variation. Because they introduce variation that is essentially random, these processes create variants that are generally nonadaptive—in many cases, *maladaptive*. Selection, according to this view, is primarily a force that conserves the adaptation of organisms to their environments by sweeping out of the population the nonadaptive, random variation introduced by mutation and migration out of the population. Only occasionally (and by chance) will a random variant actually improve the organism's adaptedness, in which case selection will retain it (that is, if it is not first lost in sexual recombination). The rate at which variation is removed depends upon the strength of selection, which is a function of how maladaptive the introduced variant is. At one extreme, a mutant allele may be lethal, in which case it is removed from the population within a generation. At the other extreme, a mutant allele may have negligible effects on fitness, in which case variation can be maintained for many generations. According to the classical view, then, a major form of genetic variation is simply "neutral variation"—variance unrelated to the reproductive fitness of the organisms. For instance, we probably differ substantially with respect to the number of hairs on our heads, and the reason we differ probably is because, within some range, our fitness is not influenced by this phenotypic variable. Theissen (1972) has argued that much genetic variation in behavior is similarly adaptively neutral—"genetic junk" produced by mutation that selection has allowed to accumulate. Given the ubiquity of genetic variance in personality traits, an implication of this view is that standardly assessed personality traits are not particularly relevant to our ability to survive and reproduce—an odd implication in view of the long-standing regard of personality as a manifestation of the organism's adaptations.

Selectionist Mechanisms

In the past several decades, population geneticists have become increasingly aware of the fact that, although selection can remove nonadaptive variation, it can *maintain* genetic variation as well. *Balancing selection* —selection which does just that—can take a variety of forms. One of the best understood forms is heterozygote superiority. When a heterozygote is more adaptive than either of the homozygotes of its constituent alleles, genetic variance in the population can be maintained. Mating of the heterozygotes and recombination of the alleles ensures genetic heterogeneity in the next generation (e.g., Dobzhansky, 1970).

A second form of balancing selection that has received a great deal of attention recently is frequency-dependent selection. Frequency-dependent selection can operate when the fitnesses of genotypes vary as a function of their frequencies within a population. When two genotypes each have frequency-dependent fitnesses, such that the fitness of each when rare exceeds that of the other, a stable polymorphism may be established for frequencies at which the fitnesses of the two genotypes equal each other.

Consider a simple example—mimicry. Suppose a species of moths comes in two forms, one that is unique to the species and one that mimics a second moth species. Furthermore, suppose the second species is distasteful to the major avian predator of the moth. If the mimic is rare, the birds will ignore it and eat the nonmimics. Over time, the mimic will become more frequent in the population and the nonmimic less frequent. As this occurs, what happens to the fitnesses of the two moths? Birds that eat the mimics will not be at such a risk, for there is less chance that the moths they eat are distasteful. Therefore, the fitness of the mimics may decrease as they become more common. At the same time, the fitness of the nonmimics may increase. To the extent that they are rare, birds who look for them as a food source may die. It is possible that at some relative proportions of mimics and nonmimics the fitnesses of the nonmimics actually equals that of the mimics. The population will be maintained in a stable equilibrium at those relative proportions.

Frequency-dependent selection may operate at several different levels of the phenotypic expression of genetic material—from the very rudimentary to the highly complex. At one extreme, some theorists have suggested that most of the genetic variability in mammalian species is due to frequency-dependent selection of basic protein codes of genetic alleles in response to attacks by parasitic micro-organisms that rely upon being adapted to the presence of proteins in their host (Rice, 1983; Tooby, 1982). This genetic variability, however, may have few or no implications for the basic design features of the organism as a complex, integrated whole (Tooby & Cosmides, in press). At the other extreme, some theorists have noted how complex patterns of social interaction are, at least in principle, prime candidates for frequency-dependent selection (e.g., Maynard Smith, 1982). The basic idea is that most mammalian species (particularly those at the K-selected end of the r-K continuum, such as humans; e.g., Chisholm, 1988; McArthur & Wilson, 1967; Pianka, 1970) live in environments with limited resources—food, shelter, mates, etc. In such circumstances, intraspecific competition is intense. Selection produces individuals who possess complex and integrated adaptive patterns of behavior—*behavioral strategies*—that allow them to compete effectively for resources. Let us suppose that a number of different strategies could, in principle, exploit available resources. Because competition is often most intense between individuals utilizing the same strategy, the effectiveness of a strategy often will be frequency-dependent. Such a situation may produce a mixture of strategies in the population whose frequencies are fixed at a stable equilibrium.

In addition to the processes just discussed, a number of other processes may produce and maintain genetic variability (see, for instance, Crow, 1986, for a good introduction to concepts and processes in population genetics). With this skeletal introduction to population genetic accounts of genetic variability, however, let us return to consider genetic variation in sociosexuality.

The Evolutionary History of Genetic Variation in Sociosexuality

What is the evolutionary history of the genetic variation in sociosexuality? Some sociobiologists (e.g., Wilson, 1978) have proposed evolutionary understandings of sociosexuality, although generally different ones have been proposed for each of the two sexes. Wilson (1978) explains the expected behavioral sex difference that purportedly follows from a fundamental biological difference between mammalian males and females:

> During the full period of time it takes to bring a fetus to term, from the fertilization of the egg to the birth of the infant, one male can fertilize many females but a female can be fertilized by only one male. Thus if males are able to court one female after another, some will be big winners and others will be absolute losers, while virtually all healthy females will succeed in being fertilized. It pays males to be aggressive, hasty, and undiscriminating. In theory, it is more profitable for females to be coy, to hold back until they can identify males with the best genes. In species that rear young, it is important for the females to select males who are more likely to stay with them after insemination. . . . Human beings obey this biological principle faithfully. (pp. 129–130)

This account does manage to explain a few facts. Thus, for instance, we have found that gender could account for about 20% of the variance in attitudes toward casual, uncommitted sex in a sample of Texas A&M students (Gangestad & Simpson, 1988b). At the same time, however, there is one glaring fact that is inconsistent with this account: a substantial proportion of the variance within the sexes is genetic variance. If we use the conservative estimate of 30% genetic variance within the sexes (Eysenck, 1976), that means about 24% of the total variance is within-sex genetic variance—more than that accounted for by between-sex differences. If, in evolutionary history, it were so adaptive for males to be hasty (i.e., unrestricted) and females coy (i.e., restricted), why hasn't selection swept out the nonadaptive within-sex variation? That is, why should there be any genetic variance within the sexes?

There are a number of potential answers to this question, some of which are more probable than others. Thus, for instance, it seems improbable that the variation is simply neutral. Neutral variation exists on features that have little or no involvement in reproductive efforts. Obviously, sex is not one of those features.

A Frequency-Dependent Model of Female Sociosexual Variation

The particular evolutionary model of sociosexual variation we have explored is a frequency-dependent one. Although we have attempted to understand variation in both male and female sociosexuality, for brevity's sake I will address only the female case here. If frequency-dependent selection has operated to establish a mixture of restricted and unrestricted females, these sexual orientations should be reflected in two strategies, each of which has been sufficiently successful to become established in the population.[1] Under such a model, each strategy must have something that the other does not. If one strategy had everything in its favor, then it alone would become fixed in the population.

Wilson (1978) and others (e.g., Trivers, 1972) have argued that a restricted female strategy should better enable a female to obtain long-term paternal investment in offspring because: (1) such a strategy forces a male partner to invest time in the offspring before its birth, which he would, from an evolutionary perspective, do well to make good; (2) such a strategy demonstrates to a male partner that any offspring the female carries is likely to be his own. To the extent that, in evolutionary history, paternal investment increased the chances of an infant's survival, restricted females should have benefited.

The fitness of a female, however, is not merely a function of the survivability of her offspring. A second factor should influence her long-term fitness: the reproductive success of those offspring. To the extent that there was any additive genetic variance in reproductive success, females in our past may have benefited (everything else being equal) by choosing to reproduce with a male who had the potential for high reproductive success. His genes may have benefited her by being passed onto her offspring—especially her male offspring (given the greater variance in male reproductive success in our evolutionary past; Alexander et al., 1979). That this additional factor should influence female choice has been referred to as "the sexy son hypothesis" (Heisler, 1981; Weatherhead & Robertson, 1979, 1981).

Would restricted sexual behavior have promoted a female's chances of reproducing with highly successful males? Not if unrestricted females were in the population. The latter do not force males to wait before mating and, therefore, should have had a competitive edge in mating with those males who were most reproductively successful. Indeed, the very benefit restricted sexual behavior provides—gaining paternal investment—may have precluded restricted females from mating with potentially very successful males: if such males had invested in a single female's offspring, they would have been less likely to be highly successful.

Our proposed model, then, suggests that restricted and unrestricted female sexuality represent two alternate reproductive strategies in evolutionary history, each having benefited in a way the other did not. Restricted females benefited from the relatively greater paternal invest-

---

[1] It may seem inappropriate to speak of two strategies given that sociosexuality is continuously distributed. In fact, however, evidence suggests that the genetic underpinnings of sociosexuality is bimodally distributed, and, therefore, it may be appropriate to speak of "two" strategies (Gangestad & Simpson, 1988b).

ment in their offspring. Unrestricted females benefited from the fact that they mated with males who possess the potential for high reproductive output and who pass their genes onto their male offspring ("sexy sons").

Could the genetic variability underlying these two strategies have been maintained through frequency-dependent selection? Pending further mathematical treatment, it appears plausible that it could. Frequency-dependent selection requires that the value of each strategy decreases as its relative frequency increases, at least across some range of relative frequency. The more unrestricted females there were, the greater would have been the competition between their sons, and, hence, the value of an unrestricted strategy should have been frequency-dependent. The more restricted females there were, the greater would have been the competition for males who would have exclusively invested in their offspring. Ultimately, there may have been enough males available for all restricted females to mate with. As their number increased, however, the average fitness of the males with whom they mated would have decreased. The value of restricted female sexual behavior should, therefore, also have been frequency-dependent.[2]

Can the Model Be Tested?

Our model perhaps makes a nice story, but how do we know that it paints an accurate picture? Ultimately, of course, scientific theories are never proven, and, therefore, we cannot expect proof for this one. Theories can be exposed to risk by entailing empirical predictions that, without the theory, we wouldn't expect to be true. As it turns out, the evolutionary model described does entail just such a prediction.

Specifically, the model suggests that, in an evolutionary sense, male and female offspring should have been differentially valuable to restricted and unrestricted females. Unrestricted females purportedly benefited from mating with reproductively successful males because the characteristics that allowed those males to bear many offspring would have been passed on to their own. These characteristics would not have benefited their daughters and sons equally, however. Sons should have benefited more for one primary reason. Because males varied more in total number of offspring than did females, reproductively more successful males produced more offspring than did reproductively successful females (Clutton & Iason, 1986). Restricted females, on the other hand, should have benefited from having relatively more daughters, given that their sons would be expected to be competing with the reproductively more successful sons of unrestricted females. To the extent that evolutionary

---

[2] I have presented the model in simple terms here. For a discussion of the intricacies of the model, as well as of various threats to the "sexy son" notion embedded in it (e.g., Kirkpatrick, 1985), see Gangestad & Simpson (1988b).

pressures can affect offspring sex ratios, we should expect that the sex ratio of offspring of restricted and unrestricted females would differ, such that unrestricted females have more sons and restricted females have more daughters.

We have attempted to test this prediction in three different studies, all of which provide support (Gangestad & Simpson, 1988a,b). In one study, a personality marker of sociosexual variation (the Self-Monitoring Scale) was correlated with the offspring sex ratio of mothers of undergraduate students. As predicted, those scoring high on the measure had more sons than did those scoring low on the scale. In a second study, nineteen occupations were ranked with respect to a personality marker of sociosexuality, and mothers appearing in *Who's Who in American Women* who worked at these occupations were identified. Occupation was found to be related to offspring sex ratio in ways predicted. The third study was the only one that used a relatively direct indicator of sociosexuality. During the late 1940's and early 1950's, Alfred Kinsey and his colleagues (Kinsey, Pomeroy, & Martin, 1948; Kinsey, Pomeroy, Martin, & Gebhard, 1953) collected a massive amount of data pertaining to various aspects of sexual behavior. In addition to asking about sexual behavior, they gathered information about respondents' offspring. To assess whether sex ratio of offspring was related to sociosexuality in the Kinsey data, we first identified the most direct behavioral marker of sociosexuality in the data base—the reported number of premarital sex partners. We then contacted the Kinsey Institute and asked them to correlate offspring sex ratio with number of premarital partners within the Kinsey samples. The weighted average for the samples (total $n = 1461$) was .07, $z = 2.67$, $p = .005$. Although this correlation may seem small, it may be about as large as one could expect, given the extent to which random factors influence determination of offspring sex. Those individuals at the 95th percentile in number of premarital partners had close to 60% boys, compared to about 50% boys for those at the bottom of the distribution —all things considered, a notable difference.

Naturally, despite the fact that plausible alternative explanations of these data may be difficult to generate, the data do not prove the evolutionary history I have painted. Additional predictions must be derived and tested. To the extent that other unique, testable predictions can be derived, however, the evolutionary history can be subjected to theoretical risk and, therefore, is, by one philosopher's criteria (Popper, 1959), testable.

Implications of the Evolutionary Understanding

If this evolutionary picture is correct, what of psychological interest can be seen in it? Certainly, it may tell us something interesting about natural history, but does it tell us anything of psychological importance? I suggest that it does.

First, it adds a dimension of understanding and meaning to the individual differences under consideration—female sociosexual variation. Specifically, it gives those individual differences a *functional* meaning. Thus, we understand not only that individual differences in sociosexuality are partly heritable, and that they emerge through some causal process involving genetic (as well as other) factors but that the individual differences have some adaptive significance. The adaptive significance can be stated in terms of different mating strategies that may have emerged from evolutionary history. Of course, a long-standing concern in personality psychology is just such an understanding of the functional and adaptive value of individual characteristics. Moreover, there are other contemporary perspectives that frame the adaptive significance in terms of means-end strategies (e.g., Cantor & Kihlstrom, 1987). Perhaps the major difference between those perspectives and the one presented here is that I have addressed strategies that, although now expressed in an environment much different than the evolutionarily-relevant one, are believed to have been specifically molded by the evolutionary process.

Secondly, given the functional significance of these individual differences, one can generate predictions about what other characteristics should cohere with them. The one prediction I have discussed involved a nonpsychological trait—sex ratio of offspring. According to the model, however, behavioral characteristics should cohere with female sociosexuality as well. One, for instance, concerns mate choice. If restricted females benefited through the investment given by the father of their offspring, they should tend to choose mates who are willing and likely to be faithful, responsible caregivers. If unrestricted females benefited by mating with partners who possessed the potential to have many mates, they should choose mates with characteristics that would have allowed them, in evolutionary history, to have had many mates. Although it is unclear what precise characteristics these are, it seems reasonable to believe that physical and sexual attractiveness would be among them. We have examined these predictions in three studies (Simpson & Gangestad, 1988b), finding support in all three. Thus, for instance, not only do unrestricted females claim to care more about physical and sexual attractiveness than do restricted females; even when their own attractiveness is statistically controlled for, unrestricted females date males who, as judged by independent raters, are more attractive than the dates of restricted females.

The process of specifying, on the basis of theory, a systematic network of distinct, covarying behaviors is a familiar one in personality psychology—it is construct validation (Cronbach & Meehl, 1955). Given that the understanding of underlying coherence, through construct validation, is a central endeavor of personality psychology, evolutionary histories should perhaps be regarded by the field as more than mere curiosities; they may assist in its most fundamental tasks.

References

Alexander, R.D., Hoogland, J.L., Howard, R.D., Noonan, K.M., & Sherman, P.W. (1979). Sexual dimorphisms and breeding systems in pinnepeds, ungulates, primates, and humans. In N. Chagnon & W. Irons (Eds.), *Evolutionary biology and human social behavior: An anthropological perspective.* (pp. 402–435). North Scituate, MA: Duxbury.

Buss, D.M. (1984). Evolutionary biology and personality psychology: Toward a conception of human nature and individual differences. *American Psychologist, 39,* 1135–1147.

Cantor, N., & Kihlstrom, J. (1987). *Personality and social intelligence.* Englewood Cliffs, NJ: Prentice-Hall.

Chisholm, J.S. (1988). Toward a developmental evolutionary ecology of humans. In K. MacDonald (Ed.), *Sociobiological perspectives on human development* (pp. 78–102). New York: Springer.

Clutton-Brock, T.H., & Iason, G.R. (1986). Sex ratio variation in mammals. *The Quarterly Review of Biology, 61,* 339–374.

Cronbach, L.J., & Meehl, P.M. (1955). Construct validity in psychological tests. *Psychological Bulletin, 52,* 281–302.

Crow, J.F. (1986). *Basic concepts in population, quantitative, and evolutionary genetics.* New York: Freeman.

Dobzhansky, T. (1970). *Genetics of the evolutionary process.* New York: Columbia University Press.

Eysenck, H.J. (1976). *Sex and personality.* London: Open Books.

Gangestad, S.W., & Simpson, J.A. (1988a). *On constructing evolutionary histories of genetic variation: The case of female sociosexuality.* Manuscript submitted for publication.

Gangestad, S.W., & Simpson, J.A. (1988b). *On human sociosexual variation: An evolutionary model of mating propensities.* Manuscript submitted for publication.

Gould, S.J., & Lewontin, R.C. (1979). The spandrels of San Marco and the panglossian paradigm: A critique of the adaptationist programme. *Proceedings of the Royal Society of London, B205,* 581–598.

Heisler, I.L. (1981). Offspring quality and the polygyny threshold: A new model for the "sexy son" hypothesis. *American Naturalist, 117,* 316–328.

Henderson, N.D. (1982). Human behavior genetics. *Annual Review of Psychology, 33,* 403–440.

Kinsey, A.C., Pomeroy, W.B., & Martin, C.E. (1948). *Sexual behavior in the human male.* Philadelphia: Saunders.

Kinsey, A.C., Pomeroy, W.B., Martin, C.E., & Gebhard, P.H. (1953). *Sexual behavior in the human female.* Philadelphia: Saunders.

Kirkpatrick, M. (1985). Evolution of female choice and male parental investment in polygynous species: The demise of the "sexy son." *American Naturalist, 125,* 788–810.

Lewontin, R. (1974). The analysis of variance and the analysis of cause. *American Journal of Human Genetics, 26,* 400–411.

Loehlin, J.C., Willerman, L., & Horn, J.M. (1988). Human behavior genetics. *Annual Review of Psychology, 38,* 101–133.

MacArthur, R.H, & Wilson, E.O. (1967). *The theory of island biogeography.* Princeton, NJ: Princeton University Press.

Maynard Smith, J. (1982). *Evolution and the theory of games*. New York: Cambridge University Press.
Pianka, E.R. (1970). On r- and K-selection. *American Naturalist, 104,* 592–597.
Plomin, R. (1986). *Development, genetics, and psychology*. Hillsdale, NJ: Erlbaum.
Popper, K.R. (1959). *The logic of scientific discovery*. New York: Basic Books.
Rice, W.R. (1983). Parent-offspring pathogen transmission: A selective agent promoting sexual reproduction. *American Naturalist, 121,* 187–203.
Rushton, J.P. (1985). Differential K Theory: The sociobiology of individual and group differences. *Personality and Individual Differences, 6,* 441–452.
Scarr, S., & McCartney, K. (1983). How people make their own environments: A theory of genotype-environment effects. *Child Development, 54,* 424–435.
Simpson, J.A., & Gangestad, S.W. (1988a). *Sociosexuality and romantic partner choice*. Manuscript submitted for publication.
Simpson, J.A., & Gangestad, S.W. (1988b). *Sociosexuality: The construct, a measure, and correlates*. Unpublished research, Texas A&M University.
Telelgen, A. (1982). *A short manual for the Differential Personality Questionnaire*. Unpublished manuscript, University of Minnesota.
Tellegen, A., Lykken, D.T., Bouchard Jr., T.J., Wilcox, K.J., Segal, N.L., & Rich, S. (1988). Personality similarity in twins reared apart and together. *Journal of Personality and Social Psychology, 54,* 1031–1039.
Theissen, D.D. (1972). A move toward species-specific analysis in behavior genetics. *Behavior Genetics, 2,* 115–126.
Tooby, J. (1982). Pathogens, polymorphism and the evolution of sex. *Journal of Theoretical Biology, 97,* 557–576.
Tooby, J., & Cosmides, L. (in press). On the universality of human nature and the uniqueness of the individual: The role of genetics and adaptation. *Journal of Personality*.
Trivers, R. (1972). Parental investment and sexual selection. In B. Campbell (Ed.), *Sexual selection and the descent of man, 1871–1971* (pp. 136–179). Chicago: Aldin.
Weatherhead, P.J., & Robertson, R.J. (1979). Offspring quality and the polygeyny threshold: The "sexy son" hypothesis. *American Naturalist, 113,* 201–208.
Weatherhead, P.J., & Robertson, R.J. (1981). In defense of the "sexy son" hypothesis. *American Naturalist, 117,* 349–356.
Wilson, E.O. (1978). *On Human Nature*. Cambridge, MA: Harvard University Press.
Zuckerman, M. (1983). *Biological bases of sensation seeking, impulsivity, and anxiety*. Hillsdale, NJ: Erlbaum.

CHAPTER 25

Levels of Explanation in Personality Theory

Jerome C. Wakefield

Personality theory, like other areas of human psychology, is an attempt to explain certain aspects of human behavior. There are currently several views of how to go about constructing such an explanation. One common position is that a person's behavior should be explained by the set of personality traits that the person possesses. For example, Allport (1961) states that "Scarcely anyone questions the existence of traits as the fundamental unit of personality," and Pervin (1984) notes that, for many contemporary psychologists as well, personality psychology is virtually synonymous with the study of personality traits. Other theorists, including cognitive, phenomenological, and psychodynamic thinkers (e.g., Baars, 1986; Erdelyi, 1985; Searle, 1983), insist that a proper explanation of behavior must involve reference to the specific meanings and experiences, in the form of mental representations, that cause an individual's behavior. The representational structure of mental states, by which they refer to outside objects, is known in the philosophical literature as "intentionality" (Searle, 1983). Still other personality theorists attempt to explain behavior in evolutionary biological terms, as resulting from naturally selected behavioral dispositions that exist because, in our environment of evolutionary adaptedness, they functioned to enhance the person's reproductive success (e.g., Buss, 1984).

To a surprising degree, the three approaches to personological explanation in terms of traits, meanings (i.e., intentional states), and evolutionary functions have been treated by their adherents as intrinsically opposed and incompatible. Consequently, the field of personality psychology often appears to consist of several subdisciplines lacking a common vision or goal, rather than as a unified and coherent scientific discipline. I argue in this chapter that much of this conflict over explanatory approaches is misplaced, because a complete personological account of any behavior must involve attention to all of the aforementioned explanatory approaches, woven into one integrated and multilayered explanation. Thus, the ideological tensions between the different approaches represent a failure by the field to achieve a metalevel understanding of the mutual dependence of the approaches in the overall personological enterprise. I will consider below what a complete or ideal personological explanation would have to include, elaborating the place of each of the three explanation types in such an explanation, and pointing to confusions between the types of explanation that are at the root of some of the misplaced explanatory dogmatism which is my target. Given the complexity of the issues and the limitations of space, my analysis here will be partial and programmatic in nature.

Action as the Domain of Psychological Explanation

To understand the nature of personological explanation, it is first necessary to establish the domain of data that is to be explained. As noted above, the consensus is that personality theory attempts to explain behavior; the common notion that psychology is the "study of human behavior" is, however, actually too inclusive. For example, physics, and not psychology, studies the physical behavior of all objects, including human beings. Biology studies the physiological behavior of all organisms, including human beings. Thus, a central conceptual challenge for psychology is to identify which bodily motions are distinctively within its domain. To make the point more vividly, consider the behavior of a "human cannonball" as he or she falls to earth in accordance with the laws of physics. The motion of the human cannonball along his or her trajectory constitutes a bodily behavior in response to the environmental stimulus of the firing of the cannon. Nevertheless, it is clear that this very substantial motion, which is the same whether the propelled object is human or inorganic, is not essentially part of the subject matter of psychology, but of physics. Yet, the relatively small motions involved in the terrified flailing of the human connonball's arms and legs as he or she plummets to earth is within the province of psychology. Clearly, behavior in the sense relevant to psychology is not simply a matter of bodily motion definable in physicalistic terms. What, then, is distinctive about the motions that are within the scientific domain of psychology?

If we accept the principle that psychology is concerned with some subdomain of behavior, then the best available answer to the problem of the domain of psychological explanation is the following: psychology is concerned in the first instance with the explanation of motivated, or intentional, behavior. 'Motivation' is often used by psychologists to refer only to some small set of ultimate drives or sources of motivational energy, but here it is used to refer to a broad range of proximal psychological causes of behavior. These causes include what are ordinarily called the "reasons" for people's behavior. Thus, if I walk to the store to get some bread, my behavior of walking to the store is motivated by my desire to get some bread, and by my belief that walking to the store is a step towards accomplishing my goal. We often describe this by saying that I intend, or my intention is, to go to the store to get some bread, and we call this sort of motivated behavior "intentional" behavior. Note that there are two different senses of "intentional" here that can easily be confused; behavior is intentional if it is intended by the person, and mental states are intentional if they are representationally structured. The two senses are very closely linked, however, because intentional behavior is behavior for which the goal is represented in certain intentional mental states. I will use the term "action" to distinguish intentional behavior from unmotivated motions of the body.

Since an action is by definition a behavior motivated by reasons, to identify a behavior as a particular kind of action one needs to identify the motivational state that caused the behavior. The motivational state constitutes the psychological meaning of the behavior to the acting person. Thus, the very same bodily motion can be described as "moving around air molecules," "a sequence of muscle firings," or "going to the store for bread," but, under usual conditions, only "going to the store for bread" is psychologically relevant because it alone labels the action in accordance with the motivation causing the behavior, and thus explains the psychological meaning of the behavior. Of course, there may be many different motivational states expressed in the same action, and, hence, several different psychologically relevant descriptions of a behavior. For example, a person may simultaneously go for bread, get some exercise, and angrily leave the house, all intentionally and all via the same behavior. It is a thorny empirical problem to determine which of all the possible motives that would explain a behavior were actually operative in a given case, and thus which action(s) a behavior actually represents.

Intentional Explanation

To claim that a behavior is an action (in the sense explained above) and not just a physical motion, such as when we label a certain bodily motion as "going to the store for bread," is already to suggest the explanation of the behavior. Thus, implicit in the very concept of action is a reference to the first explanatory level, namely, the intentional system level, by which the bodily motions that are relevant to psychology are explained. The intentional system is a system of intentional states—beliefs, desires, emotions, and so on—and each of those states consists in part of a mental representation either of what is (in the case of a belief) or what could be (in the case of a desire) (Searle, 1983). For example, a desire is, in part, a mental representation of the conditions that would fulfill it, and a belief is, in part, a mental representation of the conditions that would make the belief true. Some intentional states are idiosyncratic, but many are the shared products of a common sociocultural context (Dreyfus & Wakefield, 1988; Wakefield, 1988). These intentional states form the reasons for actions, and therefore, explain behavior.

How do reasons for actions work? The standard philosophical model (Davidson, 1963) is that actions are caused by reasons, and reasons consist of belief-desire pairs that rationalize, or make sense of, the action. Imagine, for example, that I want a drink. That desire contains a mental representation of an end state, for example, the quenching of my thirst. If, in addition, I believe that by walking to the refrigerator I can obtain a drink, the combination of the belief and the desire (along with the fact that there are no stronger countervailing factors) will cause me to walk over to the refrigerator and get a drink. Obviously, there are some mediating causal links between the reason and the action, but the belief and the desire are the directly relevant psychological links in the causal chain. Critical to the explanation of behavior in terms of reasons is the assumption that people are approximations to rational beings. On this assumption, the reason provides a plausible explanation for the behavior because it shows why the behavior is rational in light of the person's beliefs and desires. Thus, the reason-action model is able to capture succinctly the systematic relations between internal psychological states and external behavior that characterize an approximately rational being.

The belief-desire schema is extremely useful for explaining and predicting people's actions under ordinary circumstances in everyday life. Take, for example, the fact that it was known months ahead of time that the people who attended the conference at which this paper was presented were going to converge on Ann Arbor from around the country on a certain date. Imagine the difficulty of trying to predict this fact in terms of the histories of reinforcement of each of the individuals involved, or in terms of the latent unconscious meanings that the conference had for them, or in terms of any other approach to understanding action. The successful prediction, months in advance, that all of the people in question would converge at the same remote location on the same day was based simply on a few linguistic interactions with the organizers in which the attendees' beliefs, desires, and resulting intentions were expressed. It is easy to lose sight of the impressive predictive powers of the intentional explanatory schema, and of the degree to which it is tested in everyday life, perhaps due to the very frequency with which the theory is used, and its common sense origins.

In sum, intentional explanation of behavior in terms of individual meanings that form the reasons for actions is the first level of explanation to which personality theory must aspire.

Traits as Stable Dispositions of the Intentional System

Another level of explanation is the level of traits. Traits may be conceptualized as stabilities in the kind of intentional states generated by the intentional system. That is, personality traits are stable dispositions to have certain kinds of beliefs, desires, and so on. There are two features of this approach that should be emphasized. First, traits are dispositions specifically of the intentional system, so attribution of a personality trait is justified only when there is something about the nature of the intentional system itself which predisposes to a particular kind of motive. A person whose actions are consistent with the possession of a trait still may not possess the trait, because their actions may be due to special environmental circumstances. A central challenge to the personality field is to distinguish variance in actions due to traits from variance in actions due to environmental circumstances. Thus, a person might talk much more than most people, but empirical study might show that the cause lies in the person's circumstances, for example, in the kind of occupational and familial responsibilities that the person bears, and not in any special properties of the person's intentional system and its workings. If such is the case, then it is inappropriate to ascribe a personality trait of talkativeness to the person. (Of course, it is possible that further study would show that the person chose his or her circumstances in order to satisfy a constant need to talk, in which case a trait attribution might be appropriate.)

Secondly, according to the above account of traits, it is the occurrence of certain motivational states, rather than actual behaviors or actions, that form the basis for attribution of personality traits. Given that we have direct empirical access only to a person's behavior, we must always infer the existence of motivational states from behavior and any other indirect evidence that is available. Nonetheless, it is the nature of the inner motivational states, and not the behavior itself, that we are generally describing when we attribute personality traits to a person. Indeed, specific behaviors are neither necessary nor sufficient for ascription of traits. Specific behaviors are not sufficient for possession of a trait because someone might display the behaviors typically associated with a given trait but not actually possess the trait. The actions might be due to some other cause, such as a prudential desire to act as if one possessed the trait. Imagine, for example, that the Mafia has put your mother "on ice" and given you instructions to act as though you are talkative; if you comply, you still will not be a talkative person in the sense relevant to personality trait theory.

Specific behaviors are also not necessary conditions for trait attribution because possession of a personality trait in itself does not imply any particular action at all; to take an extreme case, even a totally paralyzed person possesses a personality, even though it cannot be expressed in action. Again, someone might be high on one trait but even higher on some other trait that overrides and conflicts with the expression of the first trait, so that the person does not perform the actions typically associated with the first trait despite possession of that trait. Even when someone is unable to carry out a certain kind of action, if they often have the intention to perform the relevant kind of action, we still say that they do indeed possess the related trait. For example, we would label a person "sociable," even if they never socialized, if we knew with certainty that they possessed the relevant social motivations with adequate frequency and strength, and that the reason for the lack of socializing had to do with external factors outside of the person's control. Again, a person held indefinitely in solitary confinement might be a talkative person who just happens to lack the opportunity to act in a way expressive of that trait. (I leave aside the possibility that talkativeness would be manifested in such circumstances by talking to oneself.) If my approach to traits is correct, then Buss and Craik's (1983) "act frequency approach" to traits would more accurately reflect the structure of trait explanation if it were recast as an "intention frequency approach."

Traits explain actions, but they do so indirectly, by explaining the reasons that motivated the actions. Even within the domain of reasons, however, the power of trait explanation is extremely limited. Traits can explain specific reasons or sets of reasons, but they cannot explain the entire pattern of reasons to which the trait corresponds. For example, the fact that John is a talkative person can be used to explain John's talkativeness at a particular party, or on other particular occasions. It cannot, however, be used to explain why John is talkative in general over a wide range of situations, because that overall pattern of talking constitutes John's trait of talkativeness, so the explanation would be circular. At best, a trait ascription can provide a low-level causal explanation of why someone experiences a certain kind of intentional state in a specific situation or set of situations. The trait explains specific motives in terms of a persistent and more general disposition of the intentional system to generate motives of that kind, thus subsuming the specific motive under a broader causal regularity. A further step is required to explain the causal regularity itself.

Secondary and Basic Traits

A trait is a disposition to have a certain kind of intentional state, and the existence of such a disposition calls out for explanation in terms of underlying structures that account for this property of the intentional system. One way of explaining such a disposition would be in terms of other, explanatorily deeper, mental dispositions, plus other specific intentional states. In this way, one property of the intentional system, in this case a certain trait, might be explained in terms of other properties of the intentional system, including other traits and particular intentional states. For example, a person's trait of talkativeness, which consists of a disposition to have a desire to talk, might be explained in terms of the person's belief that he or she will be better liked as a result of talking, and the person's strong desire to be liked by others. Or, it might be explained by a trait of oral libidinal fixation which generates oral cravings, and a belief that such oral cravings can be satisfied through the oral activity involved in talking.

Now, I want to make a distinction between what I call secondary traits and basic traits. A secondary trait is one that is properly explained in terms of other features of the intentional system, such as underlying beliefs, desires, and traits. For instance, as noted above, some people might be talkative because they believe that talking makes people like them, while others might be talkative because they have a craving for oral activity and talking satisfies that craving. In both cases, there are stable properties of the intentional system that cause the generation of a particular kind of intentional state, namely, the desire to talk. Thus, in both cases, the trait of talkativeness is immediately explainable in terms of other features of the mental system, and is a secondary trait. Note that the possession of a secondary trait is only as stable as the underlying intentional states that cause it. One might view certain aspects of therapy as an attempt to disconfirm ingrained beliefs underlying maladaptive secondary traits and thus to change personality.

In contrast to secondary traits, basic traits are the class of traits that are not further explainable in terms of the mental system. That is, these are the traits that provide the ground level motivational inputs into the mental system, and psychology per se cannot further explain them because the explanations lie outside the psychological domain. Examples might include certain kinds of desires that are based in biological processes, and certain basic temperamental factors that directly depend on physiological variables. For example, if Freud (1915) is correct, sexual desire arises from physiological instinctual processes; if Eysenck (1967) is correct, introversion results directly from a certain level of cortical arousal. The fact that theoreticians as divergent as Freud and Eysenck would share the strategy of ultimately explaining personality in terms of basic traits that are explainable only by nonmental processes suggests the power and apparent explanatory necessity of this approach.

In the case of a basic trait, the task of personality theory is to establish the exact nature of the intentional states initially generated in the mental system as a result of causes external to the mind, and then to map the consequences of that initial input as it interacts with other basic and secondary traits and individual intentional states to eventuate in action. All secondary traits are ultimately derived from such basic traits. A trait might be said to be deeper or more at the surface of the person's personality, depending on the explanatory distance (i.e., the number of explanatory steps) between the secondary traits and the person's basic traits. Intuitively, traits directly rooted in physiology or brain architecture are explanatorily deep, while traits dependent on a string of prior beliefs and desires, and thus distant products of the basic traits, are more at the personality's surface.

Once the basic traits have been identified, the question arises immediately as to why we possess these basic traits. One way of answering this question is by explaining the basic traits in terms of proximal physiological causes; but that does not get at the critical question of what function is served by the basic traits. It is possible that in some instances of individual differences there is no interesting answer to this question, and that personality traits, and especially individual differences, are just a form of "noise" in the genetic system. This answer to the function question, however, is utterly implausible as a general account of all basic traits. In some cases of shared traits, such as sexual motivation, their functionality is every bit as obvious as it is in the case of the eyes or the heart. More generally, personality traits, both shared features and individual differences, are such salient parts of our social interactions and play such a large role in the way we conduct our lives that it would seem they must be a part of the way we were designed by evolution to function. Thus, a further stage of personological explanation is the explanation of basic traits in terms of the function they serve. That is, why, in the first place, do we have the personalities we have, and why do they differ in the ways that they do? What beneficial role is personality supposed to play in our lives? Only through an answer to these questions do we arrive at a full understanding of the actions that derive from the basic traits. For this answer, we have to turn to another level of explanation, evolutionary biology.

Functional Explanation

Living as we do in the historical shadow of the Third Reich and its abuses of biological explanations of racial differences, contemporary psychologists have a particular responsibility to be wary of the facile use of biological explanations, including evolutionary explanations. Nonetheless, the reflexive skepticism with which the psychological community often reacts to proposed evolutionary explanations of personality appears excessive. In providing an analysis of functional evolutionary explanation below, I will argue, first, that such explanations cannot be avoided in an explanatorily complete personality psychology, and, secondly, that much of the concern over evolutionary explanations in psychology is due to conceptual confusions about the relation of functional to intentional explanations, confusions that are to some degree shared by evolutionists and their critics alike.

No matter how much about the physiology of the heart one understands, one cannot have a full understanding of the heart if one does not know that a function of the heart is to circulate the blood, and that this beneficial result of the heart's functioning partially explains the existence of hearts in our bodies. Similarly, no matter how much about the psychology of sexual attraction one understands, one lacks a full understanding of sexuality unless one understands that a function of the sexual drive is to motivate the organism to copulate and thereby to reproduce, and that this beneficial effect of sexual attraction partially explains the existence of sexual attraction as a basic motivational system. In personality theory, as elsewhere in the study of human nature, a functional understanding is mandatory for a full explanation of why we are the organisms we are.

The structure of functional explanation can be usefully elaborated as follows. Sometimes we explain the existence or structure of an organ, including a mental "organ" such as a basic trait or behavior pattern, in terms of a benefit that it provides to the organism, which we call its "function." For example, we say that a function of the heart is to circulate the blood, or that a function of sexual drive is to motivate the organism to engage in sexual activity and thereby to reproduce. Citing the function is a way of explaining the existence and structure of the organ in question, because ascribing a function to an organ is roughly equivalent to saying that the organ was "designed" for the purpose providing the relevant benefit or that the organ exists in order to provide the benefit. The source of our notion that organs can be explained functionally lies in the intuition that it cannot be accidental that so many of our organs are exquisitely adapted to provide us with what we need. The structure of the eye, the heart, or the sexual behavior system is so nearly perfect that we assume that the benefits provided by these structures must have been a causally active factor in their design. In sum, our relative perfection suggests that the very beneficiality of an organ had something to do with why it came to exist and persist in our species. A functional explanation is one that partially explains an organ by citing the causally relevant benefit.

Functional explanation is puzzling because it does not seem to conform to the usual criteria for causal explanation. A cause must always precede its effects, but a functional explanation asserts that the cause of an organ's existence is a benefit that results from and comes after the existence of the organ. At one time, this paradox was resolved by citing God's benign intentions when He created our species. This ingeniously reduces functional explanation to a form of intentional explanation. Intentional explanation is not subject to the same temporal paradox, because it is understood that an action performed in order to obtain bread is not literally caused by the later effect of possessing the bread, but rather by the preceding mental representation that constitutes the desire to obtain bread.

Today, we resolve the paradox by citing natural selection of the fittest, a nonintentional explanation of why we appear to be well-designed, even though no one actually designed us. The benefit provided by an organ can, in a sense, causally explain its structure and its existence in the population, simply because organisms that received the benefits of that organ in the past achieved greater reproductive success, and that greater reproductive success caused the organ to be retained in the population and explains why we possess that organ today. Evolutionary theory guarantees that any correct functional understanding can ultimately be exchanged for a distal causal explanation in terms of the history of the species. This guarantee allows for our tentative use of functional explanations while we are awaiting the fuller historical account.

In sum, a functional explanation is an explanation of a physical or psychological feature of an organism in terms of a benefit to the organism that caused organisms of that kind who possessed the feature in the past to have greater reproductive success, hence causing the retention of the feature in the population.

Distinguishing Functional and Intentional Explanations

It is easy to see why a confusion between functional and intentional explanation is possible. Functional explanation and intentional explanation have many features in common, and they even share much of the same teleological vocabulary. We say that the person's intention is the purpose of the action, just as we say that the function of an organ is the purpose of an organ; we say that an action is performed in order to accomplish the person's intention, just as we say that an organ exists in order to accomplish its function; we say that an action is designed to accomplish a certain goal, just as we say that an organ is designed to fulfill a certain function.

As a result of these shared features, there is endless confusion between the two forms of explanation. For example, Plato suggests, in his dialogue *Symposium,* that the goal of the desire in erotic love is reproduction. That seems wrong as a general account of the intentional content of erotic desire. Yet it is easy to see how Plato went wrong. He seems to have fallen prey to a simple confusion between the function of sexual attraction, which is or at least includes reproduction, and the intentions that constitute sexual attraction, which by no means need involve reproduction. The "purpose" of sex is reproduction in one sense but not necessarily in the other. It seems easy, however, to confuse the two senses of purpose.

In a more contemporary vein, Hogan and his associates (Hogan, Jones, & Cheek, 1985; Hogan & Sloan, in press) argue that personality traits evolved as strategies to manipulate people in order to gain personal advantage, and, therefore, that people are manipulative, selfish, and calculating in their relationships. The conclusion does not follow; it represents a confusion between a functional explanation of why certain traits exist, namely, because of the advantage that they yield to the possessor, and an intentional explanation of what kinds of motivations and representations are in our minds, namely, selfish, and manipulative intentions. The function of a personality trait might be to gain some advantage, but the intentions generated by the trait could have to do with, for example, genuine altruistic impulses, if those impulses are the ones that lead people to do the things that, in their environment, actually yield an advantage.

These examples illustrate the most common confusion between the two forms of explanation, which is to read the function of a trait into the intentions generated by the trait. This mistake is based on an intuitively reasonable strategy. If a motivational trait has the function of providing some benefit, what better way to ensure that the benefit is procured than by building in a trait that actually generates the motivation to procure the benefit? Thus, if sexual attraction is designed to achieve reproduction, it makes intuitive sense that it would work by building into our intentional systems the desire to reproduce. Plato's mistaken conclusion that sexual attraction is a desire for reproduction and Hogan's mistaken conclusion that people are calculating and selfish are examples of this sort of reasoning.

Although the direct correspondence between function and intention makes superficial sense, it is simply not how evolution works. The function of sex is reproduction, and the typical intention in sex is pleasure, and these two need not be the same because it just so happens that when people have the appropriate pleasure-seeking intentions they do precisely the things that, often quite inadvertantly, lead to reproduction. Evolutionary selection is based on such end results of motivation, which need not correspond to the intentional structure of motivation. Of course, sometimes the intention of a behavior and the function of the behavior do coincide. In intentional explanation, an action is explained in terms of a representation of the goal of the action. Functional explanation requires no representation of the functional goal of the action: the function is simply an effect of the motivation (via the actions it causes) that benefits the organism in a way that explains the maintenance of that motivation in the species. These two forms of teleological explanation are really quite independent.

The fallacy of reading a function into motivational structure leads to an exaggerated sense of the motivational implications of functional explanations, and this partially shapes attitudes towards evolutionary explanations. Psychology is specifically concerned with the mental nature of human beings, especially intentional structures that constitute motives for actions, and part of the importance of understanding motives is that they define our moral nature. Functional explanations are a part of the psychological enterprise because they help to explain where our motivations come from and what they mean in the broader biological picture. Functional explanations do not by themselves imply anything about the intentional content of motivation, however. By fallaciously reading function into intention, we attribute a power to evolutionary accounts to define our mental natures that they do not in fact possess. Thus, much of the resistance to biological evolutionary explanation in psychology may be due to the erroneous inference that the function of a trait must represent the way we are as motivated beings, and, hence, our moral nature.

Concluding Comments

Eysenck (1984, p. 237) points out that biological factors are paid only lip service in most standard personological explanations. For those who are reflexively aversive to all biological approaches to personality explanation, the upshot of my analysis of functional explanation is this: you can run from functional explanation but you cannot hide. The evolutionary history of our psychic system must be included as a level of explanation of human action in order to explain the existence of basic traits and, therefore, how the overall intentional system works. Cooperation and even collaboration between biological, trait, and intentional theorists is not merely desirable but mandatory if personality psychology is to fulfill its scientific obligations.

Let me now review the overall argument for the interconnectedness of the three forms of explanation. Psychology is about behavior, but only about behavior that qualifies as action. Action is behavior that is motivated by inner intentional states. Therefore, the very description of an action already points to the first level of explanation in terms of intentional states. We then want to explain why it is that a person experiences particular intentional states under particular circumstances, and sometimes the explanation lies in certain features of the person's intentional system that regularly generate the relevant kinds of states. That kind of stable disposition to generate a certain kind of intentional state is called a trait. Once we have explained the particular intentional state in terms of a trait, there is an immediate question of what explains the possession of the trait; that is, why is the person's intentional system such that it regularly generates intentional states of that kind? The explanation will lie in other traits and other intentional states that lie explanatorily deeper than the trait to be explained. Now, if we follow the explanatory trail down far enough, we will reach a point at which there are no more traits or intentional states to explain why a certain type of intentional state is generated; the relevant state occurs just because the body feeds that kind of state de novo into the mind. At that point we have explicated the entire nature of the intentional system insofar as it explains the action in question. For a full understanding, however, we would also like to know why it is that the person is built so as to have a biological nature that feeds in that particular sort of initial desire or other intentional state into the mental system. The answer to this question must be in terms of the function of the trait, and it must be framed in terms of evolutionary biology.

In sum, a complete explanation of a person's action would have to include at least (these are necessary but perhaps not sufficient conditions of completeness) the intentional states that caused the action, the traits that caused the intentional states, and the evolutionary causes of the basic traits that underlie the particular traits operative in the particular act. It is interesting that one of the very few personality theorists to attempt to put all these levels together in a complete personality explanation was Sigmund Freud, who interwove in his explanations the intentional level (e.g., specific conscious and unconscious beliefs and desires), the trait level (e.g., oral fixation, orderliness), and the basic trait/functional biological level (e.g., instinctual impulses aroused by bodily needs that are differentiated according to biological function). The logical comprehensiveness of Freud's approach may well be one of the features of his analysis that explains its enduring fascination, despite its many shortcomings. Contemporary personality theoreticians should be working towards a theory that is no less complete in its logical structure.

References

Allport, G. (1961). *Pattern and growth in personality*. New York: Holt.

Baars, B.J. (1986). *The cognitive revolution in psychology*. New York: Guilford.

Buss, D.M. (1984). Evolutionary biology and personality psychology: Toward a conception of human nature and individual differences. *American Psychologist, 39*, 1135–1147.

Buss, D.M. & Craik, K.H. (1983). The act frequency approach to personality. *Psychological Review, 90*, 105–126.

Davidson, D. Actions, reasons, and causes. *Journal of Philosophy, 60* (1963), 684–700.

Dreyfus, H.L. & Wakefield, J.C. (1988). From depth psychology to breadth psychology: A phenomenological approach to psychopathology. In S. Messer, L. Sass, & R. Woolfolk (Eds.), *Hermeneutics and psychological theory: Interpretive perspectives on personality, psychotherapy, and psychopathology* (pp. 272–288). New Brunswick, N.J.: Rutgers University Press.

Erdelyi, M. (1985). *Psychoanalysis: Freud's cognitive psychology*. New York: Freeman.

Eysenck, H.J. (1967). *The biological basis of personality*. Springfield, IL: Thomas.

Eysenck, H.J. (1984). The place of individual differences in a scientific psychology. *Annals of theoretical psychology, 1*, 233–286.

Freud, S. (1915). Instincts and their vicissitudes. In J. Strachey (Ed. and Trans.), *The standard edition of the complete psychological works of Sigmund Freud* (vol. 14, pp. 166–215). London: Hogarth Press.

Hogan, R., Jones, W., & Cheek, J. (1985). Socioanalytic theory: An alternative to armadillo psychology. In B. Schlenker (Ed.), *The self and social life*. New York: McGraw-Hill.

Hogan, R., & Sloan, T. (in press). Socioanalytic foundations for personality psychology. In Ozer, D.J., Healy, J.M., & Stewart, A.J. (Eds.), *Perspectives in personality:* Vol. 3. *Self and emotion.* Greenwich, Conn.: JAI Press.

Pervin, L.A. (1984). Persons, situations, interactions, and the future of personality. *Annals of theoretical psychology, 2,* 339–344.

Searle, J.R. (1983). *Intentionality, an essay in the philosophy of mind.* New York: Cambridge University Press.

Wakefield, J.C. (1988). Hermeneutics and empiricism: Commentary on Donald Meichenbaum. In S. Messer, L. Sass, & R. Woolfolk (Eds.), *Hermeneutics and psychological theory: Interpretive perspectives on personality, psychotherapy, and psychopathology* (pp. 131–148). New Brunswick, New Jersey: Rutgers University Press.

Subject Index

Accuracy, 75, 78
　circumscribed, 63
　domain-specific, 61, 63–64, 78
　global, 63
　person perception, 61, 62, 63, 64, 66, 69, 78, 79
Achievement, 33–34, 36–37
　motivation, 130–131, 135
　tasks, 47, 50–52, 57
Action, 335
Act frequency approach, 64, 338
Act tallies, 64
Adaptation, 49
Adjective Checklist, 263, 264, 265
Adjustment, 203–204
Adoption method, 296
Affect, 152, 154–156
　see also Frustration
Affiliation, 33–34, 36–37
Aggregation, 100, 110
Aggression, 99, 106
Agreeableness (A), 238, 263, 267
Anxiety, 46, 47, 49–50, 56, 139
Aschematics, 50
Aspects of Identity Questionnaire, 277
Attachment, 162, 164
Attitudes, 139, 140, 196
Attraction, 309–314
Automatic self-presentation, 204–205
Autonomy, 279

Balancing selection, 324
Behavior
　assessment, 62
　assessments of, 87
　genetics, 89
　intentional, 334, 335
　problems, 102, 103
　sexual, 322, 323
　social, 61
Behavioral correlates of personality ("behavioral prediction"), 216–219
Belief-desire schema, 336
Berkeley Guidance Study, 94
Big-Five, 262, 263, 264, 265, 267
Biography, 160, 161
Bounded rationality, 63

California Psychological Inventory (CPI), 227
California Q-sort data, 94
CAPPA (Counsellor Assisted Personal Projects Analysis), 27
Certainty ratings, 198
Change, 53, 56–57
Chaos theory, 181
Cognitive interference, 132–133
Cognitive maps, 117
Cognitive processing, 140
Cognitive strategies, 45–58

Subject Index

Competence, 129–130, 134
  valuation, 130–132, 134
Competition, 131
Complexity, 41
  of person concepts, 118, 119
Computer simulations, 199
Conceptual analysis, 227
Conditional patterns, 149–157
Conscientiousness (C), 238, 262, 263, 267
Consistency, 177–182
  coefficients, 64, 78
Construct validation, 330
Construct validity, 224–228, 230–233, 254, 255
Constructivist view of personality, 286, 292
Content validity, 223, 227, 247
Context, 110–111
Contrast effects, 310
Control, 46–47, 50–52, 143–144
Convergent validity, 224, 226–228, 232
Coping, 115
CQS factor, 241
Criterion validity, 224, 227
Cross-situational inconsistency, 292
Cue value, 129–130
Culture, 240

Dancing bears, 212
Data box, 183
Deconstruction, 140
Default processing, 313
Defensiveness, 205
Defensive pessimism, 46–47, 49–58
Developmental tasks, 86
Differential parental investment model, 310–311, 313, 317
  relationship qualified, 311
Discriminant validity, 224, 226–228, 232
Dispositional factors, 89, 90, 94, 95

Distortion, 205–206
Domain specificity, 53–55

Efficacy, 143–144, 145
Egocentrism, 117, 118
Emotional adaptation, 115–125
Emotional stability, 263, 267
Emotional stance, 116, 117, 118, 119, 120, 121, 122, 125
Errors in judgment ("attribution errors"), 211, 212, 219–220
Evolution, 308–310, 314–317
Evolutionary histories, 321, 326
Expectations, 139
Extraversion (E), 238
Extraversion-introversion, 149–152
Eysenck scales, 242

Factor analysis, 203, 207, 224, 233, 246, 247, 255
Faking (see Impression management)
Family, 141
Five-factor model, 237, 238, 240, 243, 246–253, 256
Flexibility, 53, 57–58, 205
Free description, 266
Frequency-dependent selection, 325–328
Frustration, 152, 154–156
Fulfillment, 141, 143, 145–146
Functional explanation, 340–343

Gender, 309, 314, 316, 317
  and mate selection, 309–317
Gene/environment interactions, 316–317
Generativity script, 171
Genetic influences on personality, 308–310, 313–317
Genotype, 294
Genotypic, 86

Subject Index

Goals, 32, 41–42, 143
Goldberg Adjective Scales, 240
Guilt, 279
Gynecological problems, 104, 105, 107

Happiness, 142
Health problems, 99, 104, 107
Heritability, 295, 299, 303, 320
Hierarchy, 267
Homeostatic processes, 181
Homogeneous item clusters, 251, 254–256
Hypothesis testing, 249, 252–255

Identity, 138, 145–146, 160, 161, 162, 169, 170, 171, 275, 276, 277, 278, 279, 280, 281, 282
  collective, 277
  negotiation, 286
Ideological setting, 163, 166, 167, 168, 170
Idiographic, 35, 40
Idiographic/nomothetic, 182
Idiography, 180
Illusion, 142, 144
Images, 163, 164, 165
Imagoes, 163, 169, 170
Implicit personality theory, 249
Impression management, 201, 203, 204, 206
Individual differences, 246, 247, 255, 261
Individual level of analysis, 185–186
Intellect, 262, 263, 267
Intelligence, 99, 102, 106, 139, 140, 226–228
Intentional explanation, 340–343
Intentional explanatory schema, 336
Intentionality, 333
Intentional state(s), 335, 336, 338, 339, 344, 345

Intentional system, 335, 336, 337, 338, 339
Intention frequency approach, 338
Interitem variance, 197–198, 199
Interjudge agreement, 213–216
Interpersonal conditions, 150, 155–157
Intimacy, 33–34, 36–37
  motive, 160, 161, 166, 168, 170
Intrinsic motivation, 129–135
Introversion-extraversion, 194

Language, 261, 263
L-data, 91
Lexical approach, 247–253, 255, 257
Life changes, 115, 116, 117, 118, 121, 122, 125
Life course, 85, 87, 88, 89, 90, 91, 93, 95
Life events, 88
Life story, 161, 162, 166, 168, 169, 170, 171
Life tasks, 45, 57–58, 115, 125
Longitudinal research, 85, 90, 94, 99
Louisville Twin Study, 89–90

Marriage, 141
Masochism, 140
Meaning, 138–146
  needs for, 143–145
Measurement error, 228
Mediation analysis, 131
Mental system, 339
Metatraits, 194–200
Method variance, 227–229, 231–233
Minnesota Longitudinal Studies, 87
Minnesota Multiphasic Personality Inventory (MMPI), 227
Model of personality dispositions, 61, 62, 64
  conditional model, 64, 65, 66, 68, 78

Model(s) of social judgment, 61, 62, 78
  bounded, 61, 62
  unbounded, 62
Moderator variables, 196–197, 281
Mood, 115, 118, 119, 120, 121, 123
Motivated bias, 205–206
Motivation, 160, 165, 334
Motivational processes, 130–132
Motivational state(s), 335, 337
Motives, 32–33, 41
Multi-method assessment, 239
Multitrait-multimethod matrix (MTMMM), 225–229

Narcissism, 32–38, 40–42
Narrative accounts or vignettes, 151, 153, 156–157
Narrative tone, 163, 164
NEO Personality Inventory, 237–243
  personal project correlates, 23, 24
Neuroticism (N), 238
Neutral variation, 324, 326
Nomothetic, 40
Non-conscious information processing, 315–316
nonshared environment, 295, 297–298
Nonstatic consistency, 180, 188
Nuclear episodes, 163, 167

Oakland Growth Study, 94
Observer data, 150, 157
Offspring sex ratio, 329
Openness to Experience (O), 238
Operant measures, 35–36
Optimism, 46–47, 49–58
Other deception, 203

PAC 10 units vs. Big-Five, 28
Patterns of change, 177, 179–182
Peer nominations, 101
Peer reports, 36, 38–40

Perceived competence, 130
Performance evaluation, 128–129, 132–134
Performance feedback, 128–130
Person-by-situation interactions, 135
Person perception, 141
Person-situation debate, 210
Personal fable, 167
Personal projects
  analysis, 15–29
  Big-Five dimensions, 23
  Elicitation List, 17, 18
  Open Columns, 20
  perceived efficacy, 23, 24, 25
  phrasing level and spin, 21, 25, 26
  Rating Matrices, 19
  well-being, 24
Personal strivings, 36–37, 39
Personality
  across time, 149–157
  assessment, 211
  attributes, 261
  construction, 286, 287, 289, 290, 292
  description, 286, 289, 292
    different domain of, 291
    same domain of, 290, 291
    the language of, 287, 292
  development, 155
  inconsistency, 290
  inventories (versus narratives), 151, 157
  process approach to, 181–183, 190–191
  Research Form (PRF), 243
  stability versus change, 154–156
  theory, 333, 336, 339, 341
  variables, 90
Personological explanation, 333, 340, 344
  three approaches to, 333
Perspective taking, 118, 119, 121, 123
Phenotypic, 85, 86, 94
Physical attractiveness, 281
Population genetics, 323

Positive vs. negative attributes, 204
Possible selves, 125
Power, 33–35, 36–37
Power motive, 161, 166, 168, 170
Predictive validity, 254
Primary factors, 254–256
Process-descriptive variables, 184–187
Process models, 207
Propaedeutic criteria for personality assessment, 16, 17
Proximate/ultimate continuum, 314–316
Psychiatric problems, 99, 104, 105
Purpose, 143, 145

Q-sort technique, 212

Reference groups, 280
Respondent measures, 35–36
Response format, 199
Restricted sociosexuality, 322, 327
Rewards, 129–132

Schemas, 115, 124, 125
Schematic processing, 312–314
School achievement, 99, 103, 107
SEAbank in personal projects research, 27
Second order consistency, 180–182, 188
Self, 138, 140, 144–145, 203, 204–205, 275, 276, 277, 278, 279, 280, 281, 282
  concept, 282
  consciousness, 198, 279–280
  deception, 201–209
  esteem, 196–197, 279, 281
  handicapping, 47
  monitoring, 279–280
  Monitoring Scale, 329
  other agreement, 249
  presentation, 201–209, 281
  reflection, 154
  report data, 149–151, 157
  schemas, 125, 198
Semantic similarity ratings, 291
Sense of coherence in personal projects, 29
Sexual selection, 309–312
Sexy son hypothesis, 327, 328
Shyness, 281
Simulated personality paradigm, 61, 68, 69, 76
  inverse personality, 70
  prototype aggressive personality, 70
  random personality, 70
Single trait descriptors, 287, 289
Situation (versus condition), 150, 151
Situations, 100, 110–111
Social cognition, 207, 309, 312–317
Social competence, 102, 103, 110
Social competency and project management, 26
Socially desirable responding, 201–209
Social desirability (*see* Socially desirable responding)
Social-desirability ratings, 288
Social knowledge, 61
Social learning, 309, 315–317
Social tasks, 54–55
Social time clock, 88, 92
Social withdrawal, 99, 107
Stability, 100, 140–141
Standards, 140, 142
Strange Situation paradigm, 89
Strategy effectiveness, 48–53, 56
Stream of time, 177, 187
Subjective expected utility theory, 75
Surgency, 263, 267
Symbols, 139

Task involvement, 132–133
Taxonomy, 261, 263, 269
Temporal data, 183–184

Test construction, 253, 254
Testosterone, 314, 316
Thematic Apperception Test, 35, 160
Time series, 184–186
Trait attributions, 247, 248, 250–253
Trait categories, 287
    broad, 287, 288, 289
    narrow, 288, 289
Trait category-breadth values, 288, 291
    British ratings, 288
    U.S. ratings, 288
Trait combinations, 287, 289, 290, 292
    act-contradiction, 291
    act-independence, 291
    act-overlap, 290, 291
    congruent combinations, 290
    incongruent combinations, 290, 291
    semantic similarity, 290
Trait dimensions, 268
Traited, 195, 196, 197
Trait extremity, 198, 199
Trait hierarchies, 288, 289
Trait meaning, 287, 288, 291, 292
    category breadth, 288, 289
    descriptive aspects, 287, 288, 290, 291, 292
    evaluative aspects, 287, 288, 290, 291, 292
    social desirability, 288, 289, 290
Trait pairs,
    four kinds of, 291
Trait reconciliation, 292
Traits, 32–33, 41–42, 226, 228–232, 336–340, 343, 344, 345
    as semantic categories for behavior, 287, 290
    basic, 339–340, 345
    conflicting, 290
    secondary, 339
Trait tendencies, 250, 251, 257
Transference, 155, 156
Twin method, 296

Unrestricted sociosexuality, 322, 327
Unstructured Interaction Paradigm, 89
Untraited, 195, 196, 197

Value, 144, 145, 146
Variance, 197, 198, 199, 337

Wechsler Adult Intelligence Scale (WAIS), 228